Healthcare Research

Healthcare Research

A Textbook for Students and Practitioners

Edited by

Paula Roberts
Senior Lecturer, Keele University School of Nursing and Midwifery
Keele, Staffordshire, UK

Helena Priest
Senior Lecturer, Keele University School of Psychology, Keele
Staffordshire, UK

⊛WILEY-BLACKWELL

A John Wiley & Sons, Ltd., Publication

Library of Congress Cataloging-in-Publication Data

Healthcare research : a textbook for students and practitioners / Paula M. Roberts and Helena M. Priest (editors).
    p. ; cm.
  Includes bibliographical references and index.
  ISBN 978-0-470-51932-5 (pbk. : alk. paper)   1. Medicine–Research.   2. Medical care–Research.
3. Nursing–Research.   I. Roberts, Paula M.   II. Priest, Helena M.
  [DNLM: 1. Health Services Research.   2. Research Design. W 84.3 H439 2010]
  R850.H385 2010
  610.72–dc22

                                                                            2009041777

A catalogue record for this book is available from the British Library.

Set in 10/12.5 pt Futura by Aptara® Inc., New Delhi, India
Printed in Singapore by Markono Print Media Pte Ltd

1   2010

Contents

Contributors

Sue Ashby is a Lecturer in Nursing and Co-Chair of the User and Carer Implementation Group (USIG) in the School of Nursing and Midwifery, Keele University, having previously worked as Clinical Lead for a multidisciplinary Intermediate Care Service within North Staffordshire. She has a background in nursing in primary care. She gained her Postgraduate Diploma in Clinical Leadership at Staffordshire University and is currently registered as a part time PhD student at Keele University. She was awarded a Birmingham Hospitals Saturday Travel Award in 2006 to observe older people's services in the state of Victoria, Australia. Her research interests include the interface of primary and secondary care and service user involvement in research.

Bernard Beech is a Lecturer in the School of Nursing and Midwifery, Keele University, with interests in mental health nursing, workplace violence and evidence based practice. He gained his PhD at the Institute of Work, Health and Organisations, University of Nottingham, with an evaluation of management of aggression training. His involvement in the Partnership for Older People Project (POPP) project was concerned with analysis of the quantitative data.

Roger Beech is a Reader in Health Services Research, University of Keele; Director of the Keele University Hub of the National Institute for Health Research (NIHR)'s Research Design Service; and the Academic Lead for Research, Central and Eastern Cheshire Primary Care Trust. Roger has a background in the application of quantitative approaches to health services research. He has specific interests in research to support the development and evaluation of services for older people and, in particular, those for stroke care and for promoting health and managing illness 'closer to home'.

David Bird was formerly the Health Faculty Librarian at Keele University and has worked in various public, academic and special library settings, including the Royal College of Physicians of Edinburgh and St. Thomas's Hospital Medical School. His MA in Librarianship and Information Science was awarded by Sheffield University. Research interests include historical bibliography and local history.

Mike Brough was formerly a lecturer in Computing at Keele University and is a now a University Fellow. He was one of the first School Academic Conduct Officers at Keele University and led staff workshops on student plagiarism for several years. His previous career included spells in scientific computation, medical statistics and system modelling. He has an MSc in Astronomy from Sussex University and continues his interest in astronomy, statistics and using computer software to teach maths and science. He believes that university scholarship must recognize and distinguish between the different contributions made by scholars in each discipline.

David Clark-Carter is a Professor of Psychological Research Methods and Joint Director of the Professional Doctorate in Health Psychology at Staffordshire University. He is a Chartered

Health Psychologist. He gained his PhD from Nottingham University on work into the psychology of visual impairment. His other research has included looking at the psychological consequences of long-term conditions such as pelvic pain and rheumatoid arthritis. He specializes in psychological research and statistical methods employed by psychologists. He is the former Editor and now Consultant Editor of the *British Journal of Mathematical and Statistical Psychology* and the Chair of the British Psychological Society's Mathematical, Statistical and Computing Section.

Jacqueline Collin is a Lecturer in Children's Nursing in the School of Nursing and Midwifery, Keele University. Jacquie's teaching activity encompasses the development and delivery of a range of pre- and post-registration modules across BSc and Diploma programmes. Professional and research interests include children's encounters with health professionals; she is a member of Keele University School of Nursing and Midwifery User and Carer Strategy Group, and is currently registered on a PhD programme at Manchester University focusing on the information needs of girls with Turner Syndrome and their parents. Jacqueline is a member of the Research Institute for Life Course Studies at Keele University.

Helen Combes is a Senior Clinical Lecturer at Staffordshire University on the Shropshire and Staffordshire Doctorate in Clinical Psychology Training Programme. She is also a Chartered Clinical Psychologist working in North Staffordshire. She has a particular interest in inclusive research, especially that which encourages people to connect with their local communities. She is keen that academic and health institutions should see the strength of systematic research and that these methodological skills should be shared within the wider community.

Deborah Gent is currently employed by Wigan Council as a Project Manager. Between 2006 and 2008 she managed the Partnerships for Older People Project, working closely with a number of statutory agencies and voluntary organizations to provide a range of innovative services for the over 50s. She is a qualified social care manager and social worker who has coordinated services for both older people and people with learning disabilities in the North West. During the course of her career, Deborah has managed residential services and education providers. She has developed skills in procurement, strategic planning and operational management. She is currently a member of the Voluntary Management Group of a local charity and in her spare time works with local groups to develop community resources. Deborah is currently working towards a Professional Doctorate in Health and Social Care at the University of Salford.

Mike Gibbs is a Lecturer in Learning Disability Nursing at the School of Nursing and Midwifery, Keele University. His professional background is in working with families and carers. He gained an MA in learning disability community care and is a member of Keele University School of Nursing and Midwifery User and Carer Strategy Group. Mike's teaching focus is primarily pre-registration learning disability nursing. He is the co-author (with Helena Priest) of the book *Mental Health Care for People with Learning Disabilities*. His research interests are in family carers' experiences.

Rebecca Jester is a Professor of Nursing and Head of the School of Nursing and Midwifery at Keele University. Previous appointments include Associate Dean (Taught Postgraduate Studies), School of Health, University of Wolverhampton, and Reader in Clinical Nursing at the

University of the West of England. She gained her PhD in Health Sciences from the University of Birmingham and her research interests are focused on clinical orthopaedic and trauma nursing, including Hospital at Home/intermediate care, falls risk assessment, hip fracture and associated mortality, and morbidity and spheres of practice and competence in clinical nursing.

Geraldine Lyte qualified first as a children's nurse and then as a general nurse, before specializing in children's intensive care nursing in Northern Ireland. She also spent a few years as a practicing nurse in Chicago, USA, with adults and children, before moving to Manchester, UK, to take up a senior clinical post in children's nursing. Geraldine completed a degree and an MSc in nursing and moved into a career in nurse education. As a lecturer in nursing, Geraldine developed a wide range of experience in both clinical and educational research in areas such as children's nurses' clinical judgment and decision making, child health nursing diagnoses, developing standards for undergraduate dissertation, and also a number of enquiry based learning initiatives. Geraldine's PhD focused on undergraduate nursing students' skills development and employability. She is currently the Programme Director for the Bachelor of Nursing (Hons) at the University of Manchester.

Colin Macduff is a Reader in Nursing at The Robert Gordon University, Aberdeen. He has a background in mental health nursing, general nursing and health services research. In 2007 he completed a PhD study which analysed the development of family health nursing in Scotland. Since then he has become involved in researching the dissemination of theses and dissertations in electronic format.

Sian Maslin-Prothero is Dean of the Graduate School and Professor of Nursing at Keele University School of Nursing and Midwifery. She has worked in academia, education, clinical nursing and midwifery in a variety of settings in both the United Kingdom and overseas. Her research interests include: user and carer involvement in health and social care; older people, policy and practice in the NHS; and cancer clinical trials. She works in partnership with the National Health Service, social services, voluntary services and people who access services through education, research and practice. Sian is the Associate Editor for *Nurse Education Today* and a member of the editorial board for the *European Journal of Cancer Care*.

Helena Priest (Editor) is a Senior Lecturer in the School of Psychology, Keele University, and Research Lead, Shropshire and Staffordshire Doctorate in Clinical Psychology Training Programme. Her professional background is in mental health nursing and she has worked for many years in nursing/medical education, teaching applied psychology, communication, counselling, mental health nursing and research topics. She is a Chartered Psychologist with the British Psychological Society; a member of the BPS Division for Teachers and Researchers in Psychology; and a member of the Qualitative Methods in Psychology (QMiP) section (also a member of the *QMiP Bulletin* editorial board). Her research interests are in psychology for caring, the mental health needs of people with learning disabilities and interprofessional learning in health and social care.

Sue Read is a Reader in Learning Disability Nursing at the School of Nursing and Midwifery, Keele University, Staffordshire, UK. She is currently responsible for developing research capacity and capability within the School. Her PhD involved developing a unique, specialist bereavement counselling and support service for people with learning disabilities in North Staffordshire. She has recently completed a collaborative research study with Dr. Stuart Todd, University of Glamorgan, to explore perceptions of death and dying with people with learning disabilities. She is the editor of *Palliative Care for People with Learning Disabilities,* published by Quay Books, and her most recent book is a bereavement counselling manual for people with learning disabilities, also available from Quay Books, London. She is co-author of *Living and Dying with Dignity – the best practice guide to end of life care for people with a learning disability* (Mencap, 2009). Her research interests include loss, death, dying and bereavement specifically, although not exclusively, with people with a learning disability; and aspects of user and carer engagement in research.

Paula Roberts (Editor) is a Senior Lecturer in Nursing, and Director of Marketing and Enterprise in the School of Nursing and Midwifery, Keele University. She has held various roles including: Associate Dean for the Faculty of Health, Keele University; Course Leader for Marketing and Curriculum Implementation at Keele University Medical School; Academic Conduct Officer for the School of Medicine, Keele University; Chair of the University Academic Conduct Panel; and Editor of *Nurse Researcher: The International Journal of Research Methodology in Healthcare* (RCN Publishing Company). She is a member of the Editorial Advisory Board of *Nursing Standard* (RCN Publishing Company). She gained her PhD in Marketing from Keele University, and an MA in Educational Management from the Open University. Her research interests include mental healthcare, recruitment and marketing.

David Rogers is a Clinical Effectiveness Librarian employed both by the University Hospital of North Staffordshire and The Bedside Clinical Guidelines Partnership (BCGP). He has over 35 year's experience of working in health libraries and is responsible for the evidence base underpinning the BCGP guidelines currently in use at 25 acute NHS Hospital Trusts throughout England.

Brenda Roe is Professor of Health Research at the Evidence-based Practice Research Centre, Edge Hill University. Her research interests focus on the development and evaluation of healthcare and systems for people with continuing care needs in the community, such as older people or those living with chronic conditions and disability. Organization and delivery of services, perspectives and experiences of users, clinical effectiveness, evaluation of healthcare and systems, dissemination and use of research, health policy and health promotion are also areas of expertise. She is a Fellow of the Queen's Nursing Institute and Fellow of the Royal Society for Public Health. She is an Editor of the *Journal of Advanced Nursing* and was one of the founding editors of the Cochrane Incontinence Review Group, with particular responsibility for reviews on behavioural interventions for the management of urinary incontinence. Research undertaken includes work on falls and falls prevention, a systematic review of respite care for the frail elderly, a metastudy of systematic reviews of bladder training and voiding programmes for the management of urinary incontinence, and end of life care.

Michelle Russell previously worked as a Research Assistant in the area of Health Services Research at Keele University and is now working as Development Manager for a Primary Care Trust in the UK.

Oliver Slevin lectures at the University of Ulster, where he is Course Director for the Professional Doctorate in Nursing and MSc in Nursing. Prior to his present appointment he was for a number of years Chief Executive of the National Board for Nursing, Midwifery and Health Visiting for Northern Ireland and Visiting Professor at the University of Ulster. He holds a Master's degree in Social Science from the University of Essex and a PhD in Education from Queen's University Belfast. He has served on the editorial panels of a number of journals and is currently Editor-in-Chief of the *International Journal of Urological Nursing*. His main research interests are in International Development work, primarily in the area of evaluative research in healthcare.

Tim Smale is e-Learning Fellow for the Faculty of Health, Keele University, having previously worked as a Neuroanatomy & Histology Technician at the School of Pharmacy, London. He gained his BSc Honours degree in Computing for Science with Biology at Nottingham Trent University in 2005. His research interests include virtual learning environment implementation and integration.

Susan Smith is Librarian, Joint Education and Training Library, Leighton Hospital, Crewe, Cheshire. Susan graduated from Stirling University with a degree in Biology. She has since completed her postgraduate studies at the University of Aberystwyth and been awarded Chartered Membership of the Chartered Institute of Library and Information Professionals (CILIP). Her library career started at the Dick Institute, a public reference library in Ayrshire. She also worked in the health library at the Royal Shrewsbury Hospital and as Electronic Resources Librarian for Keele University Health Library before taking up her current position at Keele University.

Ranil Tan is a Clinical Psychologist at the Psychological Therapy Service, Leeds Partnerships NHS Foundation Trust. He gained his DClinPsy from Keele and Staffordshire Universities. His research interests are in the areas of psychosis, trauma and recovery.

Michael Traynor is a Professor of Nursing Policy at Middlesex University in London. Michael studied English Literature at Cambridge and then went on to train as a nurse and Health Visitor. From 1989–1990 he worked for the South Australian Health Commission at Flinders University, working on Healthy Cities projects and on a study of the impact of a first child on Australian couples. Returning to England in 1990, he worked as Research Officer for the RCN Research Unit in London, studying the impact on nurses' job satisfaction of the 1991 'market' NHS reforms. Drawing on his background in literature, his PhD (Nottingham) focused on analysis of the language of nurses and their managers drawn from this three-year multisite study. This was published as a book by Routledge. From 1996 he worked in the Centre for Policy in Nursing Research at the London School of Hygiene and Tropical Medicine investigating research policy and research capacity building for nursing and the allied health professions. In 2004 he became Trevor Clay Professor of Nursing Policy at Middlesex University. His research interests are the evidence based movement and applying literary theory and discourse analysis to a study of policy issues. He is the European editor of *Nursing Inquiry* and Editor of *Health: an interdisciplinary journal for the social study of health illness and medicine*.

Leslie Woods' professional discipline is nursing. His research interests are varied and include the following: practice development and service delivery, nurse practitioners and advanced clinical roles, and advanced clinical practice issues such as work role transition, clinical effectiveness and role evaluation. He has twenty years experience in higher education and has taught a range of postgraduate programmes. He has considerable experience in supervising research students at master's degree and doctoral level and an established track record of publications and research grants related to his areas of research interest.

Foreword

Over the last quarter of a century research has become a key component of most undergraduate curricula in the field of healthcare. The thirst of research knowledge continues to increase as research itself continues to evolve. New and creative ways of answering key questions raised by policymakers and practitioners are evolving all the time. In the pursuit of rigour, researchers engage in debates which take a fair share of the contents of journals, books and, increasingly, of web space. It is important that experts continue to share their knowledge and experience of research in the complex field of healthcare. I believe this book achieves this objective.

Evidence based policy and practice are words which are firmly part of healthcare practitioners' vocabulary. Everyday healthcare practitioners, worldwide, take countless decisions which have implications for the lives of millions of people. Vast resources are consumed in the organization and delivery of services. Policymakers and practitioners need to know that what they do is efficient and effective. Yet for most of what they do, there is little evidence, although the pool of evidence has increased in the last two decades.

The National Institute for Clinical Excellence (NICE) was set up in the United Kingdom to provide national guidance on the promotion of good health and the prevention of ill health. To do so it relies on the expertise of practitioners and the evidence provided by researchers.

Research has the potential to contribute towards providing much needed evidence. For this to happen there needs to be a critical mass of well trained researchers capable of carrying out rigorous and clinically relevant research. The authors of this book have risen to this challenge by writing a text which simplifies research to enhance understanding and knowledge, while emphasizing the need to produce high quality studies.

There is also increasing realization that, in the context of finite resources and competing demands, research should benefit patients. As we look to the future, there are already signs that translational research and evidence of the impact of research will be predominant in the minds of those allocating research funds.

This book is written within the context of these issues. Why another book on healthcare research? There are many ways to teach and learn about research. This book provides a comprehensive coverage of the main issues, methods and approaches to research. From examining the philosophical basis of a variety of research approaches to the practical details of searching, reviewing and appraising the literature, this book will be a helpful tool to all those who want to learn about research.

Research governance is now an accepted part of the research endeavour. The increasing emphasis on ethical research and, in particular, the need to safeguard the rights of vulnerable patients, is well reflected in the content of this textbook.

Healthcare is not the monopoly of any one health profession. It is refreshing to see a book which addresses the research needs of the whole spectrum of healthcare practitioners. The authors ought to be proud of their contribution to the research enterprise in healthcare.

Kader Parahoo

Preface

Contemporary health and social care is founded upon the premise that practice must be evidence based. Practitioners in these disciplines need the skills and knowledge to be able to source evidence based information, to assess the evidence critically to determine if it is useful, valid and reliable; and then to interpret and incorporate it into their practice where appropriate. To do this, they need a sound knowledge of the different philosophical approaches underpinning research and the process of undertaking research itself.

Acquiring this knowledge and skill begins during educational preparation for professional practice, as the basic concepts are generally included in programmes that lead to registration with a professional body. Therefore, this textbook will provide invaluable support for students undertaking professional health and social care programmes. It will also help students in the preparation and presentation of course work, as it includes guidance on academic writing and preparing material for diverse audiences (including assignment markers!). It not only serves as an authoritative research methods textbook for undergraduate and postgraduate programmes, but also as an invaluable guide for health and social care professionals seeking to deliver best practice.

However, the book is not just for students. All professionals have a responsibility to deliver the highest quality of care to users of healthcare services, and thus their practice must be founded upon appraisal of best practice from the many available sources. For some practitioners, advanced knowledge will form part of continuing professional development programmes or academic programmes beyond qualification, and thus the book will be invaluable in supplementing and enhancing advanced understanding. For others, it will provide a guide to acquiring the skills and knowledge needed to develop best practice in clinical settings.

Some healthcare professionals will go on to undertake empirical research themselves, either for a postgraduate award or as part of a research team, and may eventually become a research leader as a principal investigator, leading part of a wider study or as a chief investigator, responsible for a whole research project. With a firm foundation in evidence based practice, these practitioners need additional skills to enable them to: design research proposals; undertake comprehensive literature reviews and critical appraisal; seek ethical approval for their research proposals; gather information; analyse that information; discuss findings; make recommendations; and disseminate good practice. These researchers need to have confidence in their research practice, such that their outcomes are rigorous and can be generalized if appropriate, or transferred to inform evidence based practice in their field. The chapters in this book will thus support the practise of research as well as the academic study of it. In summary, the book can be used:

(a) To support students and practitioners in academic studies that require the use of research evidence.
(b) To enable students on research methods modules and programmes to follow a learning journey from appraisal of research evidence through to conducting sound empirical studies of their own.

(c) To support health and social care practitioners wishing to find, evaluate and use research evidence relevant to their practice.

(d) To provide a starting point for practitioners wishing to conduct their own empirical research in order to enhance their practice.

The book is structured into two distinct parts. **Part One: Theory and Practice,** takes readers through a journey of knowledge and skill acquisition. Whether accessing it for the purposes of developing academic skills, or to enhance practice, or to plan an empirical research study, the book will guide the process. Chapters include **action points** and **reflection points** to help deepen knowledge and skills. Chapters 1 and 2 together provide the context and rationale for health and social care research, and thus have a more theoretical approach than the more practical chapters that follow. Chapter 1 discusses contemporary issues in good academic practice and research evidence; why we need to identify and demonstrate good academic practice; why we should appraise the quality of evidence and use research evidence in practice; and what we are trying to achieve in determining research evidence. Illustrations are provided from the field of nursing. Chapter 2 provides a historical background to healthcare research and introduces the reader to a range of research approaches including the randomized control trial, qualitative research and newer research paradigms. The chapter considers the strengths and weaknesses of different approaches and the benefits and limitations of mixing methods.

Chapter 3 explains research proposal writing, while Chapter 4 introduces readers to methods of navigating the current knowledge base of healthcare and medicine in order to identify material that will inform learning, research and practice. Chapter 5 introduces the concept of evidence based practice and considers how published research can be appraised critically in order to inform practice. Readers are guided through the process of reviewing a research article, taking a sequential approach to the appraisal of evidence from the background and design of the study; the research methods, including data collection, analysis and findings; validity and reliability; limitations; generalizability; and implications for practice. Chapter 6 considers the importance of undertaking ethical research and discusses how to seek scientific and ethical approval within the United Kingdom health and social care context. Chapter 7 describes quantitative research and enables the reader to assess the validity and reliability of published studies, while Chapter 8 describes qualitative research and enables the reader to assess the rigour of published qualitative research. Chapter 9 explores the concepts of good academic writing and referencing. The text includes worked examples of good practice, including referencing in texts and construction of reference lists, together with a section on how to reference electronic sources. The first part of the book concludes with Chapter 10, which is focused on research implementation and dissemination strategies, including suggestions for reviewing the limitations of your work, summarizing your research, writing abstracts, presenting research at conferences, and liaising with publishers and the academic press to disseminate your work.

Part Two: Research in Action, provides a range of illustrations of research with different client groups and in different care settings. Chapter 11 illustrates how methods can be combined in action research and case studies, with examples from orthopaedic care settings. Chapter 12 discusses inclusive and participatory research and illustrates with research involving vulnerable groups including those with learning difficulties and mental health problems. Chapters 13, 14 and 15 extend this theme with, respectively, illustrations of participatory research with older people, people with intellectual disabilities and children and young people. This part concludes in Chapter 16 with an illustration of mixing methods in researching health and social care organizations. All these chapters and their illustrative material focus on the active inclusion of the people who are the focus of research within that research, rather than them being passive recipients of research done 'about' them.

This textbook is aimed at healthcare students and practitioners, including nurses, midwives, physiotherapists, occupational therapists, doctors, clinical psychologists and pharmacists. However, it will also be relevant to students and practitioners in fields such as social work and other related professions and occupations. Whilst it draws predominantly upon United Kingdom policy, guidance, terminology and illustrations, reflecting the context of its authors, the general principles are applicable to an international readership.

Editors' notes

It is assumed that readers will have access to internet-enabled computers and to industry standard word-processing and presentation packages such as *Microsoft Word, Publisher* and *PowerPoint*, in order to undertake the Action Point exercises.

In keeping with the guidance presented in Chapter 9, we have as far as possible, used the publication and referencing style of the American Psychological Association (2010) throughout the book.

Paula Roberts and Helena Priest

Reference

American Psychological Association (2010) *Publication Manual*, 6th edn, APA, Washington.

Acknowledgements

The editors would like to thank all the contributing authors for their eagerness to embrace this project and for providing us with engaging illustrative material. We would also like to thank our employers and colleagues for their support. Special thanks go to Amelia Rout, Researcher, Staffordshire University, for her invaluable comments on the completed text; and to Tim Smale, Nicholas Roberts and Carrie O'Donnell for administrative and technical assistance.

Part 1

Theory and practice

1 Why Healthcare Research?

Michael Traynor

The rise of interest in research methods

If you search on Amazon.co.uk for books on research methods in health, you will find a little over 1600 titles. There are books on statistics, books on evaluation, on qualitative research, on mixed methods research, on survey questionnaires, books for clinicians and books aimed specifically at students doing work for degrees. There are books for nurses, psychologists, social workers and sports scientists, as well as for professional groups that few of us have heard of. Clearly someone – the authors and editors of these books as well as the publishers – believes that their target audiences will be interested in research enough to buy these books and, as an optional extra, read them.

Similarly, a few years ago colleagues and I studied published research which had appeared in nursing journals. The Research Outputs Database is a database of published biomedical research that can be searched by computer, developed by the Wellcome Trust. Between 1988 and 1995 the number of nursing papers appearing here rose from 0.55 to 1.29% of the database. Though small, this increase made it the fastest growing biomedical sub-field during this period (Rafferty, Traynor and Lewison, 2000). At a similar time, the United Kingdom (UK) Royal College of Nursing commissioned a review of UK nursing journals which published any research material. At that time, the study identified 27 titles published by 18 publishers. Nearly half (15 journals) of these titles had started publication within the past five years and, of these, one third had existed for no more than two years (Holdich Stodulski, 1995). Even in the mid 1990s, research was a growing enterprise amongst this section of health professionals. Today the international list of high quality research journals, ISI Web of Knowledge, contains 72 journals in its nursing subject list (http://scientific.thomsonreuters.com). Nursing is the only subject area of the Science Citation Index Expanded, on which this part of the Web of Knowledge is based, which maps on to a single professional group, so it gives a broad indication of the extent of research here.

The rise of research in the national health service: Evidence based medicine and evidence based practice

How can we account for this growing interest? Nurses and other health professionals were not taking up research for purely internal reasons. A new policy imperative within the UK National Health Service (NHS) set the context for this. Like so much United Kingdom health policy that has an impact on nursing, the chief focus of research policy from the Department of Health in the early 1990s was on problems within medicine. A House of Lords Select Committee on priorities in medical research had identified the United Kingdom's falling contribution to international research and reported that 'the NHS was run with little awareness of the needs of research or what it had to offer (House of Lords Select Committee on Science and Technology, 1988). The eventual outcome of the committee's work was the National Health Service's first research strategy, launched in 1991, with identified funding streams in priority areas for research (Department of Health, 1991). Research was to be centred around the needs of the service rather than the interests of the research community.

At its outset there were no separate funding streams for different professions, so the less politically powerful professions with less of a research background had to compete in an interdisciplinary field for research funding. Many did and some were successful. Within nursing a debate developed about the advantages and disadvantages of such an arrangement. Some argued that the profession needed to show that it had the research maturity to bid for funding on the same terms as doctors and others, while others pointed out that nursing and other health professions needed special funding to develop research capacity and infrastructure, and that the amount of research funding they presently received was disproportionately small in relation to the number of nurses delivering care. The argument was that more and better nursing research could have an enormous impact on patient outcomes and experience (Rafferty, Bond and Traynor, 2000). These arguments gained some sway and the late 1990s and early 2000s saw an unprecedented amount of research money available for these professions, from the Higher Education Funding Council for England (HEFCE) via research capacity funding jointly with the Department of Health, and major funding sources from large charities such as the Health Foundation. These were heydays, however, because not many years later such sources have diminished.

The benefit, however, was that it raised the game for research in these underdeveloped professions. (To be accurate, some of the health professions had well-established research traditions). The model of 'mainstream' scientific research, reflected in the new NHS funding streams, was one of teams of well-established experts working with large grants to solve clinical or organizational problems, possibly hiring junior research staff to collect data. The norm in nursing research, at least up to that point, was of single researchers working on areas of personal interest, often around educational issues, often for research qualifications, usually without any funding and failing to build up a body of knowledge for the profession as a whole in any coordinated way. The characteristics of the research that did appear in nursing journals reflected this model (Traynor, Rafferty and Lewison, 2001) and were atypical of biomedical research as a whole.

The final piece of background needed to understand why nursing and other health professions have become so interested in research is the emergence, along with the Research & Development (R&D) strategy in the early 1990s, of the Evidence Based Medicine (EBM) movement, later relabelled Evidence Based Practice (EBP) to reflect its ambition to include all healthcare practice. This movement made a strong challenge to traditional hierarchy and authority based practice in medicine, arguing that senior medical figures were likely to be not up to date with the latest scientific research that could be relevant for their clinical practice (Sackett, 2000). The other arguments made were that even hard working clinicians cannot hope to keep an intelligent and critical grasp on all the research that is currently published in their areas. The solutions were the development of new databases of what was considered the most rigorous and reliable research that clinicians could turn to in order to answer clinical questions, and the emergence of a great many courses, worldwide, to teach clinicians and other researchers how to make an appraisal of the trustworthiness of published research: critical appraisal (Chapter 5). Reading research was no longer sufficient. Clinicians needed to know whether it could be trusted if they wanted to base their decisions on it, or push for some change to established practice.

Understanding research in healthcare

So, to address the question, why do healthcare students and practitioners need to have an understanding of research? The first answer is because it is part of the language of healthcare today, so the practitioner who blinks and asks what EBP stands for is likely to look stupid and lack credibility. Whether all this talk of research actually makes a great deal of difference to the delivery of healthcare and the experience of patients – more than, say, the quality of managers or the amount of work to be got through – is another question. But not understanding what is being said around you is distressing and you are excluded from nice jokes about homoscedasticity, multicollinearity, or saturation. In fact, one strong impulse for nursing as a profession to take up EBP was around the desire for credibility and status. Also, as soon as talk of evidence based activity was out of the bag, it became a currency that was not likely to go away for a while. In the late 1980s and early 1990s in response to a rising managerialism and cost-containment, nurses and others were busy in efforts aimed at demonstrating their 'value for money'. Later in the 1990s, they needed to show that they were acting from a reliable scientific basis. Some looked to 'evidence' to demonstrate the value of nursing (Kitson, 1997). The danger of evidence based practice, which many clinicians were acutely aware of, was that it rendered professional decision making accessible to external evaluation. Now managers and policy makers, by collecting information on patient outcomes and having access to research based 'best treatments', even the profession's own protocols, could make penetrating judgements about effectiveness and attempt to enforce standardized treatments (Timmermans and Berg, 2003). So, the first answer is a pragmatic one. Research and talk of research is expected to be part of any credible clinical professional's repertoire.

The second answer to this question is voiced by many of the old-time researchers in nursing and is to do with a kind of intellectual restlessness. I remember the late Lisbeth Hockey (who died in 2004, aged 85), one of the United Kingdom's nursing research pioneers, telling tales of 1940s ward sisters and staff nurses exasperated by her constant demand for explanations about why things on the ward were done one way rather than another. In such stories, the justification for particular procedures given by the tired staff centres around custom rather than rationale. This fundamental confrontation between a modernizing, youthful, questioning critique and an unintelligent, status based conservatism is often staged by the proponents of research and research-mindedness. In nursing, a myth has developed that nursing practice is largely based on 'tradition, myths and rituals' (Walsh and Ford, 1989). Although traditions and rituals perhaps get unjustifiably harsh treatment, the argument is a strong one that the patients of health services would be better off receiving care and treatment from professionals who are prepared to reflect on how they do things. Being more fully conscious at work and having the nerve to ask whether things might be different may lead to an interest in research. A colleague recently told me how, as a ward sister in the early 1980s, she wrote up a kind of protocol for how each consultant on her gastroenterology ward wished their patients to be prepared for and cared for after the same surgical procedure. Predictably, they differed widely and, for a certain kind of mind, the mere act of pinning up alongside each other these lists of preferences, each with different implications for patient experience, NHS costs and presumably outcomes, would set out a research agenda.

This leads to the third reason for developing an understanding of research. The advocates of EBP point to links with revolutionary Enlightenment France, where clinicians like Pierre Louis, according to David Sackett, one of EBP's leading figures, 'rejected the pronouncements of authorities and sought the truth in systematic observation of patients' (Sackett, 2000, p. 2). Later he talks about the predicament of medical students and junior doctors who have, he says, to carry out the orders of their consultants, unaware of whether:

> . . .the advice received from the experts is authoritative (evidence-based. . .) or merely authoritarian (opinion-based, resulting from pride and prejudice). (Sackett, 2000, p. 5)

So EBP promised a kind of democratizing context where senior staff could be unsettled a little by staff who are conscientious scientists, like Pierre Louis. I think there is some evidence for this happening. In focus groups I have run with nurses over the years, I have heard repeated stories of even junior nurses claiming to have challenged doctors over particular practices with some piece of research evidence (Traynor, Rafferty and Solano, 2003). In these stories, the evidence seems to have won the day and in the process has given these nurses a new professional confidence.

Appraising the quality of research

One of the cornerstones of the Evidence Based movement has been its insistence that practitioners learn to take a critical stance toward published research, or if they cannot themselves undertake this so-called critical appraisal of research evidence, that they avail themselves of the increasing number of systematic reviews of research available in the Cochrane Collaboration (http://www.cochrane.org/index.htm) and other places (such as nursing's Joanna Briggs Institute, http://www.joannabriggs.edu.au/pubs/systematic_reviews.php). These reviews set out explicit judgements about the technical quality of the research included, or indeed excluded, so that busy clinicians can take the overall conclusions of the review with some confidence. Those involved in EBP tend not to be champions of ambiguity and subjectivity, and it is no surprise that the movement has produced a number of checklists and procedures for making judgements about the quality of an individual piece of research. Some NHS trusts run journal clubs where clinicians who are motivated to do so can be led through the questions involved in critical appraisal of papers relevant to their area of practice. Such appraisal tends to involve questions about research design; for example how randomization of participants was achieved, how completely this is described, the type of analysis undertaken and the conclusions drawn. It is possible to see such formulaic approaches to dealing with research as simplistic and authoritarian. Indeed such approaches do not encourage discussion about how the checklists themselves came into being, so can be seen as the opposite to the democratizing and empowering effect promised by EBP. However, those new to reading research, including students, can also be disempowered when instructors hand out published papers and ask them to 'critique' them without giving them a possible framework for doing this. Some students understand this as an invitation simply to criticize the work. Another problem with the democratizing potential of EBP is that, in spite of the proliferation of checklists and short courses offered to clinicians, some groups have used EBP, not necessarily consciously, as a context in which to enhance their own professional group's standing and influence. Clinical epidemiology as a previously minor medical sub-discipline (compared, for example, to surgery) stood to gain the most. Epidemiologists write:

> The main source of new knowledge for doctors in the era of evidence-based medicine (EBM) is medical research results published in professional journals. . .Nevertheless, there are numerous examples of medical studies with serious flaws in design, analysis and interpretation. It is possible to be seriously misled by taking the methodological competence of authors for granted.
>
> To critically appraise published articles, doctors should have a basic understanding of the methods of epidemiology and biostatistics. These skills are particularly needed for conducting, analyzing, and reporting results of medical research. Several studies have found that doctors are often not fully competent in basic research methods. (Novack *et al.*, 2006)

There is probably truth to this, and the practitioner who wants to consider better ways of doing what they do, and is in a position to make or recommend changes, would do well to avail themselves of the judgements of expert panels of reviewers or bring potentially useful articles to journal clubs. Some degree of familiarity with the language and concepts of research and an understanding of research design is essential, even to understand what questions to ask and this book will help clinicians who want this grounding to understand what is going on in research papers.

Why it's not so easy

Undergraduate medical and nursing curricula are crowded and only introduce their students to research at a basic level. The level of input is not necessarily sufficient for newly qualified clinicians to feel absolutely confident in the face of confidence intervals, for example (Chapter 7). Sometimes, for a similar reason of pressure and resource, undergraduate and even postgraduate research teaching and supervision is done by educators with little personal experience of research and only a partial grasp of research principles and methods. Some of those without a secure grasp of the topic can give vague or only very general advice to students and this, too, can result in perpetuating a kind of mystique around research for those trying to get to grips with it. Clinicians do not always have high levels of knowledge of and confidence around research, and this is in part a result of the structures of education in the healthcare professions.

Those who are eager to promote research in health services delivery present a picture of a process that is pleasing in its simplicity and rationality: Define and articulate a valid and important clinical question based on an uncertainty about practice, locate the evidence needed to answer it, appraise that evidence, implement it – taking into account the individual patient context – and evaluate what difference it has made. Nobody pretends this is easy and implementation is probably the most uncertain and complex and written about part of the formula. Individual nurses may find the business of changing practice more difficult than, say, a medical consultant for the obvious reason that their spheres of influence tend to be smaller. However, in many NHS trusts it is panels of clinicians, often with experts available to support them, that are involved in considering how to respond to different types of evidence and how policies about practice might be changed. There are many accounts of this kind of process and the best acknowledge the complexity of the process, how different group members may weigh different types of evidence differently for example (Dopson *et al.*, 2003; FitzGerald *et al.*, 1999; Gabbay *et al.*, 2003; Moreira, 2005). The point is that it would be a mistake to think that individuals, that is you, bear sole or even the main responsibility for this much talked about business of getting practice to change in response to research evidence. Of course it is sometimes the case that an individual might discover some highly relevant research article and may come to work promoting it to others with such energy that it is considered, but my guess would be that this is the exception.

What is quality in research?

The authors of the rest of this book will set out what we mean by quality in research in the different contexts in which research is done and from the different theoretical perspectives from which researchers work. I want only to point out here some of the very basic issues that underpin the rest. These concern asking a useful research question, letting the question determine how you answer it, telling those who read your research what they need to know and making sure that any conclusions and recommendations flow from the findings.

Most people involved in healthcare delivery have very strong feelings about some aspect of their experiences at some point in time. In a context where research is highly valued and its usefulness as a problem solving method probably overrated, many clinicians and students are persuaded to 'do some research' around some particular issue even when it is not research that is needed but some other intervention. A clue to when this might be the case is when such people say that by doing their research they 'want to show that GPs don't understand the role of health visitors or community mental health nurses' for example. It could be that what would do more good in this situation would be a leaflet campaign or a series of information giving visits rather than sending round a questionnaire. What I mean is, there is no genuine research question here. There could be, but perhaps the clinician in this case would get more satisfaction by doing something different. A successful research question in the healthcare context has to be concerned with genuine uncertainty and, in my view, have a degree of specificity. I am open to persuasion but, in my view, research questions along the lines of 'what are the experiences of' some patient group or clinicians are usually inadequately defined – at least in the context of enquiry about healthcare provision. I say this because often, under intense questioning, the authors of such questions turn out to have a much more specific interest along the lines of 'How can healthcare workers better support patients undergoing [a particular treatment]?' So, if the research question is not right, the whole enterprise is hopeless. If it is a genuine question, then so far so good.

Once we have a good research question, the way we answer it, or the method, will almost chose itself. Questions about changes over time or about prevalence or effectiveness can generally be addressed by counting or measuring something: counting admissions of patients with a certain condition in every December since 2003 and comparing it with every June in the same years; sending a questionnaire to every GP in an area and asking if they employ a practice nurse; giving one group of your patients a particular manipulation and an advice booklet and a similar group just the advice. Questions along the lines of 'why do our patients not attend outpatients appointments?' or 'why do we have such high turnover amongst our midwifery staff?' are probably best answered by asking the relevant people some questions about this. The details of different research approaches and designs that might be adopted will be covered in the rest of this book. The point is that the wrong method will not answer the question. Some research supervisors lack breadth of knowledge of research methods and advise students and new researchers to carry out 'semi-structured interviews', whatever the question.

The enterprise of science is about rigour and proof, as well as entrepreneurship, ambition, project management and having the right costume (Latour, 1987). While research in the human sciences is very different from research carried out in a laboratory, a basic feature they share is to do with replicability. The readers of a research paper need to be given enough information to judge the adequacy of what has been done, and even to be able to copy what the paper says was done and see if they get the same results. Poetic economy and elegance come second to meticulous giving of detail. It is much better to describe *how* the text of an interview was analysed than to wave an under-explained technical term around.

Finally, and following on from the notion of research being about an attempt to reduce uncertainty, the expectation of research conclusions is that they were not self-evident to everyone before the piece of research they are attached to was done.

I have just pointed out what is probably obvious to many readers. I will now leave it to the capable pens of the other writers of this book to go into more detail about the deep aspects of quality.

 Reflection Points

What is the significance/importance of implementing evidence based practice in healthcare?
In your clinical practice, what innovations/developments have been implemented which have changed practice in your area? What were the effects?

References

Department of Health (1991) *Research for Health; A Research and Development Strategy for the NHS*, HMSO, London.

Dopson, S., Locock, L., Gabbay, J. *et al.* (2003) Evidence-based medicine and the implementation gap. *Health: An Interdisciplinary Journal for the Social Study of Health, Illness and Medicine*, **7** (3), 311–330.

FitzGerald, L., Ferlie, E., Wood M. and Hawkins, C. (1999) Evidence into practice? An exploratory analysis of the Interpretation of evidence, in *Organisational Behavior in Health Care* (eds S. Dopson and A. Mark), Macmillan, London, pp. 189–206.

Gabbay, J., Le May, A., Jefferson, H. *et al.* (2003) A case study of knowledge management in multi-agency consumer-informed 'communities of practice': implications for evidence-based policy development in health and social services. *Health: An Interdisciplinary Journal for the Social Study of Health, Illness and Medicine*, **7** (3), 283–310.

Holdich Stodulski, A. (1995) RCN Study of UK Nursing Journals 1995, Royal College of Nursing, London.

House of Lords Select Committee on Science and Technology (1988) Priorities in Medical Research. 1st Report, HMSO, London.

Kitson, A. (1997) Using evidence to demonstrate the value of nursing. *Nursing Standard*, **11** (28), 34–39.

Latour, B. (1987) *Science in Action: How to Follow Scientists and Engineers through Society*, Harvard University Press, Cambridge, MA.

Moreira, T. (2005) Diversity in clinical guidelines: the role of repertoires of evaluation. *Social Science and Medicine*, **60** (9), 1975–1985.

Novack, L., Jotkowitz, A., Knyazer, B. and Novack, V. (2006) Evidence-based medicine: assessment of knowledge of basic epidemiological and research methods among medical doctors. *Postgraduate Medical Journal*, **82**, 817–822.

Rafferty, A. M., Bond, S. and Traynor, M. (2000) Does nursing, midwifery and health visiting need a research council? *NT Research*, **5** (5), 325–335.

Rafferty, A. M., Traynor, M. and Lewison, G (2000) Measuring the outputs of nursing R&D: A third working paper. Centre for Policy in Nursing Research: London School of Hygiene & Tropical Medicine.

Sackett, D. L. (2000) *Evidence-Based Medicine: How to Practice and Teach EBM*, Churchill Livingstone, Edinburgh.

Timmermans, S. and Berg, M. (2003) *The Gold Standard: The Challenge of Evidence-Based Medicine and Standardization in Health Care*, Temple University Press, Philadelphia.

Traynor, M., Rafferty, A. M. and Lewison, G. (2001) Endogenous and exogenous research? Findings from a bibliometric study of UK nursing research. *Journal of Advanced Nursing*, **34** (2), 212–222.

Traynor, M., Rafferty, A. M. and Solano, D. (2003) Between the lines. *Nursing Standard*, **18** (8), 16–17.

Walsh, M. and Ford, P. (1989) *Nursing Rituals, Research and Rational Actions*, Heinemann, Oxford.

2 Approaches to Healthcare Research

Oliver Slevin

Introduction

> Two roads diverged in a wood, and I –
> I took the one less travelled by,
> And that has made all the difference
>
> The road not taken – Robert Frost (1971).

This chapter sets the scene for the remainder of the book, contextualizing subsequent chapters that explore concepts in greater depth. It provides the historical background to healthcare research and introduces the reader to the continuum of research approaches, ranging from the randomized control trial on the one hand to examples of qualitative research on the other. Approaches to research that do not fit neatly into either the quantitative or qualitative paradigms are introduced, such as action research and participatory research methods, as are different strategies for collecting information. The concept of triangulation is introduced, and its effect on producing quality research discussed.

It is important that in these opening chapters we establish a sound foundation for proceeding to the subsequent chapters, wherein specific aspects of the research process are addressed. To achieve this firm foundation, in the current chapter we will be considering three interrelated aspects:

- the nature of research, as a phenomenon and a process;
- the historical framing of a research orientation;
- the research field, in terms of paradigms or orientations, designs and methods.

Sometimes we take as given the terminology we use. Yet, when such language is explored critically, we find that terms mean different things to different people. In the case of research, the meaning can extend from a loosely used expression meaning any attempt to explore or 'look into' something, to a very specialized technical expression whereby the term is only used to indicate a specific tightly organized process of enquiry. How we have come to see research in the latter more specialized way – as the process, in fact, of *doing* science – emerged from a range of influences over time. These historical influences shaped what we understand research to be and, consequently, shaped the very processes of research.

It is from the historically derived assumptions about research that we derive what is legitimately accepted today as research activity. Like Robert Frost (1971) in our opening quotation, we are faced with choices; about determining what research is, and how it came to be; about the type of knowledge it can create; about the right research questions to ask and about the feasibility of answering them through research.

According to how we define research, we may ask certain types of questions rather than others. On this basis, we may proceed to select certain methods of enquiry and analysis rather than others. We may then proceed to make certain knowledge claims that differ from other forms of knowledge claims in certain respects. The presentation of this knowledge must, therefore, also differ – extending from numerical formulae to framed narratives of life experiences. At each point in the way there are differences of opinion and controversies. As for Robert Frost, each road takes us on a course and nothing can be the same again. But in this chapter we can still contemplate the terrain through which each journey into research may carry us, and proceed to explore these avenues further in subsequent chapters.

Defining research: A work in progress

The notion that research should be defined in some precise way, or at least that we should continue to devote time to this issue, is not without controversy. Furthermore, it *is* indeed a 'work in progress'. What is recognized as research, both as an orientation *and* as a 'scientific' activity, has evolved over time, and indeed continues to evolve.

Knowledge is a matter of building: we can visualize clay as the basic building material from which our 'bricks' are produced (we might term this information as 'ideas'). How these ideas are then connected through propositions, just as bricks are connected by mortar (a 'binding' again produced from clay and rock), is a creative and iterative activity. From this, a body of knowledge is constructed (and we might term this a process of theorising). The application of scientific research to healthcare is quite literally often a matter of life and death. We *know* things, and on the basis of this knowledge we take *actions*. It follows that we should give some thought to the nature of such knowledge and the processes of obtaining it.

Research and science

Let us first reflect briefly on our subject. Research is associated with science. The latter term comes from the Latin term *scientia*, 'to know'. It is to do with knowledge and the construction of knowledge in a particular systematic way. This way is essentially empirical: we consider phenomena that are observable, factual and preferably measurable in some way. We submit this information ('data') to processes that will establish its validity, authenticity or truth.

These matters (validity; truth) are not without their controversies, as we shall see. For now let us take them as a means of differentiating research-derived or scientific knowledge from other forms of knowledge, such as moral positions on what is right/good/virtuous, or aesthetic positions on what has beauty. Scientific knowledge can then be taken, for now, to refer to knowledge that is shown to be factually accurate or correct (true) on the basis of the systematic examination of observations derived empirically.

It is easy to assume, because research is defined as an empirical activity, that it is simply a matter of collecting information and then interpreting this correctly. However, good research – or good science – is deemed by some to be more than this. It is seen as a highly creative and reflective activity. We contemplate phenomena in our world – objects, experiences, events or happenings. We try to describe what they are, or explain what is happening. We might even try to predict what will happen when certain events occur, when objects or events are brought into confluence in certain ways. This is a process of theorizing, involving identifying conceptual elements and the proposed links between them. Put simply, a theory is a set of concepts that are related by propositions in such a way as to describe, explain or predict phenomena (McKenna and Slevin, 2008). It is an attempt to give meaning to data.

How research is defined

The primary justification for research in healthcare is related to the matter of purpose. The purpose here is the provision of safe and effective healthcare. There is a requirement to ensure that the knowledge that informs this is the best available. Thus, we place a high premium on Evidence Based Practice, as discussed in Chapter 1. The important consideration for us, therefore, exists within the triadic relationship.

Research – theory – practice

The only knowledge of interest to us, it might be argued, is that which *transfers* into practice. It must, therefore, be *translated* into practice activities. In this sense, the most valuable research knowledge is that which we might term *applied* research. These considerations (transfer, translation and application) are worthy of note, and we return to them later. They relate to how research or its product influences practice: how it becomes theory-in-action (Slevin, 2008). Some express this as living theory, a term that in one sense infers the integration of theory into practice. The term praxis is also sometimes used to express this concept (Freire, 1964; Slevin, 2003a). It is occasionally identified as practical reasoning or (in a healthcare context) clinical wisdom (Benner, 2003; Benner, Hooper-Kyriakidis and Stannard, 1999). It comes from the synthesis of knowledge with the here-and-now doing of practice. This can be seen as going beyond a concern with cognitive 'knowing' for its own sake to the moral position of what is done with what is known. Tied in with this is a responsibility to make use of research in practice that is, therefore, not only informed but morally accepted as necessary in respect of our concern or care for others. The American nurse Jean Watson (1990) described this as *informed moral passion*.

Against a backcloth of these varying positions, the ways in which research itself may be defined also vary in often subtle ways that reflect underlying perspectives and values. This is illustrated in Table 2.1, which presents some of the definitive statements emerging from the literature.

Karl Popper (1963, 1989) took the view that absolute truth or unassailable true knowledge could, in fact, never be achieved. Rather than adopting the position that seeking verification of knowledge is possible, he proposed the idea that we accept knowledge as that which so far has not been falsified. Popper (1935, p. 280) suggested that 'the old scientific ideal of *episteme* – of absolute certain, demonstrable knowledge – has proved to be an idol ... every scientific statement must remain *tentative for ever*'.

These opposing viewpoints of verification and falsification are fundamental to the controversy surrounding what we accept as valid scientific knowledge. Later in this chapter we address the historical emergence of a movement called 'positivism', which espoused the principle of verification and the idea of knowledge as absolute truth, and postpositivist positions, as suggested by Popper (1935/1959, 1963, 1989) and others, that saw such certainty as unachievable. Consider these two opposing viewpoints in Table 2.2.

Table 2.1   Research: defining statements.

A systematic, controlled, empirical, and critical investigation of hypothetical propositions about the presumed relations among natural phenomena	Kerlinger (1986)
Diligent, systematic enquiry or investigation to validate old knowledge and generate new knowledge	Burns and Grove (1987)
An attempt to gain solutions to problems. The collection of data in a rigorously controlled situation for the purpose of prediction or explanation.	Treece and Treece (1982)
Refutes the latter. 'Not all research attempts to solve problems, and the collection of data in a rigorously controlled situation is not appropriate for all types of research'.	Hockey (1991)
(Research) ... goes beyond knowledge gained through personal experience and intuition, or second-hand through literature or tradition. It involves a *systematic collection* of *empirical information* through observation, measurement and recording, and involves *analysing* this empirical information and *reflecting on the meanings* emerging from this analysis in order to:	Slevin (1995, 2003a)

- confirm hypotheses or propositions which illustrate *relationships* or justify *predictions*; or,
- *describe* or *explain* a situation or phenomenon with *soundness*; and,
- thereby *gain new knowledge* or *verify current knowledge*.

... In simple terms, research produces sound theory, and this informs our practice.	
The study of phenomena by the rigorous and systematic collection and analysis of data.	Parahoo (1997, 2006)
Research is a systematic investigation of situations, events, objects or people and their characteristics or behaviours which may be conducted to validate old knowledge or generate new knowledge.	Porter and Carter (2000)
The root meaning of the word research is 'search again' or 'examine carefully'. More specifically, research is diligent, systematic enquiry or investigation to validate and refine existing knowledge and generate new knowledge. The concepts *systematic* and *diligent* are critical to the meaning of research because they imply planning, organization and persistence.	Burns and Grove (2001)
All sciences are concerned with the production of knowledge that is established through both reason and observation. Claims to knowledge must be verifiable by other scientists and this is achieved by undertaking a generally recognized process of research.	Mason and Whitehead (2003)
The attempt to derive generalizable new knowledge by addressing clearly defined questions with systematic and rigorous method(s).	Department of Health (2005)
Research is systematic enquiry that uses disciplined methods to answer questions or solve problems. The ultimate goal of research is to develop, refine, and expand a body of knowledge.	Polit and Beck (2007)
Research serves many purposes: at one end of the continuum it serves to generate new knowledge purely for the sake of doing so; at the other end of the continuum, research serves to solve problems ... The purpose of research is to generate knowledge and insights into our world. However, the nature of the enquiry will vary depending upon the stance that we take to view the world ... and our understanding of 'truth' as being either universal or context specific.	Watson and Keady (2008)

Table 2.2   The nature of knowledge.

Knowledge as verified absolute truth	Knowledge as tentative and provisional
Positivist	Postpositivist
Objective – empirical as impartial fact	Subjective – empirical as interpretation
Draws on the premise that things (objects, living things, structures, processes) can be directly observed – *realism*	Draws on the premise that only our experience of things, or phenomena, can be encountered through our senses - *idealism*
Testable	Untestable
Verifiable and thus unassailably true	Unverifiable and, at best, resistant to falsification 'for now'
Theory free	Theory laden
Immutable	Variable
Constant	Transient
Universal	Contextual
Transcending culture	Culture dependent or at least culture influenced
Permanent	Temporary
Absolute	Relative
Unconditional	Conditional

Not everyone would agree with these opposing listings. But even if particular positions taken are somewhere on a continuum between the two, it can be seen that the inclusion of knowledge as a goal of research is more complex than may be apparent. It is, nevertheless, the case that most people see research as a process for procuring factual knowledge.

Degrees of certainty: The concept of probability

Probability is the degree of belief in a statement, based upon the evidence available. This evidence is, more specifically, based upon empirical observations on the relative frequency of the occurrence. It is often expressed as a proportion of 1. For example, if an intervention of some sort leads to an outcome nine times out of 10, one interpretation is that there is a 10% chance that it happened by chance (or, conversely, a 90% chance that the intervention caused the occurrence); we express this as $p = 0.1$. If it occurs 99 times out of a 100, we express it as $p = 0.01$; and, if it occurs 999 times out of a 1000, we express it as 0.001. Sometimes you will see the less than symbol ($< =$ less than, $> =$ more than) used; here the term $p < 0.001$ means there is a 1 in a 1000 possibility that the intervention does not cause the occurrence.

   Action Point

At this early stage in the book we are not getting into complex statistical theory. For more detail, see Chapter 7. However, a useful starting point may be to read the following paper (which you should be able to access through your institution's Athens gateway; see Chapter 4 for information on finding literature):

Thompson, C. (2009). A beginner's guide to probability. *Evidence Based Nursing*, **12**, 67–70.

Make some brief notes as you are reading this paper, and then reflect upon how probability can help us arrive at some rational position on the 'soundness' of knowledge if we accept there is no certainty in most cases.

There is an additional thread that relates to the utility and robustness of the knowledge created. In one of the definitions presented in Table 2.1 (Department of Health, 2005), the purpose is to produce 'generalizable new knowledge'. This can be seen in an empirical sense, where it is assumed that knowledge drawn from particular situations can be taken as applying in other similar situations. This process is sometimes referred to as empirical induction, a process we return to presently. For now, we can note that the intention here is not to make a leap of faith from the particular to the general. No-one would be satisfied with applying a particular therapy to all older people suffering from dementia on the basis of it having been beneficial in one specific study of a small sample. However, if the research is repeated a number of times, the samples are large and rigorously constructed, the studies are (using the criteria we discuss above) systematic and diligent, and such findings of improvement are replicated (recur in other repeats of the study), we may feel more confident in generalizing (moving from the specific to the general), and in applying the therapy to all such individuals.

Framing the research concepts

We might, by bringing each of these elements together, construct our own definition of research. It may be useful to construct a mind map (mapping of ideas) or a more specific concept map of the ideas involved. Assuming a concept to be a cluster of linked ideas that describe a phenomenon, constructing a map of such concepts may be a more meaningful approach. Figure 2.1 reflects one possible attempt at this. As we can see, a web of linked ideas moves us towards an understanding of 'research'.

Using this, we might suggest a definition that states:

> Research is a systematic and rigorous form of inquiry using empirical methods to investigate phenomena and produce knowledge that is factually correct or true, allowing us to generalise insofar as we can assume the applicability of such knowledge in similar situations, particularly when subsequent studies replicate or confirm the original findings.

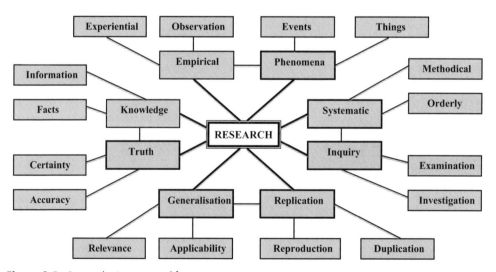

Figure 2.1   Research: A conceptual framing.

As shown in Figure 2.1, the key concepts of 'knowledge' and 'truth' reflect certain values about what these are, and terms such as information, facts, accuracy and certainty may underpin such values. Someone else constructing such a mapping may suggest different terms. Nevertheless, the above definition (and those reflected in Table 2.1) can only be accepted in terms of such language. Different conceptions of knowledge, expressed in different language within an entirely different 'worldview' or social discourse, may throw up entirely different definitions of research, as we suggest later.

Historical context

Let us reflect on the point reached. The main readers of this book are concerned with healthcare. Research is viewed as a firm foundation of modern healthcare systems. It is primarily seen (as we noted in Chapter 1) as a means of producing sound evidence that will inform practice; and thus we speak of evidence based medicine (Sackett and Rosenberg, 1995; Sackett *et al.*, 2000), evidence based healthcare, and evidence informed nursing.

From the previous sections of this chapter, we have arrived at an awareness of definitions of research, and hopefully some greater understanding of what research is. However, we must now look behind the scenes to the foundations of such assumptions. In the years up to and including the seventeenth Century, as civilization left the Middle Ages and the theological dogma rife in those times, there was an age of Renaissance (reawakening or rebirth); a return primarily to the learning of ancient Greece. In the seventeenth and into the eighteenth Century a new age emerged, one that turned civilization away from the reflective philosophies of the Renaissance to a more active engagement in the world. People could learn about this world by systematically observing it. This became known as the age of Enlightenment. One of its main elements was this turn to the real world of observable phenomena and therefore factual knowledge derived from experience that became known as empiricism. Into these times Francis Bacon (1620) brought the related concept of induction. Here, rather than moving from the generally accepted premises logically and deductively towards a specific conclusion, we move in an opposite inductive direction, making generalized claims from specific observed instances. Bacon had essentially initiated the empirical sciences, and what we today term research.

While these influences continued through the late seventeenth, eighteenth and early nineteenth Centuries, they were abated to some extent by a reaction away from an instrumental and mechanical view of the universe to one that returned to the wonder of mankind and the richness of human experience. In effect, there was a reaction against the chains of cold reasoning and an objective view of the world towards a valuing of individual freedom and the human spirit. This was yet another historical phase, the so-called Romantic era. Yet again, as the end of the nineteenth Century approached, we entered a renewed scientific age that later became known as Modernity. One important thread re-emerging here was the commitment to empirical science: we could derive factual knowledge on the basis of observation and experience of the world and the things and beings within it. Crotty (1998) suggests that this 'positing' of knowledge on such grounds became known as positivistic thought. Thus science entered the twentieth Century under the flag of Positivism.

Through various iterations of the positivist orientation, its shortcomings as a basis for how we view and use knowledge became apparent. Thus, by the late twentieth Century and into the twenty first Century, we had first (particularly during the 1960s and 1970s) a Postmodern turn that was critical of the assumptions of modernity, including its allegiance to some form of positivistic thinking, and later an emerging Late Modernity that currently adopts a more critical perspective.

The strengths of each of the earlier 'ages' or 'turns' were to some extent carried forward into the present late modernity era but, it might be argued, in a more mature and critical way that rejects naïve assumptions about science (and research) and is more open to new ways of knowing and being.

From positivism to postpositivism

Following these timelines, the end of the nineteenth Century saw the emergence of positivism. By giving primacy to empirical knowledge over all other forms, positivism at once gave precedence to knowledge gained from experience. In its extreme form, positivism excludes knowledge forms other than the empirical, and claims that empirical knowledge can be the basis of irrefutable laws; not only in respect of the physical world and things within it, but also about people.

We see in the historical story thus far this controversial and recurring theme: science is the only source of knowledge, other forms are discredited, and the quest is for verified knowledge (truth). Moving into the first 40 years of the twentieth Century, the positivistic movement became established on a more systematic basis. This was primarily influenced by the movement towards a form known as logical positivism. This was promoted by an influential group of philosophers and scientists meeting in Vienna, and known as the Vienna Circle (Ayer, 1956). This iteration of positivism held strongly to the view that true knowledge can only be achieved through either logical, reasoning processes, or empirical experience. The demise of the Vienna Circle had much to do with the rise of Nazism; however, the end of logical positivism had as much to do with the extreme viewpoint it proclaimed, which was considered as untenable as Nazism by many. As a result, a softer version of positivism known as postpositivism emerged. This was reflected in the work of such philosophers and scientists as Karl Popper, Thomas Kuhn and Michael Polanyi.

Perhaps more than any other critic of positivism and its extension into logical positivism, Karl Popper (1935/1959, 1963, 1989) advanced the killing blow. In Popper's view, the quest for verified, unassailable truth was futile. His position was essentially that no matter how tightly written our theories, or how rigorous our research, we cannot be absolutely certain that in the future further research will not refute the previous knowledge. The strength of any given piece of 'knowledge' therefore rests not on an impossible principle of absolute and permanent verification, but rather on its capacity to withstand challenges of falsification. Any such knowledge is, therefore, merely tentative; for the time being 'unfalsified'. On this basis, knowledge is advanced through processes of *conjecture* that is subject to attempts at refutation. The soundest or most valid knowledge is taken as that which withstands repeated attempts to refute it.

Kuhn's contribution emerged from a historical perspective on science. He famously put forward the idea of paradigm shift (Kuhn, 1962). A paradigm can be taken to mean an orientation, or worldview, or set of beliefs, values, theories and methodologies shared and accepted by a group (of scientists). It is, in fact, the way that a body or group of scientists approaches their discipline. Kuhn's thesis was that, within such disciplines, 'normal science' continues within the current dominant paradigm. However, a point may come when – because the dominant orientation is failing to advance knowledge or because radical new ideas emerge – that a 'paradigm shift' occurs, and a new paradigm emerges. For example, in psychology, in much of the early part of the twentieth Century the dominant paradigm was behaviourism, but this then was replaced by cognitive psychology. Kuhn did not reject the notion of science as a quest for something approximating objective knowledge entirely. But he highlighted that science is not a rigid and moribund field but rather one that does move forward – sometimes by modest development, sometimes by scientific revolutions – seeking new perspectives and new ways of advancing knowledge.

The work of Polanyi was equally radical. His argument centred on the process he described as tacit knowing (Polanyi, 1958, 1967). Polanyi's argument was essentially that objective knowledge was impossible, as even the scientist is personally engaged in the world, and influenced by it. More profoundly, he argued that the individual gains insights, and comes to know tacitly, not always thinking logically and reflectively, but sometimes through flashes of creative discovery that seem to occur intuitively. Often, the person cannot even explain how he comes to know; it is in fact a situation where 'We know more than we can tell'. Great scientists are those who are intuitively able to ask the right questions, who can gaze 'outside the box' (or paradigm), and who tacitly see in a mountain of data patterns that for them shine through. Prospective scientists are trained in the methods of research, often within a particular paradigm such as the natural sciences. Indeed, this book is an attempt to contribute to this process. However, the creative aspect of science is not so often a prominent aspect of such training.

It is recognized that the idea of postpositivism is not defined with great precision, and there is nothing like a universal agreement about when it emerged or who its main original proponents were. Those identified above (Popper, Kuhn and Polanyi) may not necessarily have labelled themselves in this way. Nevertheless, it is now generally agreed that the modern-day sciences that are often termed the physical or natural sciences – physics, chemistry, biology – and versions of the social and human sciences that model themselves on these, adopt a form of 'soft' positivism that is commonly called postpositivism. On this basis, we might see the positivistic thread within science as taking the course broadly outlined in Table 2.3.

Table 2.3 The positivist tradition.

Orientation	Core ideas	Knowledge perspective
Empiricism	Experience Observation **Induction**	Factual knowledge Generalization
Positivism	Experience Observation Induction **Objectivity**	Factual knowledge Scientific 'laws'
Logical Positivism	Experience Observation Induction Objectivity **Verification**	Knowledge as absolute truth
Postpositivism	Conjecture Experience Observation Induction Refutation **Falsification**	Knowledge as forever tentative

Insofar as dominant ideas within science and its research orientation is concerned, it is reasonable to assume that the positions reflected by positivism and logical positivism are essentially dead. One would be hard-put today to find someone in the scientific community who subscribes unequivocally to such absolutist positions. Nevertheless, the commitment within science to an empirical orientation, and a postpositivistic tentative acceptance of knowledge derived empirically that can withstand sustained attempts at falsification, are core elements in modern science. Furthermore, it is important to recognize that what scientists are prepared to state explicitly, and what is implicit in their values and activities, are often two rather different things. The oft-expressed phrase 'Research has shown ...' often contains within it both a primacy to empirical knowledge and an assumption that what follows such a phrase has been 'proven', or is 'true', in some irrefutably 'unconditional' and 'undeniable' sense.

The postmodern challenge

By the second half or the twentieth Century, a more sustained assault on positivism in any of its forms emerged. This was within a movement known as postmodernism that was in essence a wider attack on the movement or orientation known as modernism. The latter is perhaps best conceived as a movement rather than an age. Modernism, broadly speaking emerged in the early decades of the twentieth Century, is more specifically a commitment to the power of science and reason as the basis for constructing a new world. It extends across all walks of life – the arts, science, politics, architecture, industry. It champions science as the source of technology that can lead to a utopian existence. Old ways of thinking are discarded, and the old theological religions are replaced by the new orthodoxy of science and technology, with their new 'high priests' in science and medicine purveying objective knowledge, technology and certainty, rather than faith and hope.

Postmodernism was in effect a critical assault upon, and a sceptical opposition to, this orthodoxy (Lyotard, 1979). It questioned the capacity of science to be truly objective and it rejected the notion of absolute truth. All knowledge, it claimed, is in effect culture-bound and relativistic. This position cut against even the softer versions of positivism as broadly contained in the idea of postpositivism. Objectivity of any form was rejected and subjectivity as an unavoidable human characteristic asserted. Knowledge, at best, was conceived as interpretive – how people viewed and interpreted the world was culture-bound and contextual, and knowledge was, therefore, limited by the bounds of being a human 'construction'. But even attempts by those of an emerging constructivist orientation to establish a body of knowledge on this premise were viewed critically as largely interpretive and open to question.

By definition, postmodernism's unrelenting critical stance was its own undoing. Those who rejected the orientation could do so on a number of fronts. The constant rebuttal of positivism by the postmoderns was considered an irrelevance: after all, it was argued, the extremes of positivism and logical positivism had been rejected by science itself decades before. The constant and apparent obsession of postmodernism with positivism, and its strident rejection of this, was viewed as little more than jousting at windmills. Then there was the view that as all knowledge was relative, even that which recognized a constructivist or interpretive position was, by definition, suspect. No person's view of what was 'true' or an acceptable interpretation held precedence over any other person's position. This was viewed as an almost nonsensical 'anything goes' position that held no value. The problem with the postmodern orientation was that it appeared to offer no alternatives. Indeed, any proposed postmodern alternative would be negated by the extreme critical stance characterisitic of its position, or non-position: it was in effect a self-destructive philosophy. Confronted by the logical responses of the 'reasonable men' of science and philosophy, postmodernism was – just as with positivism and logical positivism before it – relegated to the graveyard of dead ideas.

Science at the crossroads: The challenges in late modernity

The postmodern orientation may well have died sometime in the latter third of the twentieth Century, but did not exactly die without trace. Like many living things, ideas often leave their own offspring that survive and have their impact on future thinking. In the case of postmodernism, this is primarily reflected in the unremitting if not indeed unrelenting critical attitude. Scepticism, the capacity to doubt that which is presented to us, no matter how much it may be vested in extensive 'proofs' or dominant social discourses, is in itself a respectable legacy. This point is made adroitly in respect of nursing and postmodernism by Watson (1999).

Research is no longer a disengaged quest for absolute truth. It no longer progresses in unidisciplinary isolation. Scientists can no longer work behind the bastions of their disciplines, viewing the focus of their inquiries through exclusive worldviews. Issues that require urgent attention – from global warming, to HIV Aids, to swine influenzas, to international terrorism – transcend national boundaries and cultures (Beck, 1992, 1999; Giddens, 1999). The paradigm walls are crumbling, and a scientific revolution that transcends this whole paradigm view is afoot. Research must adopt a truly *world* view for addressing new problems. Against this backcloth, we now proceed to outline the main research approaches available.

 Reflection Point

As we are confronted by new problems for which old solutions are inadequate, we are also confronted with a demand to consider new forms of research and new ways of doing research. Some examples of such developments are as follows:

1. As healthcare research has moved from pure to applied research, there is now a move towards *translational research,* where research is embedded in practice.
2. As globalization moves us towards our own places being multicultural environments, nursing and healthcare have increasingly adopted – in practice and in research – a *transcultural perspective*.
3. Increasingly, healthcare issues that are by nature complex and multifactorial demand *multidisciplinary research* approaches.

Consider how such developments may impact upon your own particular work and reflect upon how orthodox, traditional research approaches may fail to address some of the problems you encounter.

Research methods: Paradigms, designs and methodological orientations

Thus far in this chapter, we have hopefully established a balanced view of research as a scientific process for arriving at knowledge that may be of different forms. In the course of this journey we hope that we have also established a balanced view of what such knowledge is. Research can be a quest for factual knowledge involving empirical processes, but even here we have recognized that a narrow view of valid knowledge as absolute factual truth is too limiting. Research can also be a quest for greater understanding of experiences that are not readily accessible to the methods of the traditional quantitative sciences. We have championed a view that rejects total certainty attainable through 'method'. Although we may shy away from his reference to guaranteed truth, we have also recognized the importance of a discipline of questioning and inquiring.

This presents us with a need to consider what research processes may be involved across a wider range of knowledge possibilities. It is not our intention to provide here a detailed account of such processes. These will be considered in greater detail in subsequent chapters. However, it is useful to prepare for such comprehensive considerations of the main research approaches by considering an overview. In this context, such an overview will include quantitative and qualitative approaches, the mixing of such research processes, and the use of newer paradigms.

Researchability: The framing of a knowledge quest

Whichever orientation we are dealing with, the concept of researchability is important. That is, the extent to which a subject (topic, research question, hypothesis, posited theory, set of propositions) *can* be addressed by something we term the research process.

The research topic or issue, sometimes also identified as a research problem, is usually a descriptive statement rather than a question. Thus, the topic or interest may be 'the use of injection apparatus amongst people misusing drugs' or 'the illness experience of men with prostate cancer'. This must be clearly expressed in the research project. Usually, it should be encompassed in the title of the project. The more precise things that the research sets out to achieve must also be clearly expressed. This is most usually found in what are termed research questions. These will be statements such as 'How often do people misusing drugs share needles?' or 'What symptoms emerged within the first three months of commencing hormone therapy for prostate cancer?' From such questions, goals or objectives pertaining to how the answers will be found can then emerge. The importance of the question cannot be underestimated. What makes 'good' research is 'good' questions. Asking the right questions is not the only researchability criterion. A whole range of other issues must be taken into consideration. These include the competence of the researcher(s), the resources available and time constraints, access to research sites and subjects, and ethical considerations. Using a checklist, such as that presented in Table 2.4, all such criteria would have to be met.

In essence, the particular type of research to be undertaken is largely determined by the type of questions being asked. We must, therefore, expect that different forms of research process will emerge. Table 2.5 illustrates common examples of such research in terms of methods within different methodologies that are in turn consistent with particular paradigms or worldviews. We now briefly consider the main forms and examples.

Quantitative research

The dominant paradigm or worldview here is that of the natural or physical sciences and the paradigm case – that which perhaps best illustrates the orientation – is the experiment. The orientation consists of a particular research design intended to seek empirical information that can be collected impartially and objectively, quantified to as great an extent as possible, and analysed (usually statistically) in an equally objective way using standards of reliability and validity to test the strength or probability value of the knowledge gained.

Table 2.4   Researchability criteria checklist.

Issue	Criterion	Met or Not
Research Question/s	The question/s is/are capable of being investigated empirically	
Researcher Competence	The required knowledge and skills to undertake the identified type of investigation exist either within the single researcher or a research team if in place	
Resources	There is adequate funding to complete the study, and specialist equipment/tools needed exist *and* will be available	
Time	The study can realistically be completed within any time limits that apply	
Access	There will definitely be access to the research site. It is reasonable to assume that subjects (or other focus of enquiry) can be identified and recruited	
Ethical Considerations	The research will not breach accepted moral codes. It will not do harm to subjects. It will not breach human rights. It will not involve inhumane treatment of other sentient beings	

Common approaches within the paradigm are the experiment, the quantitative survey, the structured interview, and the Randomized Controlled Trial (RCT) common in medical research. While there may be slightly different ways of presenting the approach, and while there may be some variations in the stages of the process, it is generally a linear and sequential process that proceeds through discrete stages. These are illustrated in Figure 2.2, and such a framework is found in numerous research texts.

The example of the experiment, or perhaps more usefully the quasi-experiment, is a helpful illustration. This is essentially what the Randomized Controlled Trial used in healthcare research is – a quasi-experiment. It is *quasi* (almost, but not quite) insofar as it is not conducted under

Table 2.5   Examples of research topics and methods.

Example Research Topic	Paradigm	Methodology	Example methods
Epidemiology of a disease	Positivistic/Objective	Quantitative	Large-sample survey of family homes
Therapeutic efficacy of a drug	Positivistic/Objective	Quantitative	Quasi-experimental Randomised Controlled Trial (RCT)
Users' access to health centre services	Positivistic/Objective	Quantitative	Structured interviews
Experience of a terminal illness	Interpretive/Constructivist	Qualitative	Hermeneutic interviews
Care ethos in a healthcare facility	Interpretive/Constructivist	Qualitative	Ethnographic participant observation
Establishment of roles within a healthcare team	Interpretive/Constructivist	Qualitative	Narrative accounts
Evaluation of a healthcare programme	Mixed/Pragmatic	Quantitative + Qualitative	Quantitative survey of outcome measures Qualitative interviews exploring users' experiences

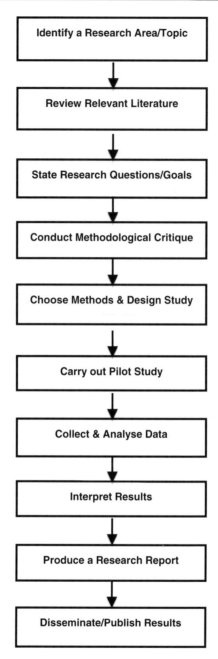

Figure 2.2 The research process.

strictly controllable conditions in a laboratory, but takes place in the real world and thus has to cope with a number of variables that are not so controllable. The purpose is to establish if an intervention (sometimes termed the independent variable) *causes* change. The object *being* changed, such as inflammation in a skeletal joint, is termed the dependent variable). It can then be suggested that some degree of predictability will apply on subsequent occasions the intervention is measured. The reader will see that the concepts of positivistic or postpositivistic thinking are starting to appear here: empirical observation, induction, verification or (withstanding) falsification, and generalization. Indeed this orientation has become the 'gold standard' for healthcare research (Bandolier, 1995; Timmermans and Berg, 2003).

In line with the natural science/positivistic/postpositivistic tradition, questions are often converted to more specific hypotheses (theories or assumptions to be tested), and this is always the case in experimental studies. For example, the question 'Does a mother's smoking affect her baby's birth weight?' would be stated something like:

> H_1: Regular and sustained cigarette smoking by mothers during pregnancy results in a reduction in newborn babies' birth weights.

Note the H_1 notation here. The H stands for 'Hypothesis' and the subscribt 1 indicates it is the research or alternative hypothesis – the one the researcher expects or anticipates will apply (as 1 it is the first, and there may be H_2, H_3, and so on. However, in modern postpositivistic research, the practice is to express the null hypothesis (that is notated H_0). This does not indicate a zero-level or nil hypothesis. Rather, it is a way of saying something similar to 'innocent until proven guilty'. Further, the assumption is that 'proven' will not come into it! The rejection of the null hypothesis will allow us greater confidence in, but not certainty of, the alternative hypothesis. The H_0 is definitely not a verification hypothesis, it is a falsification one. It is stated in null terms, as follows:

> H_0: There is no discernable difference between the birth weight of newborn babies born to mothers who are regular cigarette smokers and those born to other mothers.

Randomized Controlled Trials (RCTs)

The RCT (in line with demands of objectivity and avoidance of bias) requires that subjects are drawn from a population randomly and assigned to different groups of equal size. One or some groups are assigned to a condition (intervention) and one or some are not. They are usually described as the intervention or experimental group and the control group, respectively. Measures are taken before and after the intervention with both types of group. These are designated the pre-test and post-test measures (and they *must* be measurable by some means). It is then posited (as stated above) that differences – expressed in objective measurements – can be attributed to the condition. The attribution is expressed through statistical tests that can express the significance of differences in terms of probability (the extent to which the differences can be attributed to the condition, or alternatively attributed to chance).

This works much as follows where there are only two groups (X = Experimental Group exposed to the condition or intervention; C = Control Group not exposed to the condition/independent variable):

$$X^1 \text{(Pre-test)} \quad \text{(Condition)} \quad X^2 \text{(Post-test)}$$
$$\longrightarrow$$
$$C^1 \text{(Pre-test)} \qquad\qquad\qquad C^2 \text{(Post-test)}$$

In this case, the condition/independent variable might be something like tepid sponging the patient's body, and the dependent variable would be the patient's body temperature. The problem with such a design is that even the subjects assigned to the Control Group may exhibit changes, just by virtue of being assigned to the study and observed (in this case having their temperature taken regularly). However, assuming such bias is absent or minimal, changes in the Experimental or Intervention Group suggest the intervention has some positive (or negative) impact.

In medical RCTs it is usually the case that attempts are made to limit bias. A placebo is used with the control group to combat the biases that may exist by the mere fact of being included in a study, or if it is known that the therapeutic intervention is being withheld. This is usually (in the case of medicines) a pill of identical appearance that is in fact an inert substance or placebo. Here, bias is being combated by a process known as *blind* trialling. In *single blind* RCTs, the patient/s or subjects/participants and the clinician administering the interventions are unaware of what intervention is being applied to each subject. In *double blind* RTCs, the researcher is also unaware of which intervention is 'real' and which is placebo. Thus, the earlier configuration is modified, as follows:

$$X^1(\text{Pre-test}) \quad (\text{Therapeutic Intervention}) \quad X^2(\text{Post-test})$$

$$\longrightarrow$$

$$C^1(\text{Pre-test}) \quad\quad (\text{Placebo}) \quad\quad C^2(\text{Post-test})$$

The process outlined in this framework has an internal logic. Each stage – and they *are* viewed as sequential stages – has a purpose that allows progression to the next stage. Thus, when a particular research issue has been identified for investigation, the purpose of a Literature Review is to systematically map out the current state of knowledge on the topic, thus justifying (or otherwise) the new knowledge to be gained or current knowledge to be verified or refined. Only then can the specific research questions or goals be specified. The way in which these are expressed reflects a philosophical orientation that – broadly speaking – is in line with the postpositivistic viewpoint. Only questions that can be subject to falsification are legitimate.

While many Randomised Controlled Trials are of the above type, there are also variations. Two such examples are:

1. Extending a study vertically, beyond just two groups, with the ultimate example involving four groups and described as the Solomon Four Group Design (after the originator).
2. Extending a study horizontally, by repeating a two-group design over a long period. The classical example is the Framingham Heart Study in the USA, which has continued now since midway through the last century. The term longitudinal study is used to describe such studies.

 Action Point

Access the following sources (see Chapter 4 for help with this):

(i) Michel, Y., and Haight, B. (1996). Using the Solomon Four Design. *Nursing Research*, 45(6), 367–369.
(ii) Internet URL: http://www.framinghamheartstudy.org.

Write brief notes on each approach to the RCT.

Having identified specific questions or goals, there then occurs what is illustrated in Figure 2.2 as a 'methodological critique'. This is intended to show a quest for the best means (methods) for achieving the goals, and the best way of organizing these (design). More often than not, this stage is not even shown in illustrations or descriptions of the quantitative research process. It is taken as 'given' that if description or explanation is the level of knowledge aimed for, a survey questionnaire, interview schedule or observations study (that uses instruments to measure and record behaviour) will be used. If information of a more predictable form is required, an experiment or quasi-experiment under controlled conditions will be used. Whatever the overall design, it is a condition – in line with the philosophical underpinning – that the methods to be used allow for objective and unbiased collection of measurable data. Phenomena observed must be discrete and fully discernable; survey or interview questions must be structured and closed (only allowing specific measurable answers), rather than unstructured and open (allowing answers that are open to interpretation). The tools used must have reliability (produce the same measures in the same circumstances at different times, even if used by different observers) and validity (measure exactly what they are designed to measure).

Pilot study

Before the investigation proceeds, it is often useful to conduct a pilot study. This is a microcosm of what the complete study will be. It includes all the stages of the process identified in Figure 2.2 and is intended to identify the viability of the study and allow for any final refinements. Even where this is not undertaken, there is often an expectation that pilot testing will take place. That is, the methods to be used, such as a survey questionnaire or interview schedule are tested on a small sample.

On the basis of such testing, the research design and methods can be confirmed and the study-proper begun. Part of the design will have included the process of setting up for the next stage of the study – the data collection and analysis. This includes such matters as seeking access to research areas, addressing ethical matters such as informed consent, and identifying participants. In the latter instance, such identification in quantitative research requires objective, unbiased approaches that incorporate some degree of randomness in sampling.

At this point, as indicated in Figure 2.2, the process of collecting and analysing data can begin. This is again usually a sequential process. Data is first collected in a dispassionate, objective and unbiased way using the best and most accurate measurement tools available. It is then subjected to analysis that again is dispassionate, objective and unbiased and is usually based upon statistical procedures that treats the facts or phenomena being observed as measurable and numeric.

The interpretation and presentation of the research (in a research report, in publications and by other means) continues this trend of dispassionate, unbiased and objective accounting. How the research was undertaken, specific details of the research process and clear and honest presentation of findings must all be presented in a totally objective and unbiased manner. This ensures that the work can be rigorously critiqued, subjected to replication and further attempts to falsify the knowledge claimed, and allow for further refinement or extension of knowledge in subsequent research.

Qualitative research

This is, to all intents and purposes, the converse of the quantitative orientation. Qualitative research is concerned not with what we *know* in a cognitive, factual sense but with what we *experience* as we proceed through life. The goal has more to do with something well described by the German term *verstehen*, which broadly means 'understanding'. More specifically, the quest is for meaning rather than facts.

We do need to 'know', as health professionals, which chemotherapeutic medicines or combination of medicines will attack a malignant tumour. We also need to know what harmful effects such medication may also occasion. This ensures that appropriate clinical decisions can be made about such things as what dosages and combinations are needed to treat, and what dosages and combinations may lead to serious harm. But we also need to gain insight into what it is like to experience such drastic therapy, what it means to suffer such an assault on the person as she or he lives through it from day to day. This is the domain of qualitative research, and it is unsurprising that term such as 'verstehen', and 'understanding', and 'meaning' and 'lived experience' are used to establish its parameters.

The dominant paradigm or worldview here is that of the interpretive or human sciences and the paradigm case – one that helps to illustrate the orientation – can be taken as hermeneutic enquiry. The essential approach here draws from the ideas of phenomenology and classical hermeneutics. There is, firstly, a phenomenological concern with how things are experienced as we live from day to day. This is a concern not with epistemological knowing (which is the primary concern in the quantitative orientation) but with ontological being that relates to what we experience when we are 'thrown' into the world, when we are confronted with circumstances that impact upon us. There is, secondly, a hermeneutic concern with how such experiences (and the meanings those who experience them attach to them) can be understood. This is to do with how we interpret our own experiences and the experiences of others. There is recognition that interpretation is a problem suffused by subjective experience and personal attempts at sense-making in respect of that which we experience.

The hermeneutic approach is a suitable methodological device in such situations. Classical hermeneutics is the study of texts, particularly religious and biblical tracts, in order to establish the meanings contained within them. By moving from the whole of the text to parts of it, and from the parts to the whole, a hermeneutic circle (or circular reflexive process) is made between whole and parts as meaning emerges. In modern hermeneutic qualitative research, drawing on the philosophical interpretive hermeneutics of people such as Heidegger (1962, 1998) and Gadamer (1989), and the approaches of researchers such as van Manen (1988, 1990), Benner (2003) and Benner, Hooper-Kyriakidis and Stannard (1999), the focus of analysis may also be texts. But it may equally be any text-like alternative: a story told vocally, a dialogue undertaken, photographs, film or other media forms. Typically, the method involves open-ended qualitative interviews with participants. These tend to be discourses/conversations or dialogues rather than structured questions and answers. A characteristic of the approach is the conflation or synthesis of data (or, more appropriately, shared experience/s) and analysis.

While the transcripts of such conversations are analysed much as in the way of classical hermeneutics, even during the conversations or interviews there is an exploration of the emerging narrative; a moving in to the parts and a moving out to the whole. This process, known as the hermeneutic circle, is in effect a reflexive and iterative process that aims to uncover meaning as collection of information and coterminous analysis advances. There is often a co-creation of meaning going on here, with the researcher adopting a more involved role in the process of interpretation. This is sometimes referred to as a *fusion of horizons*, as shared existential experiences lead to an unfolding of shared meaning.

The differences between such qualitative approaches and the quantitative approaches we discussed earlier are quite radical. They not only involve different theoretical and philosophical worldviews (qualitative idealism, subjectivity, constructivism and relativism versus quantitative

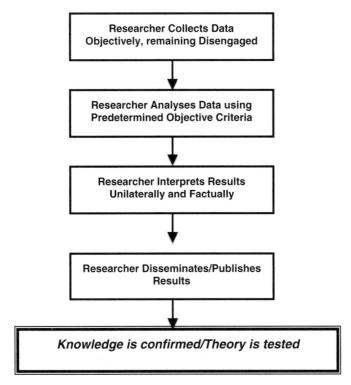

Figure 2.3 Quantitative researcher as disengaged and objective.

realism, objectivity, foundationalism, and universalism) but also differences in epistemology (the nature of knowledge or 'knowing' addressed), and the research designs and methods used. A notable variation in respect of the latter is the role of the researcher in the research process. In quantitative research, as shown in Figure 2.3, the researcher is an uninvolved observer/listener, measurer and recorder of objective information, working through a predefined and rigidly followed sequence of activities to arrive at a body of knowledge that at least tentatively can be taken to approximate truth.

In qualitative research, as illustrated in Figure 2.4, the researcher is often intimately involved in a process that is more reflexive and involves a bringing together of the elements of the research process in a more interactive way. Information collection and analysis are combined. Literature may be integrated with these processes, in effect becoming a part of the information being analysed. Researcher and research participants are often co-creating an understanding of the situation. The product is not a factual truth statement, but an interpretation that is presented for yet more interpretation by the audience. In essence, when the outcome of such research is presented, the hermeneutic process goes on.

It is this latter view of the research product in hermeneutic enquiry (and, to greater or lesser extent, in other forms of qualitative-interpretive research) that is often difficult to accommodate. Those sceptical of the approach question the usefulness of a product that makes no claim to presenting factual knowledge that has universal currency and cannot even be generalized to other circumstances. The premise that it is not even a complete 'product' but something intended to continue the interpretive process is even harder to accept. Each interpretation through pieces

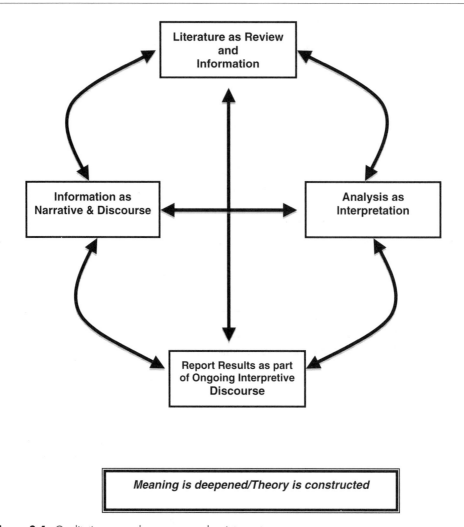

Figure 2.4   Qualitative researcher as engaged co-interpreter.

of research and individual readings of those texts is part of an emerging *verstehen*, a deepening of meaning. There is no growing body of verifiable or falsifiable knowledge here, but there is a hope that those engaged in the tale - each one an actor (patient, carer, researcher, reader) as well as interpreter – is empowered through being fellow travellers in a quest for meaning. There can be no prediction of therapeutic outcomes, either, but there can be a more insightful engagement between persons.

We must, however, add a proviso at this point. While quantitative research is a fairly structured approach so universally accepted and predetermined that it is often not even consciously scrutinized by those researchers adopting it, qualitative research is a much broader and diverse family of orientations. Not all qualitative research fits neatly under the label of hermeneutics. Indeed, many in the qualitative camp would reject such approaches. Amongst these are those who may subscribe to different viewpoints, as discussed in Chapter 8, such as using grounded theory approaches in ethnographic research (Glaser, 1992; Glaser and Strauss, 1967; Strauss and Corbin, 1997).

The case of ethnography is in fact a useful example of the diversity. The concern in classical ethnography, as its title suggests (the study of ethnic groups), is primarily with the study of culture rather than individual experience. It is unlikely that hermeneutic methods would be considered the best means of studying culture by traditional ethnographers, as opposed to other approaches such as non-participant observation. However, even here, there is increasing recognition that there is a gap between the dispassionate observer who speaks (and attempts to describe) a culture in his/her own outsider or *etic* voice, and the engaged observer who attempts to get into the insider or *emic* voice of the culture in order to fully understand what is going on. This latter form of ethnography is a mode of enquiry that embraces the concept of *verstehen* every bit as much as those undertaking hermeneutic enquiry. What is common in most of the qualitative approaches is this recognition that interpretation is the primary mode of arriving at understanding in the sense of meaning-giving, as opposed to the construction of factual knowledge.

   Action Point

Consider the following table that starts to differentiate between the two perspectives discussed above.

Quantitative orientation	Qualitative orientation
Objective	Subjective
Seeks factual knowledge	Seeks understanding
Measures phenomena	Explores meanings

Reproduce the table with at least a further nine rows. Using your reflections on the earlier sections and your further reading, add further differentiating features in the rows in each column. If any of your fellow students or colleagues are also doing this, you might compare notes and extend the table even further

---

Mixed methods and triangulation

One means of advancing more useful modes of enquiry is to mix the quantitative and the qualitative. Unfortunately, this notion can have a number of different interpretations. Indeed, it may not relate to the mixing of qualitative and quantitative approaches at all, and it is possible to mix different qualitative methods within that orientation and different quantitative methods within the quantitative orientation.

An additional area of controversy relates to the philosophical and methodological viability of mixing qualitative and quantitative approaches. One argument for adopting such a strategy is that one can enhance the other, leading to a more holistic body of knowledge. There are, however, arguments that this is a faulty premise. As one such argument runs, as one is concerned with objective factual knowledge, and the other with subjective interpretation of experience, one cannot inform the other. They speak to entirely different things. This argument brings in a concern with the concept of triangulation. The navigation concept of triangulation that uses trigonometry to plot a position on maps is used as a metaphor for treating data. In navigation, the altitude of celestial bodies (sun, stars, etc.) is used to establish a circle of position. Using circles plotted by different celestial bodies and also information on line of travel from point of origin plotted by compasses, where lines intersect gives the position from which measurements are being made (e.g. the position of a ship on the ocean). The idea in applying triangulation to research is a similar concept: if data of different types are collected, the degree to which they come into confluence increases the reliability attached to the information. But here again, as the information is of entirely different types, addressing entirely different issues, it is argued that they cannot either inform or substantiate each other.

Usually, mixed approaches relate to using different methods, and also in respect of using quantitative and qualitative research methods or tools. However, it can also imply attempts to bring together different philosophical underpinnings, different theoretical positions, and different modes of analysis. In such situations the combining of elements can become considerably complex. More often than not, researchers avoid the murky waters of philosophical differences and incompatibilities (such as the question of bringing together apparently incompatible worldviews like positivistic universalism and interpretive relativism) and proceed simply to mix their methods. Where the underpinning thinking is not confronted, there are risks that unsound research is the outcome.

The idea of mixing qualitative and quantitative methods is complex, and several understandings can be found in the literature. These are often expressed in terms of whether the methods are used sequentially or asynchronously (at different times in the study) or concurrently and synchronously (at approximately the same time in a study). It is usually found, particularly with sequential/asynchronous approaches, that different weighting is being given to one or other of the approaches. In recent times, a common notation form has been uses to indicate the degree of weighting (Creswell, 2009). Thus:

- **QUAL** indicates the qualitative predominates, while **QUAN** indicates the quantitative predominates;
- **qual** indicates the qualitative is recessive/lower-weighted, while **quan** indicates the quantitative is recessive/lower weighted;
- a plus (+) sign indicates a concurrent/synchronous design; and,
- a directional arrow (→) indicates a sequential/asynchronous design.

Using this simple device, different mixed methods designs can be outlined as follows:

Option One

qual → QUAN

Here an initial qualitative exploration (e.g. using in-depth, open-ended interviews) is used to provide information that can be used to construct and then use a quantitative survey. The arrow indicates this is a sequential/asynchronous design. While it may be an incomplete source of survey questionnaire items if used alone, it ensures there are items that are relevant in the lifeworld of subjects.

Option Two

quan → QUAL

Here an initial quantitative stage (e.g. a brief survey) identifies issues that are important, and these are then explored in greater depth using a qualitative method such as hermeneutic enquiry. This may help to identify issues or themes that (at least in numerical terms) are main or central issues. However, it also runs the risk of directing the qualitative part of the study in a biased way, rather than allowing the subject's narrative to uncover the emerging themes.

Option Three

QUAL + QUAN

or

QUAL + quan

or

Qual + QUAN

Here the two orientations (qualitative and quantitative) can have equal or unequal weighting and are being used approximately concurrently/synchronously (as indicated by the plus symbol). This is the form most often associated with the concept of triangulation discussed earlier. It is assumed that the two different forms of data will enhance the overall findings by demonstrating convergence and an overall degree of cohesiveness. It is also assumed that biases or incompleteness within one orientation will be offset by use of the other. However, as noted earlier, the fact that these approaches (according to some) address entirely different issues (one factual, objective and universal, the other interpretive, subjective and relative) means that such assumptions must be treated with caution.

As can be seen, the above three options would by no means exhaust the possible design configurations when mixing methods. The final choices, in terms of mixing methods at all, and in terms of *how* they are mixed, should always relate to the research goals or questions to be addressed. The choices must be weighed up carefully, as the decision to use mixing of methods introduces greater complexity to the research process. Matters such as modifying the overall design, how to deal with the different elements in the research process (literature review, data collection, analysis, etc.), and reporting such complex studies, are major challenges. For example, an expert researcher within the quantitative paradigm may have spent a whole career immersed in the literature on the subject, as well as the skills for reviewing such literature. However, the qualitative literature on the topic will be entirely different, and the skills of reviewing such literature in a more iterative and integrated way within and throughout the study (Figure 2.4) are entirely different. Doing one part well and the other less so is not an option and may fatally compromise the rigour of the whole project.

It is often the case, of course, that mixed methods are team projects; multidisciplinary research involving quantitative *and* qualitative researchers. However, here it is sometimes found that the different worldviews and different 'technical' language present almost insurmountable challenges – bearing witness to the criticism that mixing is an irrelevant device as the approaches in fact address entirely different things. It is important that the necessity or value added by mixing methods is established, and that the study is appropriately designed to achieve its aims.

New paradigms and the concept of bricolage

The adoption of new methods

Let us now return briefly to the diversity of qualitative research. Here, because of the complexity inherent in the human sciences, there tends to be a greater and often more creative quest for new or alternative methods. Sometimes the term new paradigm research has been used to identify such approaches. The term is not without controversy. In some instances, it is almost a 'flag of convenience' under which atypical designs and methods can 'sail', and some people in both quantitative and qualitative camps see such approaches as methodological anarchy.

In other instances, the term has been appropriated to identify what at the time of inception (though not necessarily today) were new approaches. Thus, the term has variously been used, often with lack of clarity, to label such research orientations as the more radical forms of critical theory and feminist research, and approaches deemed to be major departures in specific areas, such as realistic evaluation (Pawson, 2002; Pawson and Tilley 1997).

The most well known example of a form described as 'new paradigm' is that of action research or participatory action research introduced by Reason and Rowan (1981) and developed subsequently (Heron, 1996; Reason, 1988). Here, two core concepts largely define the orientation. Firstly, there is a bringing together of the elements of investigation and action. Rather than producing knowledge through research and then considering how this might be applied in practice, the research and practice processes are integrated: as the ongoing investigation identifies possible appropriate actions, these are integrated into and tested within the ongoing investigative process. Secondly (particularly in the form described as *participative* action research), the boundaries between researcher and participant (the researched) are broken down to the extent that on the one side the participants become co-researchers and on the other the researchers become co-policy makers/practitioners. The extent to which this aspiration can become a reality is, to a large extent, curtailed by the competencies of participants and researchers. Nevertheless, the opportunities such approaches provide for applying and indeed integrating investigation and practice can be significant. At the same time, it is in the nature of such approaches that they are ideographic (specific to the particular situation) as opposed to nomothetic (capable of generalizing to other situations) to a great extent. Action research projects are considered in Part Two of this book.

Bricolage as the ultimate adaptation

Another new way of viewing research, mainly within the qualitative worldview, is contained in the notion of bricolage. As originally proposed by Levi-Strauss (1966) and subsequently extended by qualitative researchers (e.g. Denzin and Lincoln, 2000; Kincheloe, 2001) this is a departure from older notions of mixed methods or triangulation. It draws from the French idea of *bricoleur* – a handyman who uses the materials at hand, often constructing tools from other tools to work with particular jobs. There is no exact equivalent in English, beyond the notion of handyman. However, many such workmen have in their toolkit the 'thingamabob' – a tool 'made' by the handyman himself that defies naming as it may be part screwdriver, part hammer, part punch, part wrench. A paint roller that has a flexible-necked extended handle with an automobile wing-mirror attached may defy naming to an even greater extent, but it is very useful indeed for painting around corners in restricted spaces. In a similar way, the qualitative researcher as *bricoleur* may construct a qualitative method from other methods that best fits the specific and unique nature of the enquiry.

The essential difference between mixing or triangulation and bricolage approaches is important here. Firstly, in mixed methods, different methods are used to either complement each other or validate the work. In bricolage, no such validation is primary. Secondly, mixing methods involves the use of different methods that still retain their integrity as discrete methods. Bricolage involves the construction of a *new* method from parts of other methods. The concern is to forge the method to the project rather than the project to the method. It is a drawing on tools ready-to-hand and adapting them in new ways to address current problems or issues. The challenge here is different from that in mixed methods, which involve accommodating the standards of different approaches (often quantitative as well as qualitative), including different modes of data collection, different forms of analysis, and different means of establishing rigour (such as reliability and validity tests for quantitative elements, and authenticity and verisimilitude tests for qualitative elements). In bricolage, the method itself is unique and each of these elements is in turn unique and presents its own challenges.

While using mixed methods is often viewed negatively by those who assume purist positions within particular paradigms, the notion of bricolage may be viewed with even greater caution. This is perhaps understandable, as qualitative researchers feel obliged to defend their approaches against the dominant positivistic science discourse. The idea of bricolage, flying in the face of even some positions on qualitative research standards, is seen as an almost anarchic position. Yet, in the real world, all science is much more untidy that the neat frameworks presented in the textbooks, and qualitative research, in particular, is often addressing unique and complex situations. Some would argue that each qualitative study is in certain regards different from all others. In such circumstances, there may be real strengths in a creative drawing from the qualitative 'arsenal' of tools, and even in terms of constructing new methods tailor-made for addressing particular issues.

 Action Point

In the latter paragraphs we touch briefly on the importance of research – regardless of its type – being rigorous. That is, meeting certain agreed standards. We spoke of reliability and validity in quantitative research, and equivalent tests of rigour in qualitative research.

These are matters we return to later in the book. However, in preparation for this, access the following Internet site to get you started:

http://www.bmj.com/cgi/content/full/311/6997/109.

Make notes on the main methods by which we establish how such standards are usually established. You may find it useful to save your notes in typed word processor form and retain this as an open journal that can be extended as you proceed through the book and add additional reading you undertake.

Conclusion

In this chapter we have extended the dialogue commenced in Chapter 1. There, we considered the impact of research on healthcare and, in particular, considered the case of Evidence Based Medicine or Evidence Based Practice. In the current chapter we have considered research in terms of what it actually means, how it has emerged to its present state of development through history, and how it is conducted in our modern world.

A critical and ever-doubting nature is not an unhealthy mindset when the health and well-being of others is at stake. We must remember that with all the research knowledge to guide our practice, with all the technology to transcend our senses and enhance our accuracy, humans make mistakes. In a recent investigation by the UK National Audit Commission (2005) it was found that there were 975 000 errors and near misses in 2004, approximately 10% of all patients treated. These resulted in 2182 deaths. Worryingly, the Commission considered that the latter figure may be an under-estimate of up to 15-fold (which would place such deaths at over 30 000) because of reluctance and/or absence of reporting. As humans, even cautious and vigilant professional humans, we are prone to error. An important message we have attempted to convey is that in respect of research, the evidence it produces, and our application of this in practice, we must maintain a critical and even sceptical attitude. Research must prove itself, again, and again, and even then, we must view its evidence critically and use it cautiously.

Earlier in the chapter we noted the postmodern turn away from the idea of an objective science that claims research produces universally true knowledge. At its best, postmodernism highlighted the need for a critical attitude that we must indeed bring with us into the research arena. However, at its worst it presented a petty war of attrition that did little but take pot-shots at the scientific establishment, without offering any real alternative. This we must not carry forward. Instead, we should, through the remaining chapters of this book and into the arenas of conducting research, maintain a more balanced position.

This would include continuing to refine and improve the research process. It would adopt a more critical attitude to how we undertake research and how we embed the research product in our practice. It would also involve a valuing of other ways of knowing that provide insights into healthcare delivery, and indeed help us in the important project of using research evidence in our practice. And, finally, it would help us to meet the challenges of high risk to health and survival in this era of late modernity, casting aside the fetters of narrow and restrictive scientific orientations to create new modes of enquiry for addressing new problems that past solutions cannot address.

This book endeavours to address these challenges. In the chapters that follow, we consider research that addresses the quantifiable factual world. We consider also research that engages with the need for deepening our understanding of healthcare that is qualitative and enriching. In addition, we address means by which quantitative and qualitative approaches can be effectively and creatively mixed or brought together to facilitate the exploration of real-world problems.

In his book 'The Phantom Tollbooth', Juster (1962) describes the journey of a boy, Milo, transported into a mysterious land. The book is rich in metaphor. In this strange world two nations are split apart, each ruled by an estranged brother. One brother Azaz rules Dictionopolos, where people live by the code of letters; the other brother called the Mathemagician rules Digitopolos, where it is held that numbers are supreme. The two princesses, Rhyme and Reason, attempted to broker a peace, counselling that:

> Words and numbers are of equal value, for, in the cloak of knowledge, one is warp and the other woof. It is no more important to count the sands than it is to name the stars. Therefore let both kingdoms live in peace.

There are echoes in Juster's work of the 'two cultures' of art and science, where he also hoped for a coming together of these different ways of knowing. Our book is also about researching numbers *and* words. It also recognizes the value of different perspectives and the importance of mixing these where appropriate to achieve a deepened understanding of healthcare. In so doing, we have hopefully contributed to a coherent basis upon which to build healthcare research.

References

Ayer, A.J. (1956) *The Problem of Knowledge*, Penguin, Harmondsworth.

Bacon, F. (1620) *The New Organon*. Edited by Jardine, L. and Silverthorne, M. (2000), Cambridge University Press, Cambridge.

Bandolier (1995) *Evidence Based Everything (Bandolier 12)*, Bandolier, Oxford.

Beck, U. (1992) *Risk Society: Towards a New Modernity*, Sage, London.

Beck, U. (1999) *World Risk Society*, Polity Press, Malden, MA.

Benner, P. (2003) Clinical reasoning, in *Theory and Practice of Nursing: an Integrated Approach to Caring Practice*, 2nd edn (eds L. Basford and O. Slevin), Nelson Thornes, Cheltenham.

Benner, P., Hooper-Kyriakidis, P. and Stannard, D. (1999) *Clinical Wisdom and Interventions in Critical Care: a Thinking in Action Approach*, W. B. Saunders Company, Philadelphia.

Burns, N. and Grove, S. (1993) *The Practice of Nursing Research: Conduct, critique and utilisation*, W.B. Saunders Company, Philadelphia.

Burns, N. and Grove, S. (1993) *The Practice of Nursing Research*, 2nd edn, W.B. Saunders Company, Philadelphia.

Burns, N. and Grove, S. (2001) *The Practice of Nursing Research*, 4th edn, W.B. Saunders Company, Philadelphia.

Creswell, J. (2009) *Research Design: Qualitative, Quantitative, and Mixed Methods Approaches*, 3rd edn, Sage, Thousand Oaks, CA.

Crotty, M. (1998) *The Foundations of Social Research*, Allen & Unwin, Melbourne.

Denzin, N. and Lincoln, Y. (2000) *Handbook of Qualitative Research*, 2nd edn, Sage, Thousand Oaks, CA.

Department of Health (2005) Research Governance Framework for Health and Social Care, 2nd edn, Department of Health, London.

Freire, P. (1964) *Pedagogy of the Oppressed*, Penguin, Harmondsworth.

Frost, R. (1971) The road not taken, in *Selected Poems* (ed. R. Frost), Penguin, Harmondsworth, p. 77.

Gadamer, H.-G. (1989) *Truth and Method*, Sheed and Ward, London.

Giddens, A. (1999) *Runaway World: How Globalisation is Reshaping Our Lives*, Profile, London.

Glaser, B. and Strauss, A. (1967) *The Discovery of Grounded Theory*, Aldine, Chicago.

Glaser, B.G. (1992) *Basics of Grounded Theory Analysis: Emergence Versus Forcing*, Sociology Press, Mill Valley, CA.

Heidegger, M. (1962) *Being and Time*, SCM Press, London.

Heidegger, M. (1998) On the essence of ground, in *Pathmarks* (ed. W. McNeill), Cambridge University Press, Cambridge.

Heron, J. (1996) *Co-operative Inquiry*, Sage Publications, London.

Hockey, L. (1991) The nature and purpose of research, in *The Research Process in Nursing* (ed. D. Cormack), Blackwell Scientific Publications, Oxford.

Juster, N. (1962) *The Phantom Tollbooth*, Collins, London.

Kerlinger, F.N. (1986) *Foundations of Behavioural Research*, 3rd edn, Hole, Rinehart and Winston, New York.

Kincheloe, J. (2001) Describing the bricolage: Conceptualizing a new rigor in qualitative research. *Qualitative Inquiry*, **7** (6), 679–692.

Kuhn, T.S. (1962) *The Structure of Scientific Revolutions*, University of Chicago Press, Chicago.

Levi-Strauss, C. (1966) *The Savage Mind*, University of Chicago Press, Chicago.

Lyotard, J.-F. (1979) *The Postmodern Condition: A Report on Knowledge*, Manchester University Press, Manchester.

Mason, T. and Whitehead, E. (2003) *Thinking Nursing*, Open University Press, Maidenhead.

McKenna, H. and Slevin, O. (2008) *Nursing Models, Theories and Practice*, Blackwell Publishing, Oxford.

National Audit Commission (2005) *A Safer Place for Patients: Learning to Improve Patient Safety*, Department of Health, London.

Parahoo, K. (1997) *Nursing research: Principles, process and issues*, Macmillan, Basingstoke.

Parahoo, K. (2006). *Nursing research: Principles, process and issues*, 2nd edn, Palgrave Macmillan, Basingstoke.

Pawson, R. and Tilley, N. (1997) *Realistic Evaluation*, Sage, London.

Pawson, R. (2002) Evidence-based policy: in search of a method. *Evaluation*, **8** (2), 157–181.

Polanyi, M. (1958) *Personal Knowledge: Towards a Post-critical Philosophy*, University of Chicago Press, Chicago.

Polanyi, M. (1967) *The Tacit Dimension*, Doubleday, New York.

Polit, D.F. and Beck, C.T. (2007) *Nursing Research: Generating and Assessing Evidence for Nursing Practice*, 8th edn, Lippincott Williams and Wilkins, Philadelphia.

Popper, K. (1935/1959) *The Logic of Scientific Discovery*, Basic Books, New York; first published in German, Logik der Forschung: Zur Erkenntnistheorie der modernen Naturwissen-schaft, Springer, Vienna.

Popper, K. (1963) *Conjectures and Refutations*, Routledge, London.

Popper, K. (1989) *Conjectures and Refutations*, 5th edn, revised and corrected, Routledge, London.

Popper, K. (1994) *The Myth of the Framework: In Defence of Science and Rationality* (edited by M.A. Notturno), Routledge, New York, ISBN 0415135559.

Porter, S. and Carter, D. (2000) Common terms and concepts in research, in *The Research Process in Nursing*, 4th edn (ed. D. Cormack), Blackwell Scientific Publications, Oxford.

Reason, P. (1988) *Human Inquiry in Action – Developments in New Paradigm Research*, Sage Publications, London.

Reason, P. and Rowan, J. (1981) *Human Inquiry: a Sourcebook of New Paradigm Research*, John Wiley & Sons, Ltd, Chichester.

Sackett, D.L. and Rosenberg, W.M.C. (1995) The need for evidence-based medicine. *Journal of the Royal Society of Medicine*, **88**, 620–624.

Sackett, D.L., Straus, S.E., Richardson, W.S. *et al.* (2000) *Evidence-Based Medicine: How to Practice and Teach EBM*, Churchill Livingstone, Edinburgh.

Slevin, O. (1995) Research in nursing, in *Theory and Practice of Nursing* (eds L. Basford and O. Slevin), Campion Press, Edinburgh.

Slevin, O. (2003a) Theory, practice and research, in *Theory and Practice of Nursing: an Integrated Approach to Caring Practice*, 2nd edn (eds L. Basford and O. Slevin), Nelson Thornes, Cheltenham.

Slevin, O. (2003b) Global dimensions: nursing in the risk society, in *Theory and Practice of Nursing: an Integrated Approach to Caring Practice*, 2nd edn (eds L. Basford and O. Slevin), Nelson Thornes, Cheltenham.

Slevin, O. (2008) Lost in translation. *International Journal of Urological Nursing*, **2** (3), 89–90.

Strauss, A. and Corbin, J. (1997) *Grounded Theory in Practice*, Sage, London.

Timmermans, S. and Berg, M. (2003) *The Gold Standard*, Temple University Press, Philadelphia.

Treece, E.W. and Treece, J.W. (1982) *Elements of Research in Nursing*, C.V. Mosby, St Louis.

van Manen, M. (1988) *Tales of the Field*, The University of Chicago Press, Chicago.

van Manen, M. (1990) *Researching Lived Experience: Human Science for an Action Sensitive Pedagogy*, State University of New York Press, Albany.

Watson, J. (1990) Caring knowledge and informed moral passion. *Nursing Science Quarterly*, **13** (1), 15–24.

Watson, J. (1999) *Postmodern Nursing and Beyond*, Churchill Livingstone, Edinburgh.

Watson, R. and Keady, J. (2008) The nature and language of nursing research, in *Nursing Research: Designs and Methods* (eds R. Watson, H. McKenna, S. Cowman and J. Keady), Churchill Livingstone Elsevier, Edinburgh.

3 Taking the First Step: Developing a Research Proposal

Leslie Woods, Helena Priest and Paula Roberts

Introduction

In this chapter, we discuss the early planning stages of research and, in particular, focus on the development of a research proposal. We outline what a research proposal is, why we might need to write one, what it might look like and what information it will contain. We discuss what happens to research proposals when they have been completed, and offer some suggestions for writing a proposal that will be successful in fulfilling its purpose, such as attracting research funding, or being accepted to do a research training programme, or passing an academic assignment.

There is a lot more to writing a good research proposal than perhaps meets the eye. The simplest analogy we can draw is to compare writing a research proposal to driving a car. When you have been driving a long time, the actual task of driving becomes second nature; a good driver can adapt their driving style to the road and weather conditions with little apparent effort; on the other hand, a poor driver will not take account of the varying conditions and is likely to end up in a ditch. But imagine starting out on your driving career as a learner; just sitting behind the wheel the first few times can be a daunting prospect, after all, there are so many variables to consider! Whether you are driving on a deserted motorway on a bright sunny day, or driving down a narrow, unlit country lane, in the dark during a thunderstorm, the fundamentals of good driving remain the same. And so it is with writing a good research proposal. The purpose, length, audience and so forth may vary but the basic content and structure sticks to a fundamental set of principles, which we will examine in this chapter.

To stay with the driving analogy just a little longer, to be able to adapt your driving style to the weather conditions, you need to know some theory about stopping distances, speed, car handling, such as cornering, skid technique and anti-lock brakes. If you have actual experience on top of all this knowledge, so much the better. The point we're trying to make here is that to write a good research proposal you need to have sound knowledge and understanding of the research process and research design, as covered in other chapters within this text. So while this chapter occurs toward the beginning of the book and is called taking the first steps... it could equally appear as one of the last chapters! As any strategist will tell you, the detail is in the planning! Here end the analogies, at least for the time being, so let's get started.

What is a research proposal?

A research proposal is defined as '...a document specifying the researcher's proposed study plans; it communicates the research problem, its significance, planned procedures for solving the problem and when funding is involved, how much the study will cost' (Polit and Beck, 2006, p. 507).

At its simplest, a research proposal is a plan of action. Research proposals are, therefore, future orientated. They provide accounts of how the research will be carried out so that it can achieve its aims and objectives. One way to think about research proposals is that they are intended to answer the five 'W' and 'H' questions of the research process, that is the why, what, who, where, when and how? Research proposals should provide:

- a rationale and justification for the need for the research (the why?);
- the precise aims and scope of the project (the what?);
- the participants involved in the study (the who?);
- over what period the study will take place (the when?);
- the design and methodology to be employed (the where, the what and the how?);
- the milestones to be achieved (the what and the when?);
- the resources needed (the what and the who?);
- the possible outcomes (the what?).

This may seem a simplistic formula or approach to writing a proposal, but these are exactly the sorts of questions that you need to address. A good research proposal needs to be clearly detailed, analytical and persuasive. The exact nature and extent of a research proposal will, largely, be governed by the person or organization to whom the proposal is to be submitted.

Why write a research proposal?

Essentially, no research can be undertaken without there being a research proposal in place, and reviewed and approved by others, such as academic supervisors, peers, colleagues, or research funding organizations. There are many benefits, not least being that if the proposal is well thought out and written, its contents can easily be included in the final written report of the project. (Department of Health, 1998).

Who is the research proposal for?

Research proposals can be developed for a number of purposes and audiences. As well as acting as a plan for yourself, there are probably three main reasons for developing a proposal:

- academic reasons;
- ethical reasons;
- financial reasons.

Each of these reasons will have a different audience. So whether the proposal is being developed for submission to a tutor or lecturer as an academic assignment, or to a university for an application to undertake a research degree, or to an ethics committee for ethical approval, or a submission to a funding body, the focus may be somewhat different but the essential content will be the same.

Academic reasons

Academic assignments

Many undergraduate programmes, including nursing, midwifery, medicine, social work and physiotherapy, require that students carry out a research related project, normally in the final year of the course. Increasingly, because of the requirements for project proposals to be scrutinized by a number of bodies before research can be carried out, which creates time pressures in already time-limited programmes, universities are looking to alternative methods to test students' research ability and aptitude. Sometimes, students are required to conduct a 'desk based' study such as a literature review, or produce a proposal for an audit (for more on the difference between research and audit, see Chapter 6), or, indeed, to develop and present a full research proposal for a piece of research that might be done in the future. Hence, a thorough understanding of the nature and format of research proposals is becoming increasingly relevant in higher education programmes in health and social care.

Applications to study for a research degree

These would normally be applications to study a Master of Philosophy degree or a Doctoral Programme (such as a PhD) but the range of academic programmes that include research is increasing. Some universities, for example, deliver taught Masters degrees in nursing or Professional Doctorates in health. There are a range of Professional Doctorates, such as Clinical Psychology, where doctoral level training is the normal or only route into the profession. Such programmes will normally include a research component and require the production of a research thesis. Either for admission to the programme or shortly after commencing it, a full and detailed research proposal will be required of course participants.

Ethical reasons

In simple terms, if a research proposal does not provide all the information upon which a review committee or ethical committee (Chapter 6) can make a judgement, then not only should the research not proceed, but it would be unethical for it to do so.

Financial reasons

If an organization such as a research council or a charity wants to commission and sponsor some research, and will provide finance for an appropriate project, then it is crucial that your proposal is the one that 'stands out from the crowd' in what is often a very competitive arena. Hence, the need to prepare a clearly worded, well presented and succinct account of the proposed research.

 Action Point

Write a summary of your reasons for wishing to develop a research proposal. Identify the academic, ethical and financial considerations you will need to take into account.

Support for research

Again, the amount and type of support needed to get the research off the ground in the form of a research proposal will depend on the reason for conducting the research. If you are enroled on an academic course of study, then the course tutors and lecturers are the most obvious sources of help. If you are developing a proposal in order to apply to study for a research degree, then it would be a good idea to find out the areas of research expertise and interest of the staff in your local universities within the relevant departments. If you find relevant people, you can approach them informally to find out if they are willing and able to supervise your proposed research and if they can offer you support or guidance in preparing your proposal.

If you want to conduct some clinical research, either as part of your academic studies or because, as a practitioner, you have a question about some aspect of practice or an intervention, then you will need to harness the support of your managers and colleagues. They will need to be convinced that the work is important enough to allow you the time and resources needed to carry it out. In some cases, it might be appropriate to conduct the research collaboratively amongst the team in which you work; in this case, a collaboratively prepared proposal is likely to be effective.

Whatever the purpose of your research, if you are planning to conduct research within a health or social care context you are likely at some stage to want to access patients or relatives, healthcare staff, premises, or documents such as case notes to gather information to help answer your questions. While you cannot formally approach people at this stage before the project has approval, you can 'sound out' potential sources of support who can help you to judge the feasibility of your study. Imagine that you want to carry out a survey of staff in an Accident and Emergency department, to find out how prepared they are to help patients who self-harm. It would be a good idea to talk to the clinical managers from the range of professional groups you wish to survey, to find out whether their staff are likely to respond positively to this. They can also advise on numbers of staff in the department and how best to advertise or 'sell' the idea when the research is approved, such as attending a staff meeting or putting up posters in the department.

Time spent on identifying appropriate sources of support at an early stage will pay dividends as you prepare your proposal for submission and approval to the appropriate people or organizations.

What does a research proposal contain, and how is it structured?

A typical research proposal will include some or all of the following sections, normally presented in the order shown in Box 3.1:

It is perfectly reasonable to create your own proposal, perhaps using these sections as sub-headings. The following paragraphs provide more detail on what might be included in each section, and the RD Direct organization (RD Direct, 2009) provides a clear flowchart to guide you systematically through the steps of the research process. However, funding bodies or academic institutions normally have a set format or standard application form for proposals which it would be important to follow to maximize your chances of the proposal at least being read!

Box 3.1   Research Proposal Contents

- Title;
- Summary or abstract;
- Collaboration and supervision arrangements if it is a student project;
- Introduction and rationale/justification;
- Research aims, objectives, questions and hypotheses;
- Literature review;
- Research design and methodology (including study population, research site, procedure, measures and tools, data collection, data analysis and pilot study);
- Ethical issues;
- Timescale;
- Resources and funding.

Title

This should capture and communicate readily what the proposed research is about. It is better to have a main title and a sub-title, rather than a lengthy sentence that is difficult to follow. For example, 'a qualitative study investigating the experiences of couples where one partner is suffering from cancer' might better be worded as: 'Couples' experience of cancer: a qualitative investigation'. Sometimes, both a full title and a short title are requested on proposal forms; in this instance, both the above versions might be used.

Summary or abstract

This is similar to the abstracts that precede articles published in academic and professional journals. If one is asked for, it should give the reader an overview of what the proposal contains (the why, the what, the who, the how). A maximum word limit may be given, and is likely to be no more than 300 words. In practice, the summary is likely to be written after the proposal has been completed, to ensure that all key points from the proposal are included.

Collaboration and supervision

Those judging the merit of the proposal will want to know that the research will be conducted by people who are competent to carry out all aspects of the proposed research. So, for example, if the study involves statistical analysis, it would be important to demonstrate that the team had a member who was skilled in this area. If the research is being undertaken as part of an educational qualification, then the reviewers will not expect high levels of research knowledge and experience (after all, even doctoral level study is regarded as 'research training'). They will, however, want to assure themselves that there are competent supervisors in place for the duration of the research. For these reasons, all collaborators and supervisors should be named as part of the research team.

Introduction and rationale/justification

This is the section where you make a case for doing the research in the first place. Often, in professional disciplines, the research 'problem' arises from experiences in practice. You have noticed something being done in a particular way with little effect, and you wonder if there is a better way of carrying out that task. Or you wonder what it is like to be a patient experiencing painful treatment and if there is anything that can be done to improve the treatment and lessen pain. The list of potentially researchable clinical problems is endless.

Other sources that provide the impetus for conducting research include the professional literature; for example, as a learning disabilities nurse you have read a paper suggesting that more research is needed into assessing the mental health needs of people with learning disabilities. This gets you wondering whether you could help to contribute to that knowledge base by developing and testing an assessment tool. Or, you have read accounts of research that has been done in group home settings, and you wonder whether the same findings would emerge from people living independently in the community.

Often the best research arises from someone having a 'hunch' that x or y is the case, and they set out to explore if it is so. In all cases, though, it is important to find out whether similar research has been done before and, if not, this will form part of the justification for conducting the research you are proposing. Your literature review (see below and Chapters 4 and 5) will help to establish what has been done before.

Research aims, objectives, questions and hypotheses

Depending on the format of the proposal, you may be asked to explain any or all of the following in relation to your project: aim(s), objective(s), research question(s), hypothesis(es). Each requires a slightly different approach, but all must be clearly defined and worded so that there is no ambiguity about what you intend.

Aim

This is what you, as the researcher, are hoping to achieve through carrying out the research. For example, you are working with older people admitted to hospital for short periods of respite care. Respite care is 'any intervention [such as hospital admission] designed to give rest or relief to caregivers' (Lee and Cameron, 2003). You believe that these patients' nutritional needs are not being adequately addressed on admission (in comparison to patients admitted for long-term care), and you think this may be because there is no adequate assessment tool available for short stay patients. So your research might aim to 'explore how respite patients' nutritional needs are assessed on admission and suggest improvements to the assessment process'.

 Action Point

Write a draft aim for a research project that you might be interested in conducting.

Objective

Objectives state more explicitly what will be achieved by doing the research. In the dietary needs example above, in addition to the aims, you might have an objective 'to produce and test an assessment tool for respite patients' nutritional needs'.

Action Point

Write some draft objectives for your proposed study, starting with the phrase: 'At the end of the study, the following objectives will have been achieved':

Research question

A research question provides even more precision to the aims of the project by stating exactly what it is the researcher wishes to find out. Research questions help to identify the type of information that needs to be gathered to answer the question(s), and the ways in which that information might be collected and analysed. For example, a research question might be worded as: 'How are patients' nutritional needs assessed on admission to hospital for respite care?' To find out the answer to this question, you might conduct a local observational study in your ward or a similar one, observing the admission process and noting down what is asked, by whom, in what way, what other assessments are carried out (e.g. weighing the patient), and what is done with the information. Or you might conduct a larger study whereby you send a questionnaire to nurses working with respite patients and asking for this information in writing. There are often different ways of answering the question, and deciding the best way is part of the research design process.

 Action Point

Formulate your draft research question and ask colleagues to comment on the feasibility of answering it.

Hypothesis

For some kinds of research, the question is written as a hypothesis, or prediction, that will be tested out by the research (Chapters 2 and 7). Hypotheses are normally associated with quantitative research and are often tested by means of an experiment or large scale survey. So, for example, you might conduct a nationwide survey in which you predict that: 'Respite patients are less likely to receive a thorough assessment of nutritional needs on admission to hospital than patients admitted for longer term continuing care'. In this case, you are confident of the direction that the prediction will take, that is that respite patients fare worse than continuing care patients in this respect. This is known as a 'one tailed' hypothesis. Sometimes, though, while you are sure there will be a difference, you are not entirely sure which direction it will take. This is known as a 'two tailed' hypothesis, and simply predicts that 'there will be a difference between ...' (in this example, the way in which respite patients are assessed and the way in which longer term patients are assessed).

It is usual also to write a 'null hypothesis', which allows for chance factors to have produced any observed differences. So the null hypothesis might be worded as: 'there will be no difference in the way in which respite and continuing care patients' nutritional needs are assessed'. Sometimes an additional statement is made, such as 'any differences found will be due to chance factors'. These issues are explored further in Chapter 7.

Operationalizing terms

Whether the research is exploratory or predictive, it is important that there are no ambiguous terms within research questions or hypotheses and that there is a clearly defined way of measuring all the things that you want to measure. For example, you would want to define exactly what you meant by 'respite patients', such as 'respite patients are defined as those people admitted for a period of three weeks or less to give rest or relief to their caregivers'. If you had used a term such as 'thorough assessment', you would need to say what you mean by 'thorough'; does this mean that an appropriate assessment tool has been used? Or that specific questions are asked on admission about dietary intake? Or that specific measurements are recorded, such as patients' weight and height?

Literature review

Having justified the need for the research, and explained exactly what it is you want to find out, the next step in the research process (and an important section of the proposal) is conducting a literature review. It would be unreasonable to expect a prospective researcher to have conducted a full scale review of all the relevant and available literature (including books, journal articles, official reports, unpublished material, and internet sources) before knowing whether the project will be approved or funded. Nonetheless, the prospective researcher will need to demonstrate that they have a reasonable awareness of key literature and evidence on the chosen topic in order to demonstrate that:

- this research is important;
- it is based upon a clear scientific background and rationale;
- it has not been undertaken before (or not in this way, or with this particular group of participants, or in this particular setting);
- it will provide new information;
- where appropriate, it will have a practical application.

Hence, from the outset, a broad search of the available literature is carried out, to find out whether anything similar has been done before. Searching the literature is explained in detail in Chapter 4. Following this, a selection of the most relevant literature (or all the available literature, if this is limited) is reviewed. This is important because if answers to the same or similar questions have already been established, or convincing evidence is already available, then there might be no need to undertake the project and indeed it could be unethical to do so. However, replicating research in different settings or with different populations or methods might be appropriate. We discuss how to find relevant information in Chapter 4, and ways of reviewing and critiquing the literature in Chapter 5.

One of the main purposes of the initial literature review is to justify the current research – to identify a gap in knowledge that the proposed research hopes to fill. So by looking at what is already known, this gap can be identified and communicated clearly in the proposal. Reviewers will also be able to judge, from the way that you write and structure your literature review, something about your level of knowledge, understanding and ability to communicate ideas concisely (depending on the project, you may have only one or two sides of A4 to summarize and communicate your argument). Hence, a well thought out, well constructed and accurately referenced literature review will help to convince reviewers that your proposal is worth supporting. Make sure that all the literature and documents you cite are referenced fully in a list at the end of the proposal (for more on producing reference lists, see Chapter 9).

Research design and methodology

This is one of the most important sections of the proposal. The design of the research is the broad approach to be used, such as an experiment or a survey. The methodology is the way in which that approach will be applied in your particular study; for example, the survey is to be carried to by means of a postal questionnaire.

The critical issue here is that the design and methods proposed must enable you to answer the research questions or accept or reject your hypotheses. It is not uncommon to hear people say 'I want to do a survey' or 'I would like to do some in-depth interviews', or even 'I want to do discourse analysis' (a specific approach to the analysis of interviews or texts), before they even know what it is they want to find out. We can't emphasize too strongly here: the question determines the method, not the other way round!

Having decided on the question, the design section of a research proposal will explain how the methods and procedures to be used will enable the question to be addressed. It will detail all aspects of the study design, including what will be examined under what conditions; what type of information will be collected; how information will be collected, and from whom; and what will be done with the information once it is collected. Once again, this information is provisional – it is what you propose to do. Amendments may need to be made as the research progresses and practical issues are encountered.

It would be usual to present this section of a proposal under sub-headings such as: study population, sample/participants, pilot study, sampling/recruitment, measures or tools, procedures, data analysis. It is often helpful to summarize this information in a flow chart, so that the reader can see at a glance what will be involved from the researcher and potential participants' point of view. The flow chart does not, however, replace the detailed textual description of its component parts, as follows.

Study population

Full details of participants will be included, with clear inclusion and exclusion criteria, together with details of the setting where data will be collected. There should be detail on how access to participants will be organized, and estimates of attrition (withdrawal from the study) and reasons for attrition must be provided. You should provide a justification for the selected numbers of participants, with a power analysis to calculate how many respondents are required given the chosen level of statistical significance (Chapter 7).

 Action Point

Write some inclusion criteria for the respite patients' dietary needs study, making your own decisions about things such as age group, sex, health problem and so on. To start you off, you might want to say that people can be included in your study if they are:

1. Patients admitted to Clover Ward for respite care between January 1st and December 31st.
2. Aged 65 and above.

Write some more inclusion criteria . . .

Research site or setting

This is a description of the place or places where you will carry out the research. At this stage, you may not know exactly which sites will support or host your research, so you might say something along the lines of 'one ward in a District General Hospital in the United Kingdom', or 'homes of family carers of people with Alzheimer's disease in one UK county'. Where there are multiple sites, if possible give an indication of how many, such as 'four Community Mental Health Team bases in two Strategic Health Authorities in England'. For projects that involve sites nationwide (such as a postal survey), it is adequate to say just that, that is, a nationwide postal survey will be conducted.

Whatever the precise nature of your study and the sites that you wish to access, it is important to maintain the anonymity of your proposed research sites as far as possible in your proposal, unless you have written permission to include the names of specific organizations or people.

Procedure

This should contain a clear statement of what will be done: how people will be contacted, what information they will be given, how often, what they will be asked to do, and how they will be debriefed after they have participated. The section should indicate how other information, such as biographical details, will be collected. Potential risks must be identified and details of safeguards to be put in place against any such risks outlined.

Measures/tools

Measures or tools to be used (fully referenced), and what they assess, should be described fully, including information on the range of normal scores/results and the nature of the data which will result. If tools or measures are to be developed specifically for the research, issues of reliability and validity must be addressed. Sometimes, samples of such tools are requested with the proposal, such as a validated questionnaire and evidence of permission to use it, or a self-devised questionnaire and information about how this has been/will be tested for reliability/validity, or a proposed interview schedule outlining topic areas, key questions and prompts where appropriate.

Data analysis

This section should identify the selected statistical or qualitative analysis methods to be used (Chapters 7 and Chapter 8). If hypotheses have been stated, a statistical test should be nominated with a description of exactly how the analysis will be conducted. It should show how data will be handled for analysis (for example by entering test scores into a spreadsheet or statistical package file, or by recording and transcribing interviews), whether a software package will be used, and how the analysis will be carried out (for example by using a grounded theory approach, discourse analysis, interpretive phenomenological analysis, or other method). See Chapter 7 and 8 for more information on these approaches to data analysis.

Pilot study

If applicable, details of when and with whom a pilot study will be conducted should be provided, and how the results might influence the project. In general, a pilot study is a precursor to a larger study and is used to determine certain aspects of the design and content of the full study. For example, you might want to identify an appropriate sample size for your full project, or you might wish to test out the wording of a questionnaire you have devised on a group of colleagues or on a population similar to the one you will access for the research.

Ethical issues

Key ethical issues which should be addressed in a research proposal are informed consent, confidentiality, storage of data, researcher competence, risk, safety, service user involvement, deception and debriefing. These issues are discussed fully in Chapter 6, but it is worth noting that often a participant information sheet and participant consent form(s) must be prepared and included with the research proposal. In any case, as these documents will be needed later when applying for ethical approval, it is as well to have them prepared at the proposal stage. The NHS National Research Ethics Service (NRES), which forms part of the NHS National Patient Safety Agency (NPSA) provides sample Participant Information sheets in its guidance, together with sample consent forms. These can be accessed online (NRES, 2009) and should be used/adapted in all cases of NHS research.

 Action Point

Draft Part 1 of a Participant Information Sheet for potential participants in the respite patients' dietary needs study. Refer to the template and guidance available from NRES, 2009, version 3.5, Section 6 (see: http://www.nres.npsa.nhs.uk/applications/guidance/#PIS).
   Only use the sections that are relevant to your study.

Timescale

A broad timetable for the conduct of the research is normally required as part of the proposal. At the very least, start and end dates are normally required. When planning your research proposal, it is useful to break down the project into phases or stages, and to write down the aims and methodology of each stage; this will help you to articulate clearly the process for each stage and provide an aide-memoire when writing the detailed proposal.

 Action Point

Plan a timetable for your study, using the following table, indicating the proposed stages of the study, length of time proposed for each stage, and the proposed aims, data collection and analysis method(s) of each stage.
   Study timetable

Stage of study	Dates	Aims	Data Collection Methods	Data Analysis Methods

Resources and funding

It is important that your research proposal is properly costed. If you are applying for external funding you will need to demonstrate the full costs of undertaking the research. If you work in a large organization, such as the NHS or a Higher Education Institution, your research office will be able to assist with costings. You will need to provide some basic information such as: Who will be part of the proposal? Which staff, and what will be their time commitments? For example, do you need a full or part-time research assistant? What proportion of time will the principal investigator give to the project? For example, one or two days per month? Be sure to factor in time for project team meetings on a regular basis. Everything must be costed into the proposal, such as computer equipment and software. You should consider what consumables (such as stationery and postage) you need, and how much travelling there will be to the research sites. The costings should reflect the full activity of the research proposal, including organizational running costs required. The cost of office space, lighting, heating and all the other organizational running costs have to be factored in. While your research office can help, detail of all activity needs to be specific in order to assist them in making accurate costings.

Common pitfalls and good practice in producing a research proposal

Make sure you don't fall at the first hurdle by failing to include some required information, such as the research team's Curriculum Vitae (CVs), or miss the submission deadline. When research proposals have a deadline (either as academic assignments or to obtain funding) there is a lot of pressure to finalize and submit them on time. However, a rushed submission may create problems for you later on, even if the proposal is accepted. Therefore, at the outset, you should factor in development time in order to meet the deadline.

Assuming the proposal involves more than one researcher, it is important to identify from the outset a Chief Investigator (CI) who takes the lead in developing and liaising with the others. The CI has overall responsibility for the research, including where there is more than one site. If the research will take place in more than one site, principal investigators (PIs) may need to be identified to steer and monitor the research at each site. In single-site studies, the CI and PI are usually the same person.

Liaise with potential collaborators early on, and confirm their contribution at the outset. Obtain their written consent to be included in the proposal. Specify and agree their contribution at the outset. You should also obtain their CV to include in the proposal. Do not include anyone in the proposal who has not confirmed their involvement with you directly. Do not add in anyone who someone else has recommended without having the discussions and consent of the person involved. Be cautious about including people who do not commit to the proposal during its development. Each contributor should have a specified area of responsibility for the development of the proposal. If a named contributor does not contribute during its development, for example by not attending meetings or contributing text and comments during the development of the proposal, will they contribute as agreed once they get the proposal accepted? It is important to keep copies of all documents, either in a secure computer file or printed and stored in a research folder, for the duration of the project and beyond. We discuss the ethics of data storage further in Chapter 6.

A common pitfall, when the proposal is being developed to bid for research funding, is not being sufficiently specific about the amount of time and resources required to undertake the research. This is imperative, because if insufficient funding is sought at the outset, the research team may find themselves struggling to complete the research with the time and resources available.

A useful tip is to agree that only one person works on a master file at any one time, and saves the latest working file with the date, so that when it is subsequently worked on, the next contributor saves it with the new date and e-mails it to the team and so on. In this way, there are not several versions of the same proposal under construction simultaneously, which can cause confusion.

Another tip is to use the Comment function on *Microsoft Word* to provide feedback between contributors and to provide written suggestions on each other's text.

 Action Point

Try out the Comment function on some text now. Open up *Microsoft Word*, then highlight some text you want to comment on, select the Insert menu (or Review in *Microsoft Office 2007*), and locate the Comment function. Then type your comments. When you save the document your comment will be in the margin and saved for your colleagues to see. They can then edit the comment (right mouse click, Edit Comment), add more comments, or delete the comment.

How are proposals assessed and evaluated?

Research proposals are assessed and evaluated by a number of people. Firstly, your colleagues within the research team will offer good advice in refining the proposal.

Academic assessment

Academic assessment of your research proposal is invaluable in that you will get feedback on the academic merit of your proposal. For example, an academic reviewer may suggest areas of literature to include; or help with suggested refinement of the methodology and analysis.

Peer/panel review

It is important that your research proposal undergoes peer/panel review, prior to submitting your proposal for ethical approval or funding (Chapter 6). Peer or panel reviewers have experience and expertise in the area of your research proposal. If you are submitting your proposal to a research sponsor, the sponsor may forward submissions for double-blind peer review, where you are unaware of who is reviewing your proposal and the reviewers are unaware of who the proposal authors are. This helps to eliminate review bias. The feedback gained will help you to refine and improve your proposal.

 Action Point

Draft the structure of a research proposal to explore a topic you are interested in, using the research proposal contents list in Box 3.1 to ensure you have included all necessary sections.

References

Department of Health NHS Executive (1998) Achieving effective practice: a clinical effectivenesss and research information pack for nurses, midwives and health visitors. Retrieved from: http://www.dh.gov.uk/en/Publicationsandstatistics/Publications/PublicationsPolicyAndGuidance/DH_4005638.

Lee, H. and Cameron, M. (2003) Respite care for people with dementia and their carers. *The Cochrane Database of Systematic Reviews* 1 (Art. No: CD004396). doi:

NRES (2009) Information sheets & consent forms. Guidance for researchers & reviewers. Retrieved from http://www.nres.npsa.nhs.uk/applications/guidance/#PIS.

Polit, D. and Beck, C. (2006) *Essentials of Nursing Research. Methods, Appraisal, and Utilization*, 6th edn, Lippincott, Philadephia.

RD Direct (2009) Research process flowchart. Retrieved from: http://www.rdfunding.org.uk/newsletter/Handout.pdf.

Further reading

Davis, M.B. (2007) *Doing a Successful Research Project: Using Qualitative or Quantitative Methods*, Palgrave Macmillan, Basingstoke.

Gerrish, K. and Lacey, A. (eds) (2006) *The Research Process in Nursing*, 5th edn, Blackwell Science, Oxford.

Hek, G., Judd, M. and Moule, P. (2003) *Making Sense of Research*, 2nd edn, Sage, London.

Locke, L.F., Spirduso, W.W. and Silverman, S.J. (2007) *Proposals that Work: A Guide for Planning Dissertations and Grant Proposals*, 5th edn, Sage, London.

Munhall, P.L. and Chenail, R. (2007) *Qualitative Research Proposals and Reports: A Guide*, 3rd edn, Jones & Bartlett, Boston.

Ogden, T.E. and Goldberg, I.A. (eds) (2002) *Research Proposals: a Guide to Success*, 3rd edn, Academic Press, New York.

Parahoo, K. (2006) *Nursing Research: Principles, Process and Issues*, 2nd edn, Palgrave Macmillan, Basingstoke.

Punch, K.F. (2006) *Developing Effective Research Proposals*, 2nd edn, Sage, London.

4 What Do We Know Already? Searching the Literature

Susan Smith and David Bird

Introduction

Health and ill health have been studied and written about for thousands of years. In the western world, the rebirth of scientific method coincided with the introduction of printing and provided the stimulus for a vast and ever-increasing body of literature dealing with health and medicine. Currently, more than 600 000 health-related documents are published each year (National Library of Medicine, 2008). This literature provides access to what is already known and lays the foundations for enlarging our future understanding. There is still much to investigate and much yet to learn.

Why search the literature?

Discovering and reviewing what is already known is an essential and early exercise in the research process. It provides a context and starting point for your research, helps to define and direct your own approach, and averts the dangers of potential plagiarism (Chapter 9).

The search techniques you will learn here will also help to inform best practice, such as when you need to find information about a particular health problem. For students, good searching skills are key requisites for informing academic assignments, case studies and problem solving exercises.

Where is research published?

Research is published in many ways and in many formats, both print and digital, but journals are by far the most popular vehicle for reporting research. The most effective way of finding research articles in journals is to use bibliographic databases, and because the skills and techniques required for successful database searching are so important, most of this chapter is devoted to discussing them and explaining how to use them effectively.

All other sources that report research findings will be dealt with separately, under the heading grey literature, later in this chapter. (Grey literature refers to documents that are not commercially published or readily available to the public, or which are not indexed by major databases. It includes material such as official reports, in-house drug company information, conference abstracts, theses and ongoing research).

Journals

There are several thousand journals in the fields of medicine and health, issued by commercial publishers or professional organizations. The journals appear in print and/or on-line versions at regular frequencies, commonly at monthly, bi-monthly or quarterly intervals. Only a handful of popular weekly titles are to be found in newsagents. For the vast majority of journals, annual subscriptions have to be taken out directly with the publisher or through a subscription agent. Because of their high cost (due to their specialist content and limited circulations), researchers rely on the purchasing power of libraries and other institutions to maintain and manage print and digital collections of journals.

A further distinction can be made between journals that publish peer reviewed articles and those that do not. Peer reviewed articles are those that have been sent by a journal editor for anonymous (or 'blind'), and therefore independent, critical review to one or more experts (peers) in the field. This process is designed to ensure that published papers meet rigorous standards set by the journal's editorial board. Articles not recommended for acceptance by the peer reviewers are unlikely to be published in that journal, but may be suitable for inclusion in popular or professional journals that may not require peer review.

Although journals are the key place to search for research papers, not all journal articles are necessarily research-based. Some articles may be simple descriptive accounts of case studies, for instance, or re-workings of received information, or comment on particular interventions or service provision. Spotting the difference between these and research-based papers is dealt with later in this chapter.

Occasionally, journals publish 'review articles' which survey and comment on a range of papers dealing with a specific topic. Review articles are not primary research, but they can be a very useful starting point when beginning a thorough literature search, because they may bring to light relevant papers and methodological approaches that you might not otherwise have considered.

What am I looking for?

When it comes to searching the existing research literature, your research proposal (Chapter 3) or interest provides the basis for planning the best approach. At this stage, it is important to consider your proposal carefully and to identify the key concepts involved and their inter-relationships. This will help you to frame a robust search question that is clear, precise, relevant and answerable. Your search question can then be used to develop search terms that will be used in the actual literature searching process.

To help focus your thinking, several mnemonic formulae (Table 4.1) have been devised for novice researchers. A resultant breakdown of the general topics to consider is provided in Table 4.2.

Table 4.1   Search mnemonics.

Area of research	Evidence based practice	General health	Health Management
Mnemonic	PICO	SPICE	ECLIPSE
	Patient	Setting	Expectation
	Intervention	Population	Client Group
	Comparison	Intervention	Location
	Outcome	Comparison	Impact
		Evaluation	Professionals involved
			Service
Based on:	Richardson et al., 1995	Booth, 2004	Wildridge and Bell, 2002

Table 4.2 Using the search mnemonics.

Population, Patient, Client Group	Who are the users, patients or community being affected? Consider their problems, symptoms, age, gender and any ethnic or religious aspects
Intervention (occasionally exposure)	What is being done to or for the population, for example screening, drug therapy, surgery, rehabilitation, service provision, and so on?
Comparison or control	Does your research question require a control scenario or comparative element, for example different treatment options?
Outcome, Expectation	What do you want to achieve from the study? What aspects do you wish to see measured or changed?
Setting, Location	Where is the action or intervention taking place, for example home, community or hospital?
Evaluation, Impact	How might the outcome or effects be assessed or measured?
Professionals involved	Who is involved in providing the service, for example, nurses, doctors, social services personnel?
Service	Which service provision are you interested in, for example day hospitals, outpatient service, antenatal care?

Box 4.1 is an example of how the PICO formula can be applied to a piece of clinical research that proposes to investigate the efficacy of cranberries and cranberry juice in helping to combat urinary tract infections. It is proposed to conduct clinical trials in the community with women of all ages. The initial step is to identify and consult any research studies that have been published in this area of research.

Framing a search question

Using the elements identified above, you can now formulate a single-sentence search question, such as:

> What research has been done into the effectiveness of cranberries and cranberry juice in reducing the symptoms of urinary tract infection in women?

This search question can now be analysed to pick out the key concepts central to the proposed research and which will be used to developed search terms used in the actual literature search.

Box 4.1   Applying PICO

Population/Patient/Problem. What do you know about the patient and the problem? In this case, we are dealing with women who have been diagnosed with urinary tract infections.
Intervention. What do you know about the therapeutic intervention and should alternative methods of delivery be considered? Here we shall be interested in the effects of both whole cranberries and cranberry juice.
Comparison. Do you wish to make comparisons? You may wish to compare the results against the results for non-treatment, drug therapy or other interventions. In this case, we shall not be making comparisons.
Outcome. What is the outcome for the patient? Reduction of symptoms, curing the problem and enhanced comfort are the most obvious outcomes.

Action Point

What are the central concepts in the search question above?

You may have identified terms such as research, cranberries, cranberry juice urinary tract infection and women. In more complex research proposals, you may have to frame more than one search question. The process outlined above can be applied to each question. The difference will lie in the number of key elements you identify and how the search results will be combined for each question involved.

Identifying search terms

Having identified the key concepts of your search question, it is good practice to write these down and add any alternative terms (synonyms) or similar words. As searching is a dynamic process, bear in mind that more terms may come to light when you are actually conducting the search itself or reviewing the retrieved documents.

Choosing and using search terms will be discussed in more detail when we come to look at conducting the search. Table 4.3 provides examples of some alternative terminology we may consider using in our demonstration search. By searching for all relevant terms in a systematic way, your search will be more comprehensive and effective.

Bear in mind also how these concepts relate to each other, as this will be useful later, when you are ready to combine the results of your search.

Where should I search?

Having designed your search question and identified the key concepts, you are ready to plan a search strategy. To do this, you will need to consider which search tools are available to you and which ones are likely to produce good results.

A great many resources are available for tracking down research documents, and each has its own distinctive character, positive features and limitations. Due to the vast extent of available literature and information, no single search tool comprehensively covers either all aspects of the health sciences and/or all publication media. *PubMed*, indexing about 18 million documents (and growing), comes close, but the majority of search tools cover narrower, specialist fields, for example *Midwifery and Infant Care Database; Alcohol Studies* database. Some databases restrict themselves to particular types of publications, for example the *Cochrane Library* (systematic reviews) and *mRCT* (controlled trials). Consequently, it is good practice

Table 4.3 Search Example Alternative Terms.

Concepts	Alternative terms
research	use a 'search limiter'; otherwise: study, studies, test(s), trial(s)
cranberries	vaccinium macrocarpon (scientific name)
cranberry juice	no alternatives
urinary tract infection	urination disorders
women	use a 'search limiter'; otherwise: female(s)

to select and search several likely resources. Depending on your search topic, you should also consider using the search tools of other disciplines, such as the social sciences, psychology, education, management or ethics. Although there will be some overlap of results, each resource will usually retrieve some unique and potentially valuable material.

It is also good practice to search the resources one at a time, using the index terms provided by each resource. Although it is sometimes possible to search several resources simultaneously, this is best avoided, as resources may adopt different terminology for the same concepts.

Several search tools will be discussed here, and a comprehensive selection is listed at the end of this chapter, but the best teacher is experience and practice. We shall draw examples from searching *CINAHL* – a sophisticated and well-developed database – but keep in mind that the more resources you search, the more thorough your search will be. The principles of searching are common to all the resources mentioned in this chapter.

Bibliographic databases

Bibliographic databases index current and recent journal literature and are by far the most popular starting point for identifying relevant research papers. Databases may differ in appearance and presentation but they all follow the same basic principles. An understanding of the structure and coverage of bibliographic databases will help to inform your selection choices and searching expectations.

Structure

At the heart of every database is a large collection of data or records. In the case of bibliographic databases, these records are brief descriptions of documents. Each record comprises a collection of descriptive elements, or fields, which can be systematically searched by the database's search engine. For example, the typical record for a journal article will have data fields for the name(s) of the author(s), the title of the paper, the name of the journal publishing the paper, the year it was published, volume number, issue number and page numbers. There will also be fields for subject keywords and, usually, for an abstract or summary of the article's content. Sometimes, there is a field which will link to the full text of the document.

Each database has its own search engine that is used to retrieve relevant records. Usually, you can choose either a basic search or an advanced search screen. Databases also rely on a thesaurus or structured word list of subject keywords. This standardized terminology ensures consistency in the description of data content. Finally, the results of your search will be displayed on screen. The screen display lists all the records that matched your search criteria. The records are presented as brief bibliographic descriptions and provide enough information for locating the item in a library or online collection.

Key databases

Two major databases that are a popular starting point for searching are *MEDLINE* (Table 4.4) and *CINAHL* (Table 4.5), because of their comprehensive coverage, depth and sophisticated search features. Both are currently free to NHS professionals and are available at most universities. *MEDLINE* indexes about 4600 journal titles. An additional database, *EMBASE,* concentrates more on European (rather than United States) literature, including pharmacy, although it indexes

Table 4.4   Key MEDLINE details.

MEDLINE – Medical Literature Analysis and Retrieval System Online					
Years	**1950 – date**	**Updated:**	**5 times a week**	**Thesaurus:**	**MeSH (Medical Subject Headings)**
Created by:		National Library of Medicine, USA			
Coverage:		All aspects of medicine, nursing, dentistry, veterinary medicine, healthcare systems and so on, indexing more than 5000 current biomedical journals. Abstracts are provided. Contains more than 16 million records. Many recent records are linked to free full text versions of articles.			

approximately the same number of journal titles as *MEDLINE* (see Chapter 5 for more information on EMBASE). Internet access to *MEDLINE* is also free via a number of web sites, the most popular being *PubMed* (http://www.ncbi.nlm.nih.gov/sites/entrez?db=pubmed), which combines *MEDLINE* with several other databases to provide access to 18 million records.

The Cochrane Library, although much smaller in scope, is also a popular choice because it indexes valuable systematic reviews of clinical trials literature. These three resources should be complemented by searching further databases, depending on your research topic or professional perspective, for example:

- Physiotherapy and other allied health professions: *AMED, British Nursing Index, SportDiscus, PedRo*;
- Mental health, learning disabilities, and psychology: *e-CAS, ERIC, PsycINFO, Social Service Abstracts*;
- Midwifery: *AMED, British Nursing Index, Midwifery and Infant Care Database*;
- Pharmacy: *EMBASE*.

 Action Point

Frame a search question in an area that interests you, using an appropriate mnemonic formula. Identify the key concepts and potential search terms.

Table 4.5   Key CINAHL details.

CINAHL – Cumulative Index to Nursing and Allied Health Literature					
Years:	**1982 – date**	**Updated:**	**weekly**	**Thesaurus:**	**CINAHL Subject Headings**
Created by:		Created by Cinahl Information Systems, which was acquired by EBSCO Publishing Inc. in 2003.			
Coverage:		All aspects of nursing, allied healthcare, dental hygiene, medical and surgical technology, oncology, consumer health, women's health, and so on. Currently indexes more than 1800 journals and contains about 1.3 million records, of which about 30 000 are provided in full text.			

To judge whether other databases will be useful, check their web sites for information about coverage, inclusion policy and search options. Things to look for are:

- What is the defined subject coverage?
- What sorts of publications are indexed?
- Are publications indexed cover to cover or selectively?
- Is the coverage national, international, limited to English language?
- When did the database start indexing material?
- How frequently is the database updated?
- Is there an Advanced Search option?
- Can search results be saved and combined?
- Can Boolean Operators be employed?
- Can limiters be applied to refine search results?
- Do records contain abstracts / links to full text?

Accessibility

Nearly all databases (and other search tools) for the health sciences are Internet-based. Many, including *PubMed*, can be freely accessed by anyone. However, some are available on a subscription-only basis, but these may have been purchased on your behalf by your university, college, employer or professional body.

Subscription databases are subject to license agreements that restrict access to the registered members or employees of the purchasing institution. Off-campus and off-worksite access is only possible by entering a username and password, unique to each legitimate user (via an authentication platform such as Athens). Athens is a gateway to electronic resources that can be accessed from anywhere with computer Internet access. Academic and health and social care organizations normally subscribe and give access via passwords to students and employees (see http://www.athens.ac.uk/). So, the range of subscription databases that you have access to will depend on the purchasing capacity and policy of your university or employer. Other access options are sometimes available, such as personal annual subscription and fee-based (pay-as-you-go) access.

 Action Point

Check your library's web site for details of databases and other electronic resources available to you. Library staff will also help you gain access to resources for off-site use, such as from your home or workplace computer.

Searching the database

So far, we have expressed our research topic as a search question, identified the key concepts, begun to list potential search terms, and considered which databases to search. It is now time to start searching, and it is important to do this in a systematic and unhurried way, one step at a time, in the order shown in Box 4.2 and as described below.

> **Box 4.2   Searching the Database**
>
> Conduct a separate search for each concept identified in your search question, using and combining thesaurus-term and text-word searches for each concept.
>
> THEN
>
> When you have thoroughly searched for all the concepts separately, combine the search results for each concept, using Boolean operators.

Thesaurus-term searching

To ensure the consistency of data input and the accuracy of record retrieval, the indexers who assign subject descriptors to documents refer to a thesaurus, that is a controlled list of standardized subject terms. This avoids any confusion that would be caused if indexers used different words to denote the same concept. For example, an indexer may have to make a choice between assigning the term *cranberry*, *cranberries* or the scientific name *vaccinium macrocarpon*. By consulting the thesaurus, the indexer confirms which is the preferred policy of that particular database. Identifying and using these preferred terms assists in performing an efficient search because you are assured of retrieving relevant material. Further benefits of using thesaurus searching are:

- Standardized terminology and spelling;
- Helps to clarify search strategy;
- Should ensure retrieval of relevant material;
- Allows searches to be broadened by including narrower headings ('exploding');
- Allows searches to be narrowed by selecting specific aspects of the concept (qualifying subheadings).

Thesauri vary in quality and sophistication, but *MeSH* (Medical Subject Headings), which accompanies *MEDLINE*, is probably the best known, best developed and best structured. Although the *MeSH* thesaurus is also used by a few other databases, most employ their own database-specific thesaurus. This means that different databases sometimes use different thesaurus terms for the same concept. They may also call their thesaurus by a different name, as demonstrated in Table 4.6.

Here you can see that *AMED* does not have an equivalent thesaurus term (a free text search has to be done instead), *CINAHL* offers two variant thesaurus terms, and *MEDLINE* opts for the scientific term. Consequently, it is important to browse the thesaurus of each database you search in order to confirm which thesaurus terms have been preferred for indexing.

Table 4.6   Variation in thesaurus terms.

Database (and name of thesaurus)	Thesaurus Terms
AMED (Subjects)	no term available
CINAHL (CINAHL Headings)	cranberry, cranberry juice
MEDLINE (MeSH)	vaccinium macrocarpon

Finding and using thesaurus terms

To encourage us to look up thesaurus terms before conducting a search, databases provide a link to their thesaurus on the search screen. (The thesaurus link may be labelled *Subjects*, *Subject Headings* or *Keywords*). Clicking this will open a new screen and search box which will allow you to browse the thesaurus for the terms that best describe the concept you are interested in. Entering a word or phrase in the *Browse for* box here allows us to search and browse *CINAHL*'s list of thesaurus terms. Alternatively, some databases may offer you a tick box option to 'Map to Thesaurus' when you enter your free text search term. You will be presented with a list of matching thesaurus terms, from which you can select those that you consider most appropriate. For example, entering and browsing for the word 'cranberries', will suggest Cranberry, Cranberry Juice and Fruit Juice.

By clicking the check boxes beside the term, we can choose to search for as many of these terms as we like. In our case, we would select *Cranberry* and *Cranberry Juice* to ensure a comprehensive thesaurus-term search for our 'cranberries' concept. Having selected these terms, simply click the *Search Database* button to conduct the search. Almost instantaneously, a list of search results will appear. Don't be distracted by these, as you have further searches to do yet. The results for each search conducted will be automatically saved in *Search History* and will be available to you at any time during your session. Each set of search results will be given a running number (S1, S2, etc.) and will indicate which search terms you used and how many results were retrieved. We will return to the sets of search results later in the chapter, when considering how to combine and refine them.

Note that some databases offer the option to map automatically any words you enter in the database search box to the thesaurus terms. This can be enabled/disabled by checking a tick box labelled *Suggest Subjects* (EBSCO), *Map term to Subject Headings* (OVID) or something similar.

Before we consider free-text searching, it is worth examining other features of *CINAHL*'s thesaurus which, on occasion, can prove very useful.

Tree view

The thesauri of some databases, for example *MEDLINE* and *CINAHL*, also arrange terms in a tree structure (Figure 4.1). Clicking a thesaurus term will display it in its relative context within the grand hierarchy of subjects (Thesaurus Tree). Indentations reflect the narrowing of topics

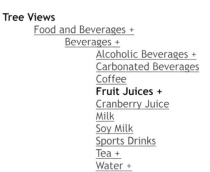

Tree Views
    Food and Beverages +
       Beverages +
         Alcoholic Beverages +
         Carbonated Beverages
         Coffee
         Fruit Juices +
         Cranberry Juice
         Milk
         Soy Milk
         Sports Drinks
         Tea +
         Water +

Figure 4.1   Tree view for Cranberry Juice in *CINAHL Headings*.

from the general to the particular (Branches). This can help if you want to consider using any broader or narrower terms associated with the concept you are interested in.

Explode

Not as dangerous as it sounds. Some thesaurus terms, depending on their place within the tree structure mentioned above, are associated with related narrower concepts. *Cranberry* and *Cranberry Juice* are quite specific terms and cannot be broken down into any narrower concepts but *Fruit Juices*, for example, is a more general concept. Clicking the term *Fruit Juices*, will reveal any narrower terms in the 'Tree View', although in this case Cranberry Juice is the only narrower option available.

The plus sign (+) indicates that there are narrower associated terms. If you were to select the 'explode' option for *Fruit Juices*, your search would not only retrieve all results for fruit juices in general, for example orange and grape juice, and so on, but would also automatically retrieve results for the narrower concept of *Cranberry Juice*. Using the 'explode' feature tends to broaden your search.

Scope

This link opens a definition of the term and can help to clarify our understanding of the concept. In the Ebsco version of CINAHL the *Scope* note for *Fruit Juices* is:

- Scope: The liquid extract of fruit. Coordinate with the specific fruit. CRANBERRY JUICE also available;
- Used for: Juices, Fruit, Fruit Juice, Juice, Fruit.

Here we can also see that if we wanted to search for the specific concept of 'orange juice', for example, we would need to combine a search for *Fruit Juice* with a separate search for *Orange*.

Major concept

If this box is ticked, the search will be restricted to records where the concept is the main topic of the article. This tends to limit the scope of the search and is best avoided at this stage of the search process.

Qualifying subheadings

Clicking individual thesaurus terms also reveals available subheadings that can be applied to qualify your chosen term, if relevant. The number of subheadings presented will vary according to the subject of the thesaurus term. Each subheading has a *Scope* note that will define its meaning. Clicking any number of the check boxes will limit your search to those particular aspects of the concept.

Administration and Dosage and *Therapeutic Use* would be relevant subheadings for our purposes, but selecting subheadings should be do with great care as the process can seriously restrict the number of search results. You don't have to select any at all. They are just an option to help you refine your search, should you want to. In fact, unless you are only interested in a very specific aspect of the concept you are searching for, it's best to leave the question of subheadings until you have completed the search process. If you then find you have too many results, you can consider returning to this screen to use some qualifying subheadings to refine your search results.

Search as keyword

At the bottom of the list of thesaurus terms in the *Browse* window, you'll notice that *CINAHL* allows you to search for the word or phrase you entered in the *Browse* search box as free text. (*CINAHL* uses the word *Keyword* to signify free text.) Click this if there is no appropriate thesaurus term or, if you feel confident enough to take short cuts, click it along with any thesaurus terms you have selected from the list. Either way, before thinking about ticking this box, make sure that you read the next section dealing with techniques required for effective free-text searching.

Free-text searching

Free-text searching is routinely used, alongside thesaurus-term searching, to ensure the most thorough search for each concept. Very occasionally, a record might be incompletely indexed, so a free-text search can also act as a failsafe. The benefits of free text searchare:

- Ensures a comprehensive search;
- Essential if thesaurus terms are not readily available, for example for new concepts, proper names or UK terminology;
- Acts as a failsafe should there be errors in database indexing.

There are also times when, in the absence of exactly-matching thesaurus terms, we may have to use free text alone in order to retrieve relevant results. In either case, simply type the word or phrase into the *Find* box on the *Advanced Search* screen and hit the *Search* button (or, if you are looking at the *Browse Thesaurus* screen in *CINAHL*, select the *Search as Keyword* option mentioned above).

There are a number of important things to bear in mind when using free text:

- Free-text searches do not search the full text of the documents themselves: they search data fields contained within the database, for example title, abstract, and so on, looking for exact matches. (A very few subscription full-text databases do, however, offer the option of searching full text);
- Common words, such as pronouns and prepositions (*a*, *the*, *it*, *on*, *to*) are ignored. These are known as 'stop words';
- The computer searches for free text in a purely mechanistic way, so be prepared to find non-relevant material amongst the results. For instance, using the free-text word *stroke*, in a search for cerebrovascular accident will also retrieve records that contain phrases such as *down-stroke*, *heat stroke*, *stroke volume*, *up-stroke*;
- Most databases emanate from North America, so it is important to consider differences in spelling and terminology. In the USA, diphthongs (two vowels rubbing shoulders) are avoided and consonants before the *-ing* and *–ed* endings are not doubled, for example

estrogen, hematology, orthopedic and *counseling*, rather than *oestrogen, haematology, orthopaedic* and *counselling*;

- Some familiar UK terminology is not used in North America and does not appear in database thesauri, for example accident and emergency, health care assistants, physiotherapy, (hospital) ward, besides terms that are specifically associated with the UK's National Health Service;
- Free-text searching is often the prefered option when looking for new or uncommon concepts, named drugs, proprietory names, acronyms, proper names of authors or institutions, for example *Aspirin, Atkins Diet, MRSA*.

Some tricks of the trade

- If searching for a phrase, place it in double quotation marks ("..."). This ensures that the computer will search only for your phrase and not for each of the words separately, for example "high blood pressure", "heart burn", "national framework". (This 'trick' can also be employed when searching other online search engines);
- Because of its mechanistic approach, the search engine will not retrieve the plural forms or slight variants of text words. However, using truncation overcomes this to some extent and saves entering a whole range of minor variations of a word. Truncation allows you to employ a symbol (*, $ or %, depending on the database) to represent any combination or number of letters at the end of a word, for example *allerg** will search for all instances of the words *allergy, allergies, allergic, allergen*;
- Similarly, a wild card symbol, for example ?, can be used to represent none, one or more letters appearing in the middle of a word, for example a free-text search for *p?ediat**, using both the wild card and the truncation functions, would retrieve all instances of *pediatric, pediatrics, pediatrician, paediatric, paediatrics, paediatrician*.

The search for our 'cranberries' concept will actually have involved several separate searches:

S1. cranberry OR cranberry juice	[two thesaurus terms selected from *CINAHL Headings*, see Figure 4.1]
S2. cranberr*	[free-text search, truncated single word]
S3. "cranberry juice"	[free-text search, phrase]

Repeating the search for the other main concept of our search question, 'urinary tract infection', will involve a further four searches:

S4. urinary tract infections	[thesaurus-term search]
S5. urination disorders	[thesaurus-term search]
S6. "urinary tract infection*"	[free-text search, truncated phrase]
S7. "urin* disorder*"	[free-text search, truncated phrase]

Later in this chapter we will describe how we consolidate and combine these sets of results and look at how *Search Limiters* can be used to further refine the search, including how our concepts of 'research' and 'women' can be accommodated in a single step.

Bear in mind that there is no single right or wrong approach to choosing search terms. Your choices will be determined by:

- the nature of your topic;
- how exhaustively you need to search;
- which databases you can access;
- how much time you have available.

Be patient and be prepared to make mistakes. You can delete individual searches that have gone wrong from your *Search History* or even clear the entire *Search History* and start afresh. Practice will develop your expertise and lead to successful results.

Combining results and using limiters

Once search terms have been identified, databases selected and each concept searched for, it is time to bring your search results together in a meaningful way which will reflect and answer your original search question. To do this, we have to instruct the database about the relationships we wish to see between our individual sets of search results. In effect, we reconstruct the meaning of our search question by combining the search results for each concept. This function is available within your Search History, which can be accessed by clicking the *Search History* tab on the database search screen.

For the database to process the combinations required, we need to select from a list of commands, known in the trade as Boolean Operators. In practice, the most commonly used Boolean Operators are OR, AND and NOT:

- **OR** is used to expand search results and is employed mostly when combining free-text and thesaurus-term searches to consolidate results for each concept (Step One below);
- **AND** is used to narrow search results and is chiefly used when combining the consolidated sets of results for each concept (Step Two below);
- **NOT** can be used at any stage of the search to further refine your results by excluding unwanted concepts.

Figures 4.2, 4.3, 4.4 and 4.5 illustrate the different actions of these three operators when applied to two separate sets of search results.

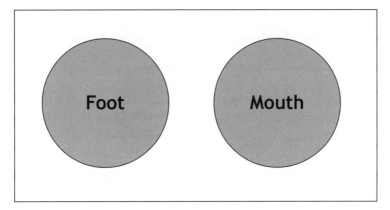

Figure 4.2 Searching for individual terms.

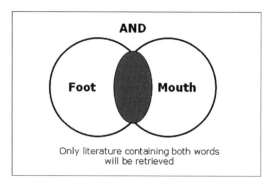

Figure 4.3 Applying the term **AND**.

These three major operators are sometimes included in drop down menus for easy application but, more often, you have to type them yourself along with the sets of results you wish to combine.

Round brackets ( ) are sometimes employed. The brackets are used to combine a complex string of discrete elements and maintain a logical sequence of actions for the computer to work with, for example (ECG OR electrocardiology) AND (children OR paediatric). Without the parentheses, this would be a very confusing command for the computer.

As mentioned, the *Search History* displays a numbered list of your searches, allocating a running line number to each set of results along with the search term(s) used and the number of articles retrieved. When you are satisfied that you have run searches for all the terms you have identified, the sets of results can then be combined. When doing this, happily, you do not have to retype the original search words or phrases, you can simply use the line number that has been allocated to that particular set of results.

Step one: Collating results for each separate concept

Let's return to our 'cranberries' question again and assume you have used a number of thesaurus terms and free-text words to search for each of the two main concepts, that is cranberries and urinary tract infection. After entering the associated terms, your *Search History* may look something like lines S1 to S7 in Table 4.7.

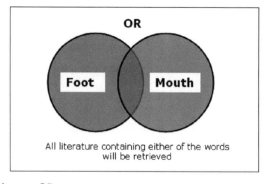

Figure 4.4 Applying the term **OR**.

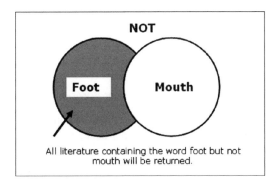

NOT

Foot   Mouth

All literature containing the word foot but not
mouth will be returned.

Figure 4.5 Applying the term **NOT**.

It is good practice now to collate the results of the multiple searches for each concept so that, instead of having to combine seven sets of results, we only have to deal with two sets of consolidated results – one set for each concept. This is done by combining the multiple search results for each concept, using **OR**. This process will also eliminate any duplicated records. For example, typing 'S1 or S2 or S3' will consolidate the results of the 'cranberry-concept' searches (line S8 in Table 4.7).

Table 4.7 Example 'cranberry' search as if conducted on Ebsco CINAHL.

Notes	Search ID	Search terms	Search options	Results
Limits applied	S11	S8 and S9	Limiters – Publication Type: Research; Gender: Female;	18
Combined topics of cranberry and urinary disorder	S10	S8 and S9	Boolean/Phrase	105
Combining all urinary disorder terms	S9	S4 or S5 or S6 or S7	Boolean/Phrase	2535
Combining all cranberry terms	S8	S1 or S2 or S3	Boolean/Phrase	246
Exact phrase (free text) using truncation	S7	"urin* disorder*"	Boolean/Phrase	551
Exact phrase (free text) search	S6	"urinary tract infection"	Boolean/Phrase	992
Free text	S5	Urination disorders	Boolean/Phrase	542
Thesaurus search	S4	(MM "Urinary Tract Infections")	Boolean/Phrase	1572
Free text with truncation (*)	S3	cranberr*	Boolean/Phrase	246
Exact phrase (free text) search	S2	"cranberry juice"	Boolean/Phrase	168
Thesaurus search	S1	(MM "Cranberry") or (MM "Cranberry Juice")	Boolean/Phrase	121

Note that search ID or line numbers are used when combining sets of results. These should be typed as they appear on screen, for example S1, and so on, in EBSCO databases; #1, and so on, in the *Cochrane Library*.

Step two: Combining the consolidated sets of search results

As we only wish to find documents that deal with both of our concepts (bearing in mind that we shall later applying Limiters to take care of the other concepts – 'research' and 'women'), we now need to run a search that combines our consolidated sets. Here, we will use the Boolean Operator **AND**.

In the *Find* box, we type:

S8 and S9.

The results of this search will appear in *Search History* against a new line number, that is S10.

The latter search will exclude any records that only deal with one of our concepts, leaving us with those records that treat both concepts in the same document. The total number of results retrieved will be drastically reduced but the document content will be more relevant to our original search question.

Table 4.7 shows how this series of searches and combinations might appear on the *Search History* screen in the *CINAHL* database. The top search in the list, S11, shows the action of applying 'search limiters', which we will consider next.

Applying search limiters

The major databases allow you to refine your search results further by selecting specific search limiters from a list. These limiters are of a general nature and can be applied to almost any search, if required. Often, they can be an important element of your search strategy, so it is worthwhile familiarizing yourself with the options on offer.

The limiters usually appear on the database's *Advanced Search* screen. You can apply them during the initial stages of searching but it is highly recommended that you revisit these options for refining your search at the last stage of the search process, for example via the *Revise Search* or *Apply Limits* links or something similar. Use limiters at the final stage of your search. Choose them sparingly and with care, as it is easy to select too many limiters and, thereby, exclude material that might be relevant. As with most things, trial and error and plenty of practice improves results. The limiters offered by *CINAHL* include the following options for restricting your search.

Full text

Checking this box will ignore records that are not directly linked to full-text versions of the documents. This limiter should be used, if at all, with great caution. Documents might be available electronically from your local library, but may not necessarily appear as a link beside the record.

It is fine if you just want a quick uncritical look at one or two articles on a particular topic but is best avoided if you are undertaking a thorough search of the literature. Limiting to full text will almost certainly eliminate vitally relevant documents.

Publication year

Here you can enter a start and end date. This will eliminate any material outside these dates. For example, entering *2005* to *2009* will retrieve papers indexed between these five years.

Author or publication

You are unlikely to want to limit your search results to one particular author or to articles that appeared in a particular publication but – should you ever want to – this feature is worth knowing about.

Research article

Restricts your search to reports of research-based studies. This is the box to tick for our 'cranberries' search question.

Publication type

This may not appear very exciting, but some of the options can usefully narrow your range of results, if relevant to your search criteria, for example *Case Study, Clinical Trial, Masters Thesis, Standards*, and so on.

Language

CINAHL (like *MEDLINE*) is an international database and indexes articles in both English and other languages. Select English if you wish to exclude documents in other languages.

Gender

The choices, unsurprisingly, are *All*, *Female* or *Male*, allowing results to be focused on a particular gender. As it is relevant for our purposes, select *Female*.

Age groups

This is a very popular feature for restricting results to a particular age group. Midwives and neonatal staff will appreciate the first option. If, for example, interest is in the prevention and treatment of pressure ulcers in neonates, this option is a handy feature for quickly focusing the search. Simply search for pressure ulcers (and variant phrases), and then apply the limiter for *Infant: Newborn 0–1 months*. If older people are the area of research interest, choose the limiters *Aged, 65+* or *Aged, 80 and over*.

As with options on other drop-down menus, different age groups can be combined by holding down the shift key on the keyboard while making your choices. For children of school age, select the two options: *Child, 6–12* and *Adolescent, 13–18*.

Different databases and search interfaces will use different limiters; these are generally self-explanatory. Common sense should dictate which are the most relevant to your search.

Example search strategies are shown in Case Examples 4.1, 4.2 and 4.3.

Case Example 4.1: Using thesaurus-term, text-word and truncation search

A second-year physiotherapy student was looking for any research about the feeling of abandonment experienced by stroke patients during rehabilitation.

Selecting thesaurus terms and text words for stroke was straightforward. However, of the major databases, only *PsycINFO* employed a thesaurus term for the concept of abandonment, so it was important to use free text when searching for this concept in other databases. The truncated form 'abandon*' was used. Simplified, the search process looked like:

PsycINFO
S1. Cerebrovascular Accidents [thesaurus term].
S2. stroke [free text].
S3. S1 or S2.
S4. Abandonment [thesaurus term].
S5. abandon* [free text].
S6. S4 or S5.
S7. S3 and S6.

MEDLINE
S1. Cerebrovascular Accident [thesaurus term].
S2. stroke [free text].
S3. S1 or S2.
S4. abandon* [free text].
S5. S3 and S4.

CINAHL
S1. Cerebral Vascular Accident [thesaurus term].
S2. stroke [free text].
S3. S1 or S2.
S4. abandon* [free text].
S5. S3 and S4.

This uncomplicated strategy retrieved relevant and manageable sets of results, helping the student to submit an informed and successful assignment.

 Action Point

Try running the search yourself, based on the following question:

Has there been any research conducted about the feeling of abandonment experienced by stroke patients during rehabilitation?

Case Example 4.2:   Using the PICO formula and setting limiters

A group of nurses considered undertaking some local research to find out which cleaning agents and germicides might be the most effective in combating an outbreak of *clostridium difficile* in their hospital's surgical units.

They decided first to search the literature to find out what research had already been published in this area. Because of the clinical nature of the issue, the PICO formula was used to define a straightforward search question: *How effective are hospital cleaning agents and germicides against epidemic Clostridium difficile strains?* The search was restricted to English language articles published in the last five years:

MEDLINE
S1. *Clostridium difficile* [thesaurus term].
S2. Spores, bacterial [thesaurus term].
S3. c. difficile [free text].
S4. S1 or S2 or S3.
S5. Anti-Bacterial Agents [thesaurus term].
S6. Disinfectants or Disinfection [thesaurus terms].
S7. Detergents [thesaurus term].
S8. germicides [free text].
S9. "cleaning agent*" [free text].
S10. S5 or S6 or S7 or S8 or S9.
S11. S4 and S10.
S12 .S4 and S10 + Limiters: Date of publication: 2004–2008; Language: English.
The search was also run on *CINAHL* and *EMBASE*. Although the nurses abandoned thoughts of conducting a local research project, they applied (with considerable success) the findings of the recent research studies identified by their literature search.

   Action Point

Try running the search yourself, based on the question:

How effective are hospital cleaning agents and germicides against epidemic *Clostridium difficile* strains?

Case Example 4.3:   Using alternative databases

A relationship counsellor is considering starting a new, safe, dateline service for people with learning difficulties. Initially he wishes to identify some background material on similar services that may already exist.

The counsellor is aware that this is an area of research where terminology quickly changes. Phrases that may today be considered offensive started out as official medical terms. This search is complicated because of the different types of relationships that can exist and because sometimes, expressed feelings are interpreted as challenging behaviour rather than being channelled appropriately and encouraged:

PsycINFO
S1. Social Dating or Romance [thesaurus terms].
S2. Marriage [thesaurus term].
S3. Dating or romantic or romance or marr* [free text].
S4. S1 or S2 or S3.
S5. Mental Retardation [thesaurus term].
S6. Learning Difficulties [thesaurus terms].
S7. mental adj retard* [free text].
S8. intellectual* adj (disabilit* OR disorder* OR challeng*) [free text].
S9 learning adj (disabilit* OR difficult* OR disorder*) [free text].
S10. S5 or S6 or S7 or S8 or S9.
S11. S4 and S10.
S12 .S4 and S10 + Limiters: Language: English.
The search would need to be modified considerably to be run on alternative databases, for example marr* returns married in PsycINFO but on a more clinically orientated database may return bone marrow.

Viewing results and modifying your search

Once your search sets have been combined, it's time to look at the retrieved records to see if they match your expectations. Effective searching is a dynamic process and, even by this stage, you may already have developed your search strategy and modified your choice of search terms. Reviewing the results of your search now provides further opportunity to modify, refine and enhance your search. Before discussing this, let's take a look at how the results of your search are displayed.

Presentation of results

Results are displayed as a list of brief citations. Usually, the most recently indexed documents appear first, although there are options for customizing the display, for example sorting results by relevance, author or source. A typical citation (from *CINAHL*) looks like:

> *Cranberry juice in the prevention of urinary tract infection* (includes abstract) Stephens G; Journal of the Association of Chartered Physiotherapists in Women's Health, 2005 Autumn (97): 3–14

(journal article – research, systematic review, tables/charts) CINAHL AN: 2009119577 *Cited References (38)*
    PDF Full Text

This citation is made up of the following elements:

- Title of the article with hypertext link to full details, abstract, thesaurus terms, and so on: *Cranberry juice in the prevention of urinary tract infection*;
- Name of the author: *Stephens G*;
- Title of the journal in which the article appeared: *Journal of the Association of Chartered Physiotherapists in Women's Health*;
- Where to look in the journal to find the article, that is in issue 97, Autumn 2005, pages 3 to 14: *2005 Autumn (97): 3–14*;
- Type of publication: *(journal article – research, systematic review, tables/charts)*;
- Unique identification tag: *CINAHL AN: 2009119577*;
- Number of documents cited by the author in this article (with link to details): *Cited References (38)*;
- Full text available, depending on database subscription: *PDF Full Text*.

Too few results?

Don't feel disappointed if your search retrieves few or even no results. Most searchers will find that, for some questions, they will have to repeat or modify the search process. Here are some tips on broadening your search to capture more results:

- Use free-text searching as well as thesaurus-term searching;
- Incorporate synonyms, using OR;
- Use the thesaurus *Explode* option, if available;
- Avoid using subheadings to qualify your concepts;
- Look for additional search terms in any relevant articles already retrieved;
- Consider running the search on other databases;
- Try full-text searching if this is featured on the databases you have access to.

It may just be, of course, that few or no research papers have been written or published in your area of interest.

Too many results?

If you retrieve large quantities of results, some of which seem irrelevant, try to narrow your search:

- Use thesaurus terms only, the more specific the better;
- Think about incorporating more terms and concepts, combining these with AND (this will reduce the number of results);
- Apply 'search limiters';
- Qualify your search terms with subheadings, if available;
- Consider searching document title and abstract only.

Using search engines

As previously mentioned, bibliographic databases are the preferred method for conducting a literature search. The inclusion of a thesaurus and the ability to refine the results makes it the ideal tool. We don't always want to conduct an in-depth literature search when looking for more generalized material or non-researched based information; for example, you would not go to a bibliographic database to search for information on local bereavement support groups in your area. Sometimes you just want a quick overview of material to give you an idea of where to start when formulating your full search strategy. In these instances, it is helpful to use an Internet search engine.

As with bibliographic databases, you can find different types of search engines designed for different purposes. General search engines like Google (www.google.co.uk) and Yahoo (www.yahoo.co.uk) are good places to search for grey material. What most people don't realize is that very little of what is online is indexed by search engines. Fallows (2005) states that only a fraction of the tens of billions of pages available on the Internet are indexed by the major search engines (Google indexes approximately 8 billion [Coughran, 2004]). In short, there is too much information out there! Most of the information is held on the dark or hidden web; that is, behind databases, password protection, and web site content that is not indexed. The number of irrelevant search results and the sometimes questionable quality of the information returned can often prove more time consuming to sift through than a well conducted search on a bibliographic database. However, there are a number of specialized search engines and gateways that can help us retrieve better results.

Google scholar: http://scholar.google.co.uk/

A *Google* search engine designed to search for scholarly articles. Use with caution as the content is not always current and the ranking system favours older papers. Page indexing is compiled by non-health professionals.

Scirus: http://www.scirus.com

This is Elsevier's free version of the *Scopus* resource. As a search engine it is better adapted for more complex health searches and will suggest additional keywords to help refine your search.

Google health directory: http://www.google.com/Top/Health/

This is a customized search tool that lies beneath *Google*. When you enter selected health-related terms you may see a group of subheadings available at the top of your search including topics such as Treatment, Test/diagnosis, For patients, From medical authorities and so on.

   Action Point

1. In *Google Scholar*, run a search for ~pediatrics. This should also search for synonyms but note that whilst 'hospital', 'medicine' and 'pediatrics' are highlighted, the term 'paediatrics' is omitted.

2. Further examples to try on *Google*-based search engines:

   Compare searches for pediatrics and paediatrics.
   Browse results for child health using *Google Health* Directory.
   Compare searches for ~pediatrics against pediatrics or paediatrics.
   Search for obesity children site: www.dh.gov.uk then later add filetype:pdf to your
   search.

The current contributor list is strongly biased towards North American organizations or individuals. This bias is reflected in the search results, and makes it unsuitable for United Kingdom specific queries.

Intute: http://www.intute.ac.uk/healthandlifesciences/

This is a specialist search engine dedicated to Health. Using *Intute* will greatly reduce the number of results obtained from a search and will only return content that has been evaluated. The *Virtual Online Training Suite* offers excellent online tutorials.

NHS evidence: http://www.evidence.nhs.uk/

This is a gateway to numerous quality-checked resources, covering a range of different specialties and hub areas for search-specific content, for example images, evidence based reviews, clinical guidelines and care pathway finder.

 Action Point

- On the NHS Evidence web site: Use *Search Resources* to look for *Guidance* on Influenza;
- Use *Search Resources* to find evidence for Bandage use in Leg Ulcers;
- Using the *Images* hub, search for pictures of Diabetic Foot;
- In the *For Patients* section, search for information on Smoking by the British Heart Foundation;
- Find a current awareness update using Really Simple Syndication (RSS) feed search for modernization and management;
- Using *Health Libraries tab*, search for how many health libraries are within 10 miles of your local University, and note the phone number of the Health Library.

Search tips

You can use search engines for:

- Quick answer queries;
- General information;
- Grey literature (including conference proceedings, charity reports and governmental documents).

Table 4.8 *Google* advanced search terms.

Command	Searches for ...	Example
"" (standard in most search engines)	Exact phrase	"cranberry juice"
~	Synonyms	~child
define:	Provides online dictionary definitions	define:otolaryngology
site:	Searches within a specific web site	site:dh.gov.uk
filetype:	Locates specific files types	Filetype:pdf
lnurl: or allinurl:	Searches for one word or more than one word in the web address respectively	allinurl:gov uk
intitle: or allintitle:	Searches for one word or more than one word in the web page title respectively	allintitle:stroke treatment

They are not suited for complex health-related queries.

When using search engines it is still necessary to frame a search question and select the terms to use. Most search engines are capable of using Boolean Logic but automatically insert the word 'AND' between search terms. Some advanced search options may provide a couple of search lines to help build a slightly more complex search, but the documents aren't indexed in the same way as a database, making it difficult to differentiate between Dr Field the author and field of research or a field in the country.

The best way to think about building up your search is by using the Telegram method (Clarke and Wentz, 2000). This is where you think about the fewest possible words to get your message across. From our earlier example, we might use the search terms: **Cranberries urinary tract**. Some search engines also have commands to help improve your search (Table 4.8). For further search tips, visit www.googleguide.com.

Better results are usually retrieved by using a combination of Boolean logic and commands: (cranberry or '*Vaccinium macrocarpon*') 'urinary tract'.

 Action Point

Try this (or your own search) in the different search engines, and compare the information found.

Short-listing and managing results

Once your search has been refined to a manageable number of citations, the next step is to select which articles should be short-listed. Some of the records retrieved may not be totally relevant to your search, so short-listing allows you to identify the most appropriate publications that you will need to locate and critically appraise. When short-listing, it is important to remember that quality is superior to quantity.

Here are some tips of what to look for when short-listing your results. However, this advice must be taken as guidance only, as some degree of personal judgement is required.

How appropriate is it to your needs?

Simply checking the title is sometimes sufficient to identify whether the document is relevant to your search question, but it is best to look at the abstract for fuller detail. You may be more interested in studies that are readily applicable in the country or region in which you are based. You may have a preference for documents containing helpful images, graphs or illustrations that clarify the text.

Is the title in brackets or in a foreign language?

It is worth remembering that although the abstract of an article is published in English, the full text of the original article may be in a different language. A title enclosed in brackets generally denotes that it has been published in a foreign language. This is no reflection on the quality of the work, but common sense should be used. It is not worth spending time and effort on locating an article if you are unable to translate it. Of course this depends on your circumstances. A good systematic review should attempt to include all relevant items, irrespective of language. If time allows, you may wish to find some means of translating an article.

What kind of journal is it from?

Obscure titles may be more difficult to obtain, especially at short notice. This can be especially true if the article is noted as an e-publication or ahead of print. Abstracts are often published in advance of the complete article and there may be lengthy delays before the article goes to print or before an embargo on access is lifted. Sometimes, it is possible to identify these articles by an 'e' prefixing the article page numbers, or by noting whether page number details are omitted.

What is the article length?

If the article is only one or two pages long, then it is likely to be an abstract, poster presentation, letter or comment. In some instances, it may be necessary to include this kind of material, especially if you are looking for information about a new area of research, but it is better practice to follow the research hierarchy (Figure 4.6) wherever possible.

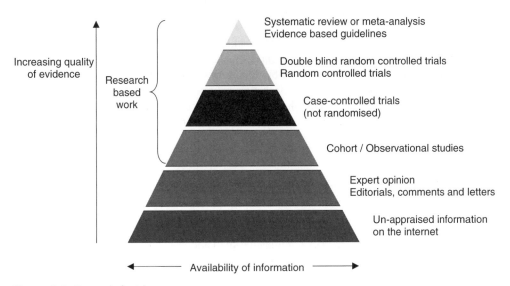

Figure 4.6 Pyramid of evidence.

Does the citation refer to a piece of research?

Applying the 'search limiter' for *Research*, where available, will have filtered out any articles that are not research based, but there are occasions when you may have to exclude non-research based documents manually. Sometimes, the full citation (click on the title to see this) may indicate the type of publication, for example *research, clinical trial*. If not, the trick is to look at the abstract and check for words and numbers that suggest research methodology and research findings. Common expressions are: *study, trial, test, questionnaire* – the sort of language you'll become familiar with from reading this book.

How current is the article?

Evidence based research continually drives the health system to question its practice and improve its services. As a result, papers can quickly become out of date as new evidence is discovered. Unless researching a rare condition or historical paper, as a rule of thumb, all evidence should have been published within the last ten years or, preferably, five years.

Collating and managing your short-listed citations

When viewing your list of search results, you will see a check box next to each citation title. Tick these boxes to select the citations you wish to short-list and save. Often, items ticked in this way will be automatically added to a search folder that you can open, edit and manage in other ways. The options available depend on the database used, but the principles are the same.

Display styles

Citations can be displayed in one of three styles:

- Short/Brief – basic citation details only;
- Medium/Brief and abstract – basic citation with abstract and thesaurus terms;
- Full/Detailed – this contains all the bibliographical information associated with indexing.

The recommended style is citation and abstract. This will provide you with enough information when deciding whether to locate and review the document.

The order of citations is chronological by default (most-recently indexed items come first) but you can usually change this if you wish, for example sort by relevance, source, title or author. You may also be able to modify the citation style, such as APA (American Psychological Association), Vancouver, and so on. (see Chapter 9 for advice on referencing and citation styles).

Storage options

Your short-listed citations can now be stored in a number of ways:

- as a printed paper copy;
- saved to a portable storage device, for example a memory stick;
- e-mailed as an attachment to your nominated e-mail address;
- exported to a software package that manages citations, for example *Endnote, Reference Manager, RefWorks*.

These options are available from your *Search Folder*, where you can also further refine which results you wish to save. In addition, some search platforms allow you to bookmark and share your *Search History* results through social networking sites such as *Facebook, Delicious, Windows Live* or *Twitter*. Look out for bookmark or share options when conducting your search.

Saving your searches

Once you are satisfied that your refined search strategies have produced useful and relevant results, it is often prudent to save the search strategy itself, in case of any mishap. This a separate process from saving the results of your searches (citations) discussed above. Saving search strategies can be valuable for a number of reasons:

* Insurance against loss of information;
* Re-running a search can pick up recently published research if displayed chronologically;
* Acts as a reminder of your search strategy;
* Small sections of frequently run searches can be saved and re-run as filters (some good suggestions are available from InterTASC Information Specialists' Sub-Group from the Centre for Reviews and Dissemination (http://www.york.ac.uk/inst/crd/intertasc/filters.htm)).

Normally, your work on a database will be lost once you end the session or have been 'timed out'. To avoid this, many databases offer a facility for creating a personal account where you can save and name your searches, retrieve them, edit them and re-run them. Look for the link on the *Search History* screen. You are asked to register for this service and select a user name and password that will allow you to access your saved files.

Grey literature

Valuable as they are, bibliographic databases tend to focus closely on indexing articles from easily-accessible high-quality professional journals, neglecting other forms of reported research, such as official reports and documents, open-access repository material, academic dissertations and theses, in-house reports of local small-scale studies, conference presentations, symposia and information about research in progress. This less accessible material is generally known as grey literature.

Happily, grey literature has its own range of search tools and finding aids but search options are often less sophisticated than those found in bibliographic databases. The American Academy of Medicine maintains a fairly comprehensive finding aid:

Current Grey Literature Report: http://www.nyam.org/library/pages/current_grey_literature_ report

Commissioned research reports

Research is sometimes reported in separate free-standing publications or monographs. In this format, research is usually presented in much more detail than in papers prepared for publication in journals. Such studies are usually commissioned by government departments, professional bodies, commercial enterprises, charitable foundations or other agencies. Here is an example:

Cancer prevention: Knowledge, attitude and behaviours of people in mid-life (2006).

This is a 90-page report of a research project commissioned by the Ulster Cancer Foundation and undertaken by a team of researchers at the University of Ulster; http://www.science. ulster.ac.uk/inr/pdf/full_report_2007.pdf.

The web sites of research-funding organizations often list the projects which they have sponsored, for example:

- UK Clinical Research Network Study (UKCRN) Portfolio Database: http://public. ukcrn.org.uk/search/ (Covers 'ongoing and recently completed research projects funded by, or of interest to, the United Kingdom's National Health Service'.);
- Funded activities (Wellcome Foundation): http://www.wellcome.ac.uk/fundedactivities.

Some of the databases listed at the end of this chapter index research monographs as well as research published in other formats, for example *Department of Health Publications, PEDro, Research Findings Electronic Register* and *Social Care Online*. Other sources of monograph literature, although not always easy to search, are the catalogues of major libraries, such as

- The National Library of Medicine (USA): http://locatorplus.gov;
- The Library of Congress (USA): http://catalog.loc.gov;
- The British Library: http://catalogue.bl.uk.

Open-access repositories

A growing trend is to place pre- and post-publication research papers in online open-access repositories that can be freely visited by any Internet user. OpenDOAR (http://www. open-doar.org/) is a directory of such repositories worldwide, while the SHERPA web site offers a list of United Kingdom repositories and service providers (http://www.sherpa.ac.uk/repositories/). One of the best tools for searching across all open-access repositories is *OAIstar* (http://www.oaister.org/), which catalogues about 14 million digital resources, including dissertations, theses and other material from open-access repositories.

Dissertations and theses

Dissertations and theses are primarily undertaken to fulfil academic award requirements and, although the content may only involve small-scale studies, they can provide both valuable source material and models of methodological approach. There are comprehensive subscription resources for tracking down academic research but you will need to check if these are available at your local institution or library. For example:

- Dissertation abstracts online (covers US, etc. 2 million+ records);
- Index to theses (covers Great Britain and Ireland: 500 000+ records).

Some free finding aids, besides *OAIstar* mentioned above, are also available:

- EThOS (Electronic Thesis On Line System) (British Library): http://ethos.bl.uk/ (a charge may be levied for items not yet digitized);
- Dissertations (NDLTD): http://www.ndltd.org/find;
- Directory of dissertations in progress (Canada and USA): http://www.lib.utulsa.edu/databases/descriptions/HISTDISS.asp.

Conference and symposia proceedings

Research undertakings are often reported verbally at conferences or symposia and may later be written up and published in a relevant volume of 'proceedings'. The British Library holds almost half a million conference proceedings and these can be searched separately by selecting the 'catalogue subset search' of the library's integrated catalogue: British Library: integrated catalogue http://catalogue.bl.uk/

Two important subscription services, if available to you, are also valuable for tracing 'proceedings':

- ISI Proceedings (science and technology), adds the proceedings of more than 1100 conferences every three months;
- Scopus, one of the largest abstract and citation databases of research literature, also indexes 500+ conference proceedings.

Research in progress

It is important to find out if anyone else is undertaking any unpublished research closely related to your area of interest. You may even wish to contact and discuss matters with the researcher involved. There are two useful starting points:

- metaRegister of Controlled Trials (mRCT): http://www.controlled-trials.com/mrct/ (Covers 13 registers of ongoing research, including updates from the Medical Research Council, National Institutes of Health, NHS Trusts, UK Clinical Trials Gateway, the Wellcome Trust, etc.);
- UK Clinical Research Network Study (UKRCN): Portfolio Database: http://public.ukcrn.org.uk/search.

Individual institutions, such as charitable foundations and universities, often list and describe their ongoing research activities on their web sites.

Clinical trials

One of the more comprehensive search tools for clinical trials is the already-mentioned *mRCT*. In addition, several search tools are available for specific conditions or interventions, for example:

- Stroke Trials Registry: http://www.strokecenter.org/trials (A continuously updated registry of randomised clinical trials relating to stroke and cerebrovascular disease.);

- The Trials Register of Promoting Health Interventions (TRoPHI): http://eppi.ioe.ac.uk/webdatabases/Intro.aspx?ID=5 (A searchable register of randomised and non-randomised controlled trials relating to public health and health promotion interventions).

MEDLINE has special limit filters (in the 'Publication Types' drop-down menu) for restricting searches to *Clinical Trials* or even to specific phases (I, II or III) of clinical trials.

Systematic reviews

Although not primary research papers in themselves, systematic reviews can provide a very useful starting point during an initial survey of the research area you are interested in and may suggest documents and approaches that you might not otherwise have considered.

The Cochrane Library

Covering most areas of healthcare, this is the most popular free UK source for identifying full-text systematic reviews and protocols (reviews in progress). The library is a collection of five different databases that focus on systematic reviews and clinical trials. The databases can be searched simultaneously or individually and systematic reviews can be browsed by topic.

On the *Cochrane Library* home page (www.thecochranelibrary.com), click the *Cochrane Advance Search* link. This option allows you to search for and enter *MeSH* terms or free text in separate search boxes. You can combine these as necessary by selecting AND or OR operators from a drop-down menu. You can narrow searches by restricting them to the abstract or title field, or limit to a specific date range. Searching *Full text* will obviously broaden your search.

Results are returned and displayed for each database separately, indicating the number of hits retrieved. Cochrane reviews are displayed by default, but to view results from the other databases, you need to click the database name. In the *Search History*, search line numbers are preceded by the hash symbol – #. Remember to use this when combing sets of search results, for example #1 or #2 or #3. Searches can be saved.

Managing online information

The options for managing citations drawn from the Internet vary, depending on the host web site. It is often quicker to enter references manually into your stored list of citations. Some web sites allow instant uploading of the citations to specific reference management sites or software. However, the format options are usually very limited.

One solution is to use social book-marking sites such as *CiteULike*, *Connotea* and *Zotero*. These sites allow you to set up a list of your favourite citations, link to access (where available), and promote the allocation of tags to help you identify your articles and share the information with others.

CiteULike (http://www.citeulike.org) A powerful package, currently hosted by the University of Manchester. Citations can be entered manually or added by searching *PubMed* or specific publishers. A toolbar button can be downloaded to allow one-touch saving of citations once they have been located. *CiteULike* deals mainly with supported sites to limit spam and controls the quality of information displayed. Entries can then be edited and notes attached.

There is also an option for attaching your own personal copy of a PDF version of the article, making it accessible from any computer.

Members of the *CiteULike* community can also set up specific groups for sharing their favourite resources. Once pages of interest have been identified, they can be 'watched' to alert you of any added information. *CiteULike* is compatible with *Bibtex* and *Endnote* reference management systems.

Connotea (http://www.connotea.org) Similar to *CiteULike* but isn't as adept at handling PDF files. Articles can be added using the Digital Object Identifier (DOI) reference for greater precision. This will identify and fully cite your reference ready for the addition of tags. Embargoes can be placed on citation lists to control when they are made accessible to share.

Searching citations in *Connotea* can be limited to your own library, by user or by exact tag, making it easier to share and search group work. By using *OpenURL* technology, it may also be possible to locate quickly and easily the reference through your local library holdings. Other features include:

- the ability to identify yourself as an article author, providing an easy way of tracking your publication record;
- 'geotagging' which will display a map showing the distribution of the places of publication in relation to any tagged group of citations.

Zotero (http://www.zotero.org/) Free reference management tool download, which can be attached to the Mozilla FireFox browser allowing you to add citations direct from the web site. Additional tools are available to allow you to enable the Cite While You Write function when using word documents and saving your browser settings to a USB stick to create a portable version.

Locating and obtaining material

Having identified the material to be viewed, the next challenge is to locate and obtain copies of what you want to see. You may be able to do this directly yourself (via web-based text) or through a third party (library service or the author).

Immediate access

When you run a literature search, the retrieved citations may contain a link indicating that the full text of the document is immediately available. Clicking the link will either open the full text in a new window or take you to a related link, for example the publisher's web site. Happily, many journal articles and other documents in the health sciences field are freely available. However, most require some form of subscription or payment.

Not all freely available information will be automatically linked into citation databases or citation searching software. Consequently, it is sometimes worth searching for the document title on a general Internet search engine. To ensure an exact match, it is best to place the title in quotation marks " ".

If the citation is an article published in a subscription journal, a personal or institutional subscription is required. If your library uses a 'link resolver' software package, the full text of articles from e-journals that the library subscribes to will be automatically linked to citations in its bibliographic databases. Otherwise, you will have to check the e-journal or paper journal holdings of your library through its online catalogue. In some libraries, electronic holdings and print copies are assimilated into a single list, but often there will be two different online listings to check.

Once you have found an online article, there is often a choice to be made between displaying it in Portable Document Format (PDF) or HTML. As the name suggests, PDF files are self-contained files that can be easily stored or e-mailed. PDF is an image of the printed document and is, therefore, ideal for printing: line illustrations, graphs, and tables retain their original layout. However, PDF is unable to support multimedia content and many older PDF documents, which have been simply scanned from the original, may display some loss of image quality, which can be an important factor when seeking high-resolution images such as X-ray scans.

HTML is designed to be read on a computer and can make full use of its multimedia capabilities. Images can be enlarged or media files can provide accompanying video footage. Designed for the online environment, HTML can also incorporate hyperlinks that take you directly to further information, relevant web sites, and so on.

Using libraries and requesting material

If you are unable to access the required literature directly from the computer, other options are at hand:

- Visit your home library, if it holds a paper copy, and obtain a photocopy;
- Use your home library to make an interlibrary request;
- Order a copy from the British Library;
- Visit other libraries;
- Contact the author;
- Purchase the material.

Visiting your local library

Most libraries have online catalogues which include their holdings of paper journals, and so on. The catalogue will also give details of the years/volumes held and indicate whether they are on the open shelves or kept in store. (Older volumes are sometimes held in a store room and have to be asked for at the library counter.) If the library has the item(s) you are looking for, check the opening times and allow yourself sufficient time to locate and photocopy what you need. (Most libraries have self-service photocopiers: some take coins, some require a pre-paid card that can be purchased at the library counter.) If you need advice or help, ask a member of library staff.

Making an interlibrary request

All libraries offer some form of interlibrary request service, as it is impossible to store all possible reading material under one roof. Reciprocal agreements exist between libraries for the exchange of information, to give people broader access to material. Journal articles are supplied as PDF print copies or photocopies. Books, reports, dissertations and theses can also be obtained and borrowed, which is why the service is often called an interlibrary loan (ILL) service. You will need to make a request for each item you require and enter its full details on an online or paper request form.

Copyright law governs all aspects of document provision and restricts what can be ordered. You are legally required to sign a copyright declaration for each item (unless covered as part of an institutional license) to ensure that you understand how the copy may be used. For more information on copyright, ask your local librarian or check the Copyright License Agency's web site (http://www.cla.co.uk/).

The charge for interlibrary requests varies from library to library, as does the length of time it takes to obtain a copy of the document. Interlibrary request are usually received within 1–7 days, the time interval depending on a number of factors:

- Ready availability of the item;
- Size and set up of the library service;
- Article format;
- Internal postal policy.

If the library receiving the request has a PDF scanner, then it is a relatively quick process to scan and e-mail the document as a PDF file to the requesting library. Unfortunately, the expense of such scanners prohibits smaller libraries from doing this and results in many requests being satisfied with photocopies delivered by post. It is vital not to leave things to the last minute when submitting requests. Paper journals may have been sent out of the library for binding. Similarly, a book, and so on, may be out on loan.

British library

The British Library is the main national repository for British publications, but also carries an extensive collection of print journals and books from around the world. *British Library Direct* (http://direct.bl.uk) provides access to the library's e-journals (last five years only) offering a direct download service for a fee. This service is instant once the payment has cleared, but requires the registration of a credit card and the successful enablement of your computer to accept encrypted files.

Visiting other libraries

Why not check other local libraries, by visiting their web sites or checking on *WorldCat* (http://www.worldcat.org)? *WorldCat* helps you to locate where a book is held near you. Not all libraries are listed, but it can be a good first place to look. Remember to find out if you are eligible to join the library and have borrowing rights. Most health libraries are closed libraries, but may allow access for reference purposes on proof of work or student identification. It is essential to phone the library in advance before arranging a visit. A joining fee may be required if you wish to borrow material.

Students can also apply for access to other academic libraries through the *SCONUL Access* scheme (http://www.sconul.ac.uk/). Visit your home library to register.

Contacting the author

If you wish to see unpublished material, for example poster and conference presentations, 'abstract only' publications, ongoing research, and so on, you should consider contacting the author or research group directly. Contact details are frequently made available in the citation or abstract of unpublished work. If no contact information is given, check the web site of the author's affiliated organization.

Purchasing material

It is now commonplace for journals to offer downloadable copies of articles for a fee. Many articles have restrictions placed on them; for example, the downloaded file may become inaccessible after a specified number of days. This is an expensive method of accessing articles and not universally available from all publishers. Remember to check the full details and format being offered before purchasing online.

Grey literature publications are usually unpriced and often unobtainable from commercial book suppliers. Fortunately, the full text of much recent grey literature is freely available online, for example Department of Health and Health Technology Assessment publications. If this is not the case, use the Internet to contact the issuing body or author to enquire about the availability of priced or free copies.

Finding statistical data

Official statistical surveys provide rich sources of raw data that researchers often employ to provide a context for their work or to underpin statements in their study.

Official statistics monitor the health of the nation's population and are collected specifically to inform policy, debate, research and management decisions at national and local government level. Monitoring public health is the chief concern; for example, in the United Kingdom it is mandatory to report certain notifiable diseases, such as anthrax, measles, meningitis and small pox, but statistics are also collected to help monitor healthcare provision, interventions and hospital activity.

Collecting statistical data can be time-consuming and costly. Consequently, official statistics are not gathered out of idle curiosity, so don't be disappointed if none have been collected for your particular area of interest. When using statistics, ask yourself:

- Who has collected this data?
- Why was the survey undertaken?
- Might there be bias?
- What geographic area is covered?
- What population group was surveyed?
- What criteria were applied?
- Are there any special exceptions?
- How current are the data?
- Are the data comparable with other data?

Fortunately, statistics are more accessible and easy to use than they once were. A representative selection of free Internet sources, ranging through international, national, regional, local and topical data is given at the end of this chapter. A general Internet search might be helpful if the statistical data you need does not appear on one of the official web sites. Be aware, though, that there is no guarantee that data has ever been collected for the topic that you are researching.

/ **Action Point**

Try to answer the following questions:

1. **How many people in my local area suffer from a long-term health problem or disability?**
   Using *Neighbourhood Statistics* (http://www.neighbourhood.statistics.gov.uk/dissemination/), type your post code in the search box and select 'Ward'. In the list of *Topics*, select *Health and Care*, then choose *Limiting Long-term Illness*. Explore other statistics available for your Ward and/or click the links at the bottom of the screen for your Local Authority, Primary Care Organization or Health Authority.
2. **Are alcohol-related deaths increasing in the UK?**
   Visit the *UK Statistics Authority* web site (http://www.statistics.gov.uk/), go to the *Virtual Bookshelf* and open *Advanced* search (top right of screen) and type in 'alcohol death'.
3. **What are the latest comparative statistics for UK deaths from lung cancer?**
   A good source for cancer statistics is Cancer Research UK (http://www.cancerresearchuk.org/). On the home page, locate and click the link to *Cancer statistics* under *News and Resources* in the left-hand panel.

Keeping up to date

For research projects, dissertations, professional development and personal interest, it is always worth keeping up to date with the latest information. Many databases allow you to set up an alerting service that will automatically e-mail any new results from your saved searches. In *CINAHL*, this is accessed via the *Saved Search/Alerts* link or by using the orange RSS icon. By default, the new results are e-mailed to you on a daily basis, but this frequency can be customized. To learn more about this, and how to set up the alerting service, read *Saving a Search as an Alert* in *CINAHL*'s help notes. You can also set up an e-mail alert to notify you automatically each time a new issue of a selected journal title becomes available. *CINAHL* and many other databases, including *PubMed*, also support the creation of RSS feeds for search alerts and journal alerts.

Really Simple Syndication (RSS Feeds) is an excellent means of bringing the latest information from many sources (databases and web sites) directly to you in one place. Besides news and current affairs sites, RSS feeds are offered by learned and professional societies, institutional web sites and commercial publishers.

In order to view feeds, you must first register with an RSS Reader. This can be a stand-alone reader such as *NewsGator* (www.newsgator.com) or *Google Reader* (http://www.reader.google.com). They may also be included as part of a customisable web site such as *MyLibrary*, hosted by NHS Evidence (http://www.evidence.nhs.uk/, accessible to those with NHS Athens access), or *iGoogle* (http://www.google.com/ig).

Help

Librarians can be your best allies when seeking what is already known. Your local health library will probably offer hands-on training in literature searching, specifically geared to the databases and search tools that you have local access to. Skilled library staff may also be available to provide you with personal one-to-one support. Search tools are constantly developing, so it's worthwhile updating yourself with a training session, even if you had one only a few years ago. Telephone, e-mail or ask at the library Help Desk.

The best databases and search tools have on-screen links to supporting information and assistance. The links may be labelled *Help*, *Search Tips*, *How to Search*, and so on. These help notes are written specifically for the search tool in question and should be consulted to clarify any uncertainties you may have, for example, what symbols are used for truncation or wild-card searching.

A variety of guides, online tutorials and search tips are freely available on the Internet, some aimed at users of specific database hosts:

http://support.dialog.com/ for *Dialogue* users
http://support.epnet.com/training/ for *EBSCO* users
http://www.ovid.com/site/help/documentation/owg.jsp?top=28&mid=30&bottom=55 for
   OVID users
http://www.nlm.nih.gov/bsd/disted/pubmed.html for *PubMed* tutorial
http://www.library.nhs.uk/help/hdas for *Search 2.0* users

Many individual libraries also provide online user guides to locally-accessible databases.

 Action Point

Explore some of the databases in the list of specialist healthcare databases, run some sample searches and compare results. Note the strengths and weaknesses of different databases.

References

Booth, A. (2004) Formulating answerable questions, in *Evidence-based Practice for Information Professionals: a Handbook* (eds A. Booth and A. Brice), Facet, London, pp. 61–70.

Clarke, J. and Wentz, R. (2000) Letters: Pragmatic approach is effective in evidence based health care. *British Medical Journal*, **321** (7260), 566. Retrieved from: http://www.library.nhs.uk/help/hdas.

Coughran, B. (2004) Google's index nearly doubles. *The Official Google Blog*. Retrieved from: http://googleblog.blogspot.com/2004/11/googles-index-nearly-doubles.html.

Fallows, D. (2005) *Search Engine Users*, Pew Internet & American Life Project, Washington. Retrieved from: http://www.pewinternet.org/pdfs/PIP_Searchengine_users.pdf.

National Library of Medicine (2008) Factsheet: MEDLINE. Retrieved from: http://www.nlm.nih.gov/pubs/factsheets/medline.html.

Richardson, W.S., Wilson, M.C., Nishikawa, J. and Hayward, R.S.A. (1995) The well-built clinical question: A key to evidence based decisions. *ACP Journal Club*, **123** (3), A12–A13.

Wildridge, V. and Bell, L. (2002) Brief communication. How CLIP became ECLIPSE: A mnemonic to assist in searching for health policy/management information. *Health Information & Libraries Journal*, **19** (2), 113–115.

Further reading

Asking the question

Akobeng, A.K. (2005) Principles of evidence based medicine. *Archives of Disease in Childhood*, **90** (8), 837–840.

Armstrong, E.C. (1999) The well-built clinical question: the key to finding the best evidence efficiently. *Wisconsin Medical Journal*, **98** (22), 25–28.

Bandolier (no date) Glossary of diagnostic terms. Retrieved from: http://www.jr2.ox.ac.uk/bandolier/booth/diagnos/glossary.html.

Booth, A. and Dixon-Woods, M. (2004) How to do a literature search [PowerPoint presentation]. *ESRC Research Methods Festival, St Catherine's College, Oxford. 1–3 July 2004*. Retrieved from: http://www.ccsr.ac.uk/methods/festival2004/programme/Sat/pm/D/Documents/Booth_000.ppt.

Booth, A. and Brice, A. (eds) (2004) *Evidence-based Practice for Information Professionals: a Handbook*, Facet Publishing, London, pp. 65–66.

Centre for Clinical Effectiveness (2006) *Evidence-based Answers to Clinical Questions for Busy Clinicians*, Monash Institute of Health Services Research, Melbourne, Australia. Retrieved from: http://www.mihsr.monash.org/cce/pdf/ebpworkbook2007.pdf.

Centre for Evidence Based Medicine (CEBM) (2000) *Asking Focused Clinical Questions*, CEBM, Oxford. Retrieved from: http://www.cebm.net/index.aspx?o=1036.

Cooke, A. (2001) *A Guide to Finding Quality Information on the Internet: Selection and Evaluation Strategies*, 2nd edn, Facet Publishing, London.

Doig, G.S. and Simpson, F. (2003) Efficient literature searching: a core skill for the practice of evidence-based medicine. *Journal of Intensive Care Medicine*, **29** (12), 2119–2127.

Dorsch, J. (2005) Formulating Patient Centered Questions, University of Illinois, Chicago 's Library of the Health Sciences, Peoria. Retrieved from: http://www.uic.edu/depts/lib/lhsp/resources/pico.shtml.

Ely, J.W., Osheroff, J.A., Ebell, M.H. *et al.* (2002) Obstacles to answering doctors' questions about patient care with evidence: qualitative study. *British Medical Journal*, **324** (7339), 710–713. Retrieved from: http://www.bmj.com/cgi/content/full/324/7339/710.

Maslin-Prothero, S. (ed.) (2005) *Baillière's Study Skills for Nurses and Midwives*, 3rd edn, Baillière Tindall, Edinburgh.

Oxman, A.D. Sackett, D.L., Guyatt, G.H. and the Evidence Based Medicine Working Group (1995) How to get started. Based on: Users' guides to evidence-based medicine. *JAMA*, **270** (17), 2093–2095. Retrieved from: http://www.cche.net/usersguides/start.asp.

Ridley, D. (2008) *The Literature Review: A Step-by-Step Guide for Students*, Sage, London.

Scott Memorial Library (2006) Evidence-based Medicine: The Well-Built Clinical Question, Thomas Jefferson University, Philapdelphia. Retrieved from from: http://jeffline.tju.edu/Ask/Help/Handouts/EBM_PICO.pdf.

Straus, S.E., Richardson, W.S., Glasziou, P. and Haynes, B. (2005) *Evidence-based Medicine: How to Practice and Teach EBM*, 3rd edn, Elsevier Churchill Livingstone, Edinburgh.

Wyer, P.C., Allen, T.Y. and Corrall, C.J. (2004) Finding evidence when you need it. *Evidence-based Cardiovascular Medicine*, **8** (1), 2–7.

Xiaoli, H., Lin, J. and Demner-Fushman, D. (2006) Evaluation of PICO as a Knowledge Representation for Clinical Questions. AMIA Annual Symposium Proceedings, pp. 259–363. Retrieved from: http://www.pubmedcentral.nih.gov/articlerender.fcgi?tool=pubmed&pubmedid=17238363.

Accessibility

Blackwell Synergy (2007): Online journals for learning, research and professional practice. Retrieved from: http://www.blackwell-synergy.com.

Biomed Central Ltd. (2007) Biomed Central. Retrieved from: http://www.biomedcentral.com.

Department of Health (2007) Department of Health Homepage. Retrieved from: http://www.dh.gov.uk.

Internet searching

Bergman, M.K. (2001) The deep web: surfacing hidden value. *The Journal of Electronic Publishing*, **7** (1). Retrieved from: http://quod.lib.umich.edu/cgi/t/text/text-dx?c=jep;view=text;rgn=main;idno=3336451.0007.104.

Blachman, N. (2007) Google guide: making searching even easier. Retrieved from: http://www.googleguide.com/.

Brophy, J. and Dawden, D. (2005) Is Google enough? Comparison of an internet search engine with academic library resources. *Aslib Proceedings: New Information Perspectives*, **57** (6), 498–512.

Dess, H.M. (2006) Database reviews and reports: Scopus. *Issues in Science and Technology Librarianship*, **45** (Winter), Retrieved from: http://www.istl.org/06-winter/databases4.html.

Fingerman, S. (2005) SCOPUS: profusion and confusion. *Information Today*, **29** (2), 36–38. Retrieved from: http://info.scopus.com/docs/fingerman_online_marapr05.pdf.

Fox, S. (2006) Online Health Search 2006, Pew Internet & American Life Project, Washington. Retrieved from: http://www.pewinternet.org/PPF/r/190/report_display.asp.

Giustini, D. and Barsky, E. (2005) A look at Google Scholar, PubMed, and Scirus: comparisons and recommendations. *Journal of the Canadian Health Libraries Association*, **26** (3), 85–89. Retrieved from: http://pubs.nrc-cnrc.gc.ca/jchla/jchla26/c05-030.pdf.

Giustini, D. and Barsky, E. (2005) Using Google Scholar(TM) in Health Research: Comparisons with PubMed. CHLA/ABSC Conference –Toronto, 1 June 2005. Retrieved from: http://www.chla-absc.ca/2005/Presentations/0601/GiustiniBarsky_CHLA2005.pdf.

Google (2006) Google announces healthcare search clustering [Internet]. *E-Health Insider*. Retrieved from: http://www.e-health-insider.com/news/item.cfm?ID=1880.

Health on the Net Foundation (HON) (2006) HON's partnership with Google [Internet] Geneva: HON. Retrieved from: http://www.hon.ch/Project/GoogleCoop/.

Henderson, J. (2005) Google Scholar: a source for clinicians? *Canadian Medical Association Journal*, **172** (12). Retrieved from: http://www.cmaj.ca/cgi/content/full/172/12/1549. doi:10.1503/cmaj.050404

Jacso, P. (2005) As we may search – Comparison of major features of the Web of Science, Scopus, and Google Scholar citation-based and citation-enhanced databases. *Current Science*, **89** (9), 1537–1547. Retrieved from: http://www.ias.ac.in/currsci/nov102005/1537.pdf.

Jasco, P. (2005) Google Scholar (Redux) [Internet]. *Péter's Digital Reference Shelf* June 2005. Retrieved from: http://gale.cengage.com/servlet/HTMLFileServlet?imprint=9999&region=7&fileName=reference/archive/200506/google.html.

Kiley, R. (2003) *Medical Information on the Internet: a Guide for Health Professionals*, 3rd edn, Churchill Livingstone, Edinburgh.

Lawrence, S. and Giles, C.L. (1998) Searching the World Wide Web. *Science*, **280**, 98–100.

Regazzi, J.J. (2004) The Battle for Mindshare: a Battle Beyond Access and Retrieval [Presentation]. Miles Conrad Memorial Lecture, 46th NFAIS Annual Conference, 23 February 2004. Retrieved from: http://www.nfais.org/publications/mc_lecture_2004.htm.

Tenopir, C. (2004) Is Google the competition? *Library Journal*, **4** (January). Retrieved from: http://www.libraryjournal.com/article/CA405423.html.

Yang, K. and Meho, L.I. (2006) *Citation Analysis: a Comparison of Google Scholar, Scopus, and Web of Science*. Proceedings 69th Annual Meeting of the American Society for Information Science and Technology (ASIST), 43 (ed. A. Grove), Austin (US). Retrieved from: from: http://eprints.rclis.org/archive/00008121/01/Yang_citation.pdf

Social bookmarking

Chillingworth, M. (2005) Pointing your peers in the right direction. *Information World Review*, **Nov**, (218), 40–41. Retrieved from: http://www.iwr.co.uk/information-world-review/features/2147772/pointing-peers-right-direction.

Gordon-Murnane, L. (2006) Social bookmarking, folksonomies, and Web 2.0 tools. *Searcher*, **14** (6), 26-38. Retrieved from: http://pqasb.pqarchiver.com/infotoday/results.html?QryTxt=id(1061344611)).

Hannay, T., Hammond, T., Lund, B. and Scott, J. (2005) Social Bookmarking Tools (I). *D-Lib Magazine*, **11**(4). Retrieved from: http://www.dlib.org/dlib/april05/hammond/04hammond.html.

Lund, B., Hammond, T., Flack, M. and Hannay, T. (2005) Social bookmarking tools (II): A case study – Connotea. *D-Lib Magazine*, **11** (4). Retrieved from: http://www.dlib.org/dlib/april05/lund/04lund.html.

Rethlefsen Melissa, L. (2006) Product pipeline: Social reference managers. *Library Journal*, 15 October 2006 (suppl Net Connect), 14–16. Retrieved from: http://www.libraryjournal.com/article/CA6375468.html.

Resources

Databases

Alcohol and other drug-related databases (mostly free): An extensive list of databases focusing on alcohol and substance abuse. http://etoh.niaaa.nih.gov/Databases.htm

Alzheimer's Disease Education and Referral Centre (free): Clinical trials, including trials in progress. http://www.nia.nih.gov/alzheimers

AMED – Allied and Complementary Medicine (subscription): Covers complementary medicine, occupational therapy, palliative care, physiotherapy, rehabilitation, podiatry, rehabilitation, speech and language therapy. Indexes about 600 journals (mainly European) and includes abstracts for most post-1995 records. Updated monthly. Currently free to NHS professionals and members of the Chartered Society of Physiotherapy.

BioMed Central (free): Full-text peer-reviewed research articles in all fields of biological sciences and clinical medicine. http://www.biomedcentral.com/search/bmc/

CAS online (subscription): Contains references to over 40 000 journal articles, books and research covering all aspects of learning disabilities. Updated monthly.

Child Abuse, Child Welfare and Adoption (free registration): 42 000 + records. http://www.nisc.com/frame/freeaccess-f.htm

ClinicalTrials.com (free): Registry of more than 140 000 clinical trials across the world. http://www.clinicaltrials.gov/

CRISP (free): Database of federally-funded biomedical research projects conducted at universities, hospitals and other research institutions in the USA. http://crisp.cit.nih.gov/

ERIC (free and subscription): The Educational Resources Information Centre database covers all aspects of education, including medical education, counselling and learning disabilities. Contains about 1.3 million records, derived from more than 2000 journals, books, theses, conference papers, curricula and standards, dating back to 1966. Although available from major database vendors, a free version can be accessed at: http://www.eric.ed.gov/

ETHXWeb (free): Journal articles, book chapters, bills, laws, court decisions, reports, and so on, relating to bioethics and professional ethics. http://bioethics.georgetown.edu/databases/ETHXWeb/

Evidence Base (free): An information resource developed by the former Health Development Agency. It consists of evidence briefing papers and evidence reviews across a range of topics, identifying gaps in the research base and making recommendations for future research. http://www.nice.org.uk/aboutnice/whoweare/aboutthehda/evidencebase/evidence_base.jsp

Maternal and Child Health Library (free): Offers five databases in this field. http://www.mchlibrary.info/databases/about_databases.html

Midwifery and Infant Care (subscription): Covers the midwifery profession, pregnancy, labour, childbirth, postnatal care, neonatal care and the first year of an infant's life. Contains 120 000+ records drawn from more than 550 English-language journals, books and grey literature. Updated monthly.

NARIC Databases (free): REHABDATA (1956–) contains approximately 69 000 abstracts of books, reports, articles and audiovisual materials relating to disability and rehabilitation research. The NIDRR Project Database (1993–) collects information about all projects funded by National Institute on Disability and Rehabilitation Research. http://www.naric.com/research/

National Cancer Institute (free): Search 5000+ clinical trials. http://www.cancer.gov/

PEDro (free): The Physiotherapy Evidence Database provides details and abstracts of randomized controlled trials, systematic reviews and evidence-based clinical practice guidelines in physiotherapy. Most trials are rated for quality. http://www.pedro.org.au/

POPLINE (free): Major bibliographic database for reproductive health, covering family planning issues, population law and policy and primary healthcare, including maternal/child health in developing countries. More than 350 000 records (journal articles, monographs, technical reports and unpublished works), updated monthly. http://db.jhuccp.org/popinform/basic.html

PsycINFO (subscription): Besides core psychology topics such as personality and mental health, this major database covers the behavioural sciences in related disciplines, for example healthcare, education, organizational behaviour, consumer behaviour, and so on. More than 2150 journals are indexed and the databases contains over 2.4 million references to journal articles, books, book chapters, technical reports and dissertations published in more than 50 countries. Updated weekly.
Created and maintained by the American Psychological Association. Fixed-fee subscription for Internet access is available from all the major database vendors. Access is currently free for NHS professionals.

Search the studies at NIH (free): Database of clinical studies conducted by the National Institutes of Health, USA. http://clinicalstudies.info.nih.gov/index.html

Social Care Online (free): Provided by the Social Care Institute for Excellence. http://www.scie-socialcareonline.org.uk/

Social Services Abstracts (subscription): Covers current research in social work, human services and related areas. It includes topics such as community and mental health services, crisis intervention, family and social welfare, gerontology, poverty and homelessness, professional issues in social work, social and health policy, social services in addiction, social work practice, support groups/networks, violence, abuse, neglect and welfare services. The database contains 140 000 + records and indexes about 1500 serial publications. It includes abstracts of journal articles and dissertations. Updated monthly. Published by Cambridge Scientific Abstracts.

Springer Link (free): Searchable database of abstracts from hundreds of scientific journals, including life sciences and medicine. 3.6 million records. http://link.springer.de/search.htm

TOXNET (free): A cluster of 14 searchable databases, including TOXLINE which covers all aspects of toxicology, including hazardous chemicals, pharmaceuticals, pesticides, environmental pollutants and safety, mutagens and teratogens. Provides bibliographic citations and abstracts from journal articles, monographs, technical reports, theses, letters, meeting abstracts, papers and reports. Produced by the US National Library of Medicine. http://toxnet.nlm.nih.gov/

TRIP Database (free): *Turning Research into Practice* aims to support research amongst primary care teams in Wales. Search results (mostly full text) are sorted by evidence-based practice, peer-reviewed articles and clinical guidelines, and so on. http://www.tripdatabase.com/

Global and collected national data

United Nations Statistics Division: http://unstats.un.org/unsd/sitemap.htm
A comprehensive source for social indicators, including data about population, child-bearing, fertility patterns, youth, elderly populations, education, human settlements, literacy, water supply and sanitation, income and economic activity, housing, unemployment and health.

United Nations Population Information Network (POPIN): http://www.un.org/popin/data.html
Publishes a broad range of global statistics, indicators and projections, including information and data about population trends, ageing, HIV/AIDS, contraceptive use, marriage, children and fertility patterns.

The World Health Organization Statistical Information System (WHOSIS): http://www.who.int/whosis/en/
Issues global health data on a range of health issues. Includes an online version of *World Health Statistics Annual* – the most recent statistics gathered from WHOs 193 member states.

WHO regional offices: http://www.who.int/about/regions/en/index.html
Links to the WHO's six regional offices.

Demographic and Health Surveys: http://www.measuredhs.com/
Collects, analyses and disseminates accurate and representative data on population, health and nutrition through 200+ surveys in 75+ countries.

The CIAs World Factbook: https://www.cia.gov/library/publications/the-world-factbook/index.html
A regularly updated source for general statistical data about individual countries. Includes demographic and public health information (major infectious diseases and HIV/AIDS).

Europe

WHO Regional Office for Europe: health topics: http://www.euro.who.int/healthtopics
An extensive set of statistics for European Union countries, arranged by topics (A–Z).

Eurostat: http://europa.eu.int/comm/eurostat/
Statistical data collated by the European Commission, including public health and ageing population issues.

UK national, regional and local data

UK Statistics Authority: http://www.statistics.gov.uk/
The official UK statistics site, providing a wide range of statistical data gathered by the Office of National Statistics and government departments. The UK Snapshot data is grouped by themes, including *health and care*, *population and migration* and *social and welfare*. Statistical tables are searchable and are also listed alphabetically.
Virtual Bookshelf: http://www.statistics.gov.uk/onlineproducts/default.asp
Provides quick links to full-text versions of popular statistical publications, for example *Focus on Health, Health and Personal Social Services Statistics, Health Statistics Quarterly, Mortality statistics, Regional Trends, Social Trends*.
Association of Public Health Observatories (APHO): http://www.apho.org.uk/
Amongst other things, the APHO produces data to inform health care planning by health authorities, primary care groups and local authorities in Wales, Scotland, Ireland and the English regions.
Health Protection Agency: http://www.hpa.org.uk/
Data reflects the HPAs concern with the surveillance of infectious diseases. An English site but has links to similar agencies in Northern Ireland, Scotland and Wales.
HSE Statistics: http://www.hse.gov.uk/statistics/index.htm
Statistics on work-related ill-health, injuries, dangerous occurrences, and so on.
Neighbourhood Statistics: http://www.neighbourhood.statistics.gov.uk/
Detailed demographic and social information for individual electoral wards in England and Wales, provided by the Neighbourhood Statistics Division of the Office of National Statistics.

England

Department of Health: Statistics: http://www.dh.gov.uk/en/Publicationsandstatistics/Statistics/index.htm
The main source for health statistics in England, with search and browse options. The *Health profile of England* is a helpful survey of the nation's health.
Statistical work areas: http://www.dh.gov.uk/en/Publicationsandstatistics/Statistics/StatisticalWorkAreas/index .htm
Lists statistics by topic area.
Performance data and statistics: http://www.dh.gov.uk/en/Publicationsandstatistics/Statistics/Performancedata andstatistics/index.htm
Collates performance assessment of the NHS and social care provision in England.
Hospital Activity Statistics: http://www.dh.gov.uk/en/Publicationsandstatistics/Statistics/Performancedata andstatistics/HospitalActivityStatistics/index.htm
Provides activity data (in Excel format) for individual NHS organizations in England.
Various **annual reports** also contain important data: http://www.dh.gov.uk/en/Publicationsandstatistics/ Publications/AnnualReports/index.htm
The *Chief Executive's Report to the NHS* describes recent NHS activity and performance, backed up by a very useful *Statistical Supplement*. The *Annual Report of the Chief Medical Officer* highlights contemporary trends and health concerns, supported by statistics and graphs.
Association of Public Health Observatories: http://www.apho.org.uk
Useful small-area community health profiles for local authorities and health services aimed at highlighting and comparing health issues across England. The profiles are designed to show where there are important problems with health or health inequalities.
Hospital Episode Statistics (HES): http://www.hesonline.nhs.uk/
Presents data about patient care provided by individual NHS hospitals in England with a helpful link to *Understanding the data*.
Confidential enquiries
Confidential enquiry into maternal and child health http://www.cemach.org.uk/

National confidential enquiry into patient outcome and death http://213.198.120.192/

National confidential enquiry into suicide and homicide by people with mental illness http://www.medicine.manchester.ac.uk/suicideprevention/nci/

Healthcare Commission: http://www.healthcarecommission.org.uk/guidanceforhealthcarestaff/nhsstaff/annualhealthcheck.cfm

England's healthcare watchdog that inspects standards and the performance of NHS and independent healthcare organizations. Enter the most current *Annual Health Check*, then follow the *Performance ratings* link for detailed information.

Northern Ireland

Department of Health, Social Services and Public Safety: Statistics and Research: http://www.dhsspsni.gov.uk/index/stats_research/stats-activity_stats-2.htm

Northern Ireland Statistics and Research Agency (NISRA): http://www.nisra.gov.uk/

Scotland

The Scottish Government: Statistics: http://www.scotland.gov.uk/Topics/Statistics/Browse/Health

Covers *Health of Scotland's Population* and *Health Service Provision*.

ISD Scotland: http://www.isdscotland.org/

Information Services Division (ISD), NHS National Services Scotland, provides comprehensive and detailed statistical data about health and health services in Scotland.

Scottish Neighbourhood Statistics: http://www.sns.gov.uk/

Wales

NHS Wales: Health Statistics: http://www.wales.nhs.uk/page.cfm?pid=739

Collates the statistical data available about the health of the population of Wales and Welsh health and care services.

Welsh Assembly Government: Health Statistics Wales: http://new.wales.gov.uk/topics/statistics/theme/health/?lang=en

Commonwealth countries

Australian Institute of Health and Welfare: http://www.aihw.gov.au/

Canadian Institute for Health Information: http://secure.cihi.ca/cihiweb/splash.html

Statistics Canada: http://www40.statcan.ca/z01/cs0002_e.htm

India Health Statistics: http://www.indiahealthstat.com/

Government of Pakistan: Federal Bureau of Statistics: http://www.statpak.gov.pk/depts/fbs/statistics/social_statistics/social_statistics.html

USA

National Centre for Health Statistics: http://www.cdc.gov/nchs/

Extensive statistical data on public health in the USA.

CDC Wonder: http://wonder.cdc.gov/

Public health information collated by the Centers for Disease Control and Prevention, including

Morbidity and Mortality Weekly Report: http://www.cdc.gov/mmwr/

Current public health data and information (USA).

Data on specific topics

Bear in mind that many of the above sources also provide thematic access or can be searched for specific health topics. Sometimes the data is collated and reworked and can be found on the web pages of special-interest agencies, for example:

Action on Smoking and Health (ASH): http://www.newash.org.uk/.
Arthritis Research Campaign: http://www.arc.org.uk/.
Cancer Research UK: http://www.cancerresearchuk.org/.
CancerMondial: http://www-dep.iarc.fr/.
European Surveillance of Congenital Anomalies: http://www.eurocat.ulster.ac.uk/.
Royal Society for the Prevention of Accidents: http://www.rospa.com/.
UK Creutzfeldt-Jakob Disease Surveillance Unit: http://www.cjd.ed.ac.uk/.
United Kingdom Transplant Support Service Authority: http://www.uktransplant.org.uk/.

5 Can We Trust the Evidence? Critically Reviewing a Research Paper

David Rogers

Introduction

Your literature search (Chapter 4) may have found a few (up to a dozen or so) or many (a hundred or more) references. Exactly how many will depend on the question asked and the sensitivity (how many *potentially* useful references *might* be retrieved) or specificity (how many *definitely* useful references *have* been retrieved) of your search strategy.

The next step is to make a value judgement – a critical appraisal – about the quality of the research reported in those papers, and thus to identify which ones are best suited to answering your clinical question reliably. Why should this be necessary? Surely any paper published in a reputable journal, especially a peer reviewed journal, should be of acceptable quality? (A peer reviewed journal is one in which papers are critically reviewed, normally 'blind', by at least one person from a similar academic or professional community to the author.) Although most papers accepted for publication by such journals are of reasonable quality (especially in the last few years since critical appraisal has been widely adopted for use as a screening tool), some still slip through that contain significant errors of one sort or another.

One of the tasks of critical appraisal is to identify these at an early stage in the process of answering a clinical question. A paper published in JAMA (*Journal of the American Medical Association* (Altman, 2002), made the following observation: 'Peer review can and should weed out serious methodological errors. However, expert methodological input is in short supply. Only a third of high-impact journals reported statistical review of all published manuscripts. The vast majority of research is published in low-impact journals, where peer review is undoubtedly less thorough'. In an earlier paper (Altman, 1994) the same author had put forward the view that the poor quality of much published research was directly due to the 'publish or perish' climate that was prevalent amongst the medical profession throughout the world. Having papers published was seen as a vital addition to the CV of any doctor wishing to progress along a career path, and this emphasis on quantity necessarily resulted in a dropping-off in quality. The author concluded that, 'The manufacturing industry has come to recognize, albeit gradually, that quality control needs to be built in from the start rather than the failures being discarded, and the same principles should inform medical research.'

Historical background

Critical appraisal is usually defined as 'the process of systematically examining research evidence to assess its validity, results and relevance before using it to inform a decision' (Hill and Spittlehouse, 2001). It is an integral part of practising evidence based healthcare, the origins of which may, arguably, be traced back to a conversation between two epidemiologists in Wellington, New Zealand, sometime in 1976. One was Kerr White and the other was Archie Cochrane, the founder of the Cochrane Collaboration. According to the account given on the ScHARR web site (www.shef.ac.uk/scharr/ir/percent.html), Kerr White suggested that 'only about 15–20% of physicians' interventions were supported by objective evidence that they did more good than harm'. Cochrane responded: 'Kerr, you're a liar! You know it isn't more than 10%.' Critical appraisal aims to help identify this small minority of key studies.

What is critical appraisal?

Taking the three key words from Hill and Spittlehouse's definition (validity, results and relevance), we can begin to form a clear idea about the purpose and methodology of critical appraisal. Firstly, validity, which can be defined as 'closeness to the truth'. Note that the word 'truth' here has not been given a capital 'T'. We are not talking about that great Truth that the X Files says is 'out there' somewhere. In the context of research, 'truth' means 'the extent to which these findings can be held to apply to most people in this situation, most of the time'.

Secondly, results. The results section of any research paper is where we would expect to find the key findings of the author's work; the section to which we ought to be giving our closest attention. It is here that we must be alert to the possibility of *bias* creeping in to affect the author's findings, and also to whether mistakes have been made in calculations of any sort.

Thirdly, relevance. A piece of research may have been carried out perfectly and fulfilled every criteria for a well-conducted study, but if its findings cannot be directly applied, or reasonably extrapolated, to the patient group that we have in mind in our clinical question, it is of no use to us. For example, the findings of a study carried out amongst a mixed population in the United States could reasonably be applied to an equivalent population in the United Kingdom. If, however, the population studied consisted solely of Pima Indians from Southern Arizona, that might no longer be the case.

What is critical appraisal for?

We have already established that critical appraisal is a tool by which papers may be screened out that are poorly designed, that have invalid results or that are irrelevant to finding an answer to a particular clinical question. Another use might be to compare the strengths and weaknesses of papers on the 'short list' of those you are considering. In this way, a 'league table' can be drawn up, with only the three or four papers at the top being given a thorough examination, while the rest can be looked at more briefly. In an ideal world, equal time would be given to every paper on the short list, but in the real world there is seldom time available to do this. Another bonus of subjecting papers to critical appraisal is that, with a little practice, it becomes apparent that some mistakes occur repeatedly. These mistakes, once identified, can then be avoided in any research that you may carry out on your own behalf.

How is critical appraisal carried out?

Most critical appraisal is carried out with the help of checklists that typically present a list of questions to answer (mostly with 'yes', 'no' or 'don't know'). The organization 'Critical

---

Box 5.1   Types of Research Paper for which CASP Provides an Appraisal Checklist

- Systematic Reviews;
- Randomized Controlled Trials (RCTs);
- Qualitative Research;
- Economic Evaluation Studies;
- Cohort Studies;
- Case Control Studies;
- Diagnostic Test Studies.

Appraisal Skills Training' (CASP) provides freely available checklists covering a range of types of research papers (Box 5.1).

Screening questions

The initial questions in the CASP checklists are termed 'screening questions' and are designed to help you decide quickly whether or not a paper is worthy of full appraisal.

In the case of randomized controlled trials (Chapter 7), for example, the first of these screening questions asks 'Did the paper ask a clearly focused question?' This may seem quite fundamental but is, nonetheless, very important. The clearer the question asked, the more likely it is that a good literature search will have been carried out, that the methodology used for the study will have been an appropriate one, and that the author's conclusions will be borne out by the results and will support the stated aims of the study.

The second screening question in the case of randomized controlled trials asks whether or not randomization was used in the study. Randomization is a key technique used to eliminate bias in the design of clinical trials. If those running the trial were given a free choice of whether to assign a patient to a group receiving an active treatment or to another group receiving a dummy drug or placebo, the temptation to influence the results by deliberately placing those patients with the best chance of a positive outcome into the active treatment group would be very strong. Randomization means that it is left purely to chance which group individual patients are entered into. In the early days of clinical trials, numbered envelopes were often used to assign patients to groups, but most trials now randomize using a computer program to generate random numbers. The paper by Altman referred to earlier (Altman, 2002) found that 68% of 206 studies in obstetrics and gynaecology journals and 52% of 80 studies in general medical journals failed to report an adequate method for generating random numbers. Any paper that fails one or both of the screening questions is put to one side and not given the full appraisal.

Appraising the literature search

Assuming that both screening questions have been passed, the next thing to consider is whether or not the author has carried out a good enough literature search to identify any papers that have previously researched the question being addressed. Too often, no details at all are given of the search strategy (if any) employed by the author. In a random selection of four papers published in the BMJ during 1993, Jones *et al.* (1994) found one claiming that 'to our knowledge . . . no previous reports have assessed illness in diabetic patients in relation to social deprivation' (a literature search by the authors revealed at least three), and another claiming that 'no study has investigated the nature of backache after childbirth' (two were identified, although the relevant section was 'hidden' in one and not immediately obvious from the title of the paper). It is also not uncommon to read something along the lines of: 'We searched the MEDLINE database using the keywords A, B and C.'

Two alarm bells should be ringing if this is the case. Firstly, only one database, MEDLINE, has been searched. Although MEDLINE indexes about 4600 journal titles, it is very far from being fully comprehensive, as over 12 000 different journals are currently being published in the world's biomedical literature. EMBASE, although it indexes approximately the same number of journal titles as MEDLINE, concentrates more on European (rather than US) literature and is stronger than MEDLINE on indexing papers about drug trials. A literature search should ideally have been carried out on both MEDLINE and EMBASE as a minimum, with additional databases being searched if the study is in a specialist area (e.g. PsycINFO for psychiatry or psychology).

Secondly, it is not always clear what the author means by 'keyword'. It may refer to the specialized word list or thesaurus used by the indexers of a database (e.g. MeSH for MEDLINE and EMTREE for EMBASE), but more commonly means a significant word occurring in the title or abstract of a paper. It is very important that *both* approaches have been used in the search strategy. If only title/abstract words are searched, great care must have been taken to include any synonyms, acronyms or abbreviations that may have been used in the original paper. MeSH and EMTREE, although designed to bring all possible variations of a term under a single heading, also have their weaknesses and should not be relied upon in isolation. Indexers can and do make mistakes and may use headings inconsistently or inaccurately. Furthermore, recent papers are included on most databases before they have been assigned thesaurus headings (Chapter 4), and these will have been missed unless the searcher has managed to retrieve them in another way (usually by title/abstract word searching).

Other factors to consider in evaluating an author's search strategy are:

- Were reference lists from retrieved papers followed up? Additional references are very often identified in this way;
- Were non-English-language papers considered? Although translation costs may be high, an English language abstract is often available and may be sufficient to decide whether or not a paper is a key one. This can be especially important if few relevant papers have been retrieved by the initial search;
- Was the 'Grey Literature' searched? Grey literature refers to documents that are not commercially published or readily available to the public, or which are not indexed by major databases. It includes material such as official reports, in-house drug company information, conference abstracts, theses and ongoing research. A Google search (especially using Google Scholar, which filters out any hits not from specifically academic sources, for example sites that exist purely for commercial reasons to sell a particular product or promote a single idea or cause) is a good way of finding such material; but see also resources described in Chapter 4.

Appraising the results

The next step brings us to the three key questions in any critical appraisal:

- What are the results?
- Do the results match the conclusions?
- Will the results be useful locally?

As mentioned earlier, the *validity* or *closeness to the scientific truth* of the results is of paramount importance. How can validity be assessed? Each of the following points should be considered:

- Was the trial randomized? This has, of course, already been addressed in the first of the screening questions, but at this stage it should be established that the randomization was carried out properly, for example by the use of a randomized number generation computer program rather than any other method that might be vulnerable to interference;
- Was blinding used? Ideally, both those carrying out the study and those receiving any treatment (whether an active one or a placebo) should be unaware of who is in which group. This is known as a double-blind study and further helps in reducing any possible bias. Double blinding may not always be possible, as in a drug trial where the active treatment has a distinctive taste or smell that cannot be accurately replicated by a placebo, or in a 'hands-on' treatment where it is obvious to a patient whether they are receiving it or not. There may be ingenious ways of getting around such problems, as in 'sham acupuncture' which uses a needle with a retractable point to simulate a genuine treatment. A study in which only the patient or the investigator (but not both of them) knows who is receiving what treatment is known as a single-blind study. Altman (2002) found that 51% of 506 studies in cystic fibrosis journals, 33% of 196 studies in rheumatoid arthritis journals and 38% of 68 reports in dermatology journals failed to state whether blinding was used;
- Were the study and control groups similar? Well designed studies will take great pains to match the two groups as closely as possible, in terms of, for example, age range, gender distribution, social class, education and even average annual income. The more similar to each other the two groups are, the less likely it will be that any measurable differences will have been due to factors other than the efficacy (or otherwise) of the treatment being studied;
- Were the two groups treated equally? Were they, for example, followed up at the same time intervals? Again, the more similar the treatment of the two groups, the better;
- Did the numbers add up? Were there any apparently missing patients unaccounted for by the author? If so, why? It is always worthwhile counting up the numbers beginning and completing a study and checking that all drop-outs have been accounted for.

The greater the number of affirmative answers to these questions, the more likely it will be that the results of the study are valid.

In all of this, there are two possible explanations for the appearance of apparent anomalies in research papers. Sometimes, a mistake or omission has been entirely innocent and accidental, usually due to bad practice or poor design. Alternatively, an error has been introduced intentionally in order to deceive or confuse. It is often difficult to distinguish between the two.

Looking at the results themselves, four important questions need to be asked:

- How *large* was the treatment effect? When considering this, it is necessary to distinguish between a statistically significant difference (Chapter 7) between the treatment and control groups and a clinically significant difference. Depending on the statistical test used, very small differences may be detected between two groups. What might appear to be quite a large effect statistically may result in no apparent clinical benefit to the patient. In this case, there is no clinically significant difference;
- How *precise* was the estimate of the treatment effect? This is often expressed in terms of a Confidence Interval (Chapter 7), for example 95% CI 0.99–1.43. This means that 95% of the results fell somewhere in this range. The wider the range, the more *imprecise* are the results, the narrower the range, the more *precise* are the results;
- Could bias of one sort or another have influenced the results? This can happen if, for example, randomization was not applied, if blinding was not done, or at any stage in the research process where errors have remained undetected or unacknowledged;
- Were the conclusions adequately supported by the data? Eagerness to support a pre-conceived theory sometimes leads authors to reach a particular conclusion when their results are insufficiently clear to justify this.

Even if the paper satisfies all these criteria, it must still be rejected if the results cannot be applied to the patient population to which your question relates. Any benefits of an intervention must also be balanced against the costs, both economic and in terms of potential harm to the patient. All drug treatments carry the risk of side effects; some of these may be serious or even potentially life-threatening and thus outweigh any benefits. Altman (2002) found that 61% of 192 reports in seven different medical specialties contained inadequate information on the possible harmful consequences of interventions.

The perfect paper?

No paper can be expected to achieve 100% perfection. It is, therefore, unrealistic to reject every paper because it has some fault or other – if something needs to be done for the patient, the best treatment available, even if less than perfect, is preferable to doing nothing. Therefore, we have to have something with which to work. It is human nature to want to believe in some things and not to believe in others. This may be called 'intuition', but intuition is sometimes used to justify prejudice: 'We tend to look harder for flaws in research that defies our personal intuition and beliefs' (MacCoun, 1998). As long as you are aware that you may be influenced by your own prejudices and beliefs when conducting a critical appraisal, you will be on your guard against allowing this to influence your judgement.

Using the checklist approach for critical appraisal

CASP (the Critical Appraisal Skills Programme) has a number of checklists, referred to earlier, that are available for download at: http://www.phru.nhs.uk/Pages/PHD/resources.htm. These checklists typically consist of up to 12 questions, the first of which are known as 'screening questions'. These help you to decide quickly whether or not a paper is worthy of a full appraisal – if the answer is 'no' to any or all of them, the paper can be discarded, at least for the time being. Tick boxes for 'yes', 'no' and 'can't tell' are provided for all of the screening questions, and for most of the others. For our purposes, a 'can't tell' is as bad as a 'no'.

Using the 'randomized controlled trial' checklist as an example, the questions are as follows (the first three are the 'screening questions'):

1. *Did the trial address a clearly focused issue?*
   Although this might seem to be a fundamental point, it is not uncommon for the authors of a paper to fail to describe clearly the patient population(s) included in the study, what intervention(s) they received, and whether all of the stated outcomes have been addressed. If any or all of these are not readily identifiable in the introduction to the paper (or in the abstract), there is little chance that the results will be in any way useful or able to be generalized. Why, if this does prove to be the case, should this be so?

2. *Was the assignment of patients to treatment randomized?*
   If not, why not? And if randomization was carried out, was it done appropriately (i.e. by using an electronic random number generation system, rather than, for example, sealed envelopes, which may be vulnerable to interference or tampering).

3. *Were all of the patients who entered the trial properly accounted for at its conclusion?*
   Were all of them assessed at the appropriate follow-up intervals, as well as at the trial's conclusion? Was all analysis of patient data carried out within the same groups to which they had been randomized?

   All subsequent questions, are described as the 'detailed' questions. The first of these asks:

4. *Were the patients, health workers and study personnel 'blind' to what treatment each group received?*
   The more 'blinding' that is possible within a study, the less likely it will be that observer bias might be a possibility.

5. *Were the groups similar at the start of the trial?*
   The two groups should be as close as possible with regard to age, gender and social class. Other factors that may be taken into consideration include education, annual income and any other aspect of lifestyle that could be relevant in the context of the study in question.

6. *Were the groups treated equally, apart from the experimental intervention?*
   Any degree of unequal treatment (e.g. one group receiving more attention during follow-up) might have an effect on results.

7. *How large was the treatment effect?*
   Was it both statistically and clinically significant?

8. *How precise was the estimate of the treatment effect?*
   Remember that wide confidence intervals do not inspire confidence in the results.

9. *Can the results be applied to the local population?*
   If the study population is too dissimilar to your own situation, it is unlikely that the results can be extrapolated.

10. *Were all clinically important outcomes considered?*
    If some were not (why not?), does this affect the usefulness of the study?

11. *Are the benefits worth the harms and costs?*
    This question is unlikely to have been addressed by the authors and it may be that you have to make a subjective judgement based on your own experience and local situation. All drug treatments have side effects, which in some cases may be worse than the condition that

they are designed to alleviate. Cost effectiveness also has to be considered, in the context of a cash-strapped health service.

Worked example: Quantitative research

 Action Point

Using the example of the 'randomized controlled trial' checklist from CASP, work through what to look for in the following trial:

Hickson, M., D'Souza, A.L., Muthu, N., *et al.* (2007). Use of probiotic *Lactobacillus* preparation to prevent diarrhoea associated with antibiotics: randomised double blind placebo controlled trial. *British Medical Journal,* **335**, 80–4

(This paper is freely downloadable from the BMJ web site at: http://www.bmj.com/cgi/reprint/335/7610/80).

If you wish, and if you have access to the paper copy of the journal, you may find it more convenient to work from a photocopy. If not, download a pdf (portable document format) version of the paper from the web site and print off a copy, along with a copy of the checklist for randomized controlled trials at: http://www.phru.nhs.uk/Doc_Links/rct%20appraisal%20tool.pdf.

One advantage of having an electronic copy of the paper on the computer screen whilst the appraisal is being carried out is that the 'find' and 'find next' functions of the pdf format can be used to quickly identify and highlight key words, rather than having to repeatedly scan through a print copy.

This paper addresses an increasingly common and worrying problem for the NHS, that of diarrhoea (particularly that associated with *Clostridium difficile*) in hospitalized patients, caused by treatment with antibiotics. Remember that the first three questions are the 'screening questions' and that if the paper fails any of these, there will be no point in subjecting it to the full appraisal.

Did the trial address a clearly focused issue?

The abstract of the paper states that the main objective of the trial is 'To determine the efficacy of a probiotic drink containing *Lactobacillus* for the prevention of any diarrhoea associated with antibiotic use and that caused by *Clostridium difficile*'. This is clear, simple and unequivocal, so we can safely answer 'yes' to the first question.

Was the assignment of patients to treatments randomized?

Both the title of the paper and the description of the trial's design in the paper's abstract state that randomization was used. This is clear enough, but was the randomization carried out in a proper manner? Entering 'Randomization' into the pdf 'Find' box leads us to the appropriate section of the paper, which states that 'An independent statistician generated the random allocation sequence'. Although the actual name of the software used is not given, we may reasonably assume from this statement that randomization was carried out appropriately and that an added safeguard against bias was used, in the form of a statistician who was not part of the study team. So we can also answer the second question with a 'yes'.

Were all the patients who entered the trial properly accounted for at its conclusion?

The authors of this paper have provided a flow chart detailing the numbers of patients initially assessed, those actually enrolled, the allocation to probiotic or placebo groups, those lost to follow-up (with reasons why this happened) and the final numbers available for data analysis. The answer to the third and final screening question is, therefore, also 'yes' and we can proceed to the 'detailed' questions. It might be worth noting at this stage, however, the large number of patients ($n = 1625$) excluded from enrolment in the trial, most of whom were deemed not to have met the inclusion criteria. Perhaps these criteria were excessively stringent? If so, for what reason?

Were patients, health workers and study personnel 'blind' to treatment?

The patients in the study were randomized to receive either *Actimel* (probiotic drink) or *Yazoo* (longlife sterile milkshake). *Actimel* is sold in 100 g white plastic bottles and *Yazoo* in 200 ml white plastic bottles. The authors maintain that patients and researchers were blind to which drink was used as they did not see the bottle in which the drink was originally packaged (nurses dispensed the drinks in 100 ml cups and were not told which bottles contained which drink. The bottles had their commercial labels removed and replaced by generic labels). Do you think that blinding was adequate, or less than adequate?

Were the groups similar at the start of the trial?

Table 1 of the paper describes the baseline characteristics of the study participants. Remember that the more similar the two groups are in as many respects as possible, the more likely the results will be able to be generalized. In most respects, the two groups are very similar (a sign of effective randomization), but in one aspect, the number of smokers, there is a substantial difference in numbers. Given that smoking has been shown in some studies to provide some protection against the effects of inflammatory bowel disease, do you think that this could be significant in the context of this study?

Aside from the experimental intervention, were the groups treated equally?

In the 'Study plan' section, the authors state that both groups of patients were followed up four weeks after finishing the course of antibiotics. Both groups were also telephoned at weekly intervals to ask about any episodes of diarrhoea and whether they were continuing to take any prescribed antibiotics they had been given on discharge from hospital. Can any other areas be identified in which the two groups were or were not treated equally?

How large was the treatment effect?

Table 2 of the paper can be studied alongside the results section in order to assess the size of the treatment effect. It appears that the treatment effect was quite substantial – only seven of the 56 patients taking the probiotic experienced diarrhoea, compared to 19 of the 53 control patients. A 'P value' of 0.007 is given for this result. The P value (which is expressed as a value from 0 to 1) indicates the probability that results could have occurred by chance. The value generally held to be acceptable is 0.05, or a chance of 1 in 20. As the P value given here is much smaller than 0.05, this means that we can be reasonably confident that these results did *not* occur purely by chance. (See Chapter 7 for further information on statistical significance of results.)

How precise was the estimate of the treatment effect?

In the results section, we read that the absolute risk reduction for occurrence of antibiotic associated diarrhoea was 22% (95% confidence interval 7–37%). As noted earlier, this means that 95% of the results fell between these two values and that the 'true' result could be anywhere along this spectrum. Do you think that this is an acceptable range in the context of this study?

Can the results be applied to the local population?

A number of points could arise out of this question:

- Hospitals vary widely in their reported incidence of both antibiotic related and *C diff* associated diarrhoea. Would hospitals with rates that were not similar to the three London hospitals from which patients were recruited for the study show similar results from treatment with probiotics?
- Of 1760 patients screened for the study, 135 actually took part. Of these, 113 were followed up for evidence of diarrhoea. Was this (less than 7% of the potential target group) still a truly representative population sample?
- Risk of antibiotic associated diarrhoea increases with the duration of hospital stay. The study population had median hospital stays of just over a week. Were they, therefore, an atypical group?
- Treatment with more than one antibiotic is very common in the older adult hospital population and increases the risk of associated diarrhoea. The majority of the study subjects received a single antibiotic. Does this make them unrepresentative?
- Was the exclusion of patients with 'bowel pathology that could result in diarrhoea' important?

Were all clinically important outcomes considered?

An easy question to answer this time, as there were only two outcomes under consideration: The occurrence of antibiotic associated diarrhoea (primary outcome) and how much of this was caused by *C diff*. Both were accounted for in the results and conclusion.

Are the benefits worth the harms and costs?

Any intervention, however apparently benign, may have side effects in some people. A case study in two paediatric patients (Land *et al.*, 2005) found that probiotic treatment could, in rare cases, have the potential for causing bacteraemia and sepsis in susceptible individuals. Might older people with weakened immune systems also be at risk? The authors of this paper estimate the costs of probiotic treatment to be £50 to prevent one case of antibiotic associated diarrhoea and £60 for *C diff* diarrhoea. Compared to an estimated £4000 in additional costs associated with the latter in UK hospitals, this suggests that impressive financial savings might be possible.

Additional points for discussion

- Was a suitable placebo treatment selected? The placebo group received 'a longlife sterile milkshake'. Was this product likely to have been part of a typical diet for a hospital in-patient? Might a milk-based product in itself be capable of causing diarrhoea in some patients?
- Where did the funding for the study come from? Had any of the authors any kind of affiliation with the funding bodies? Could this have resulted in any bias?

Worked example: Qualitative research

 Action Point

The second article that we shall consider as a practical example for critical appraisal is a qualitative study:

Phillips, R., Amos, A., Ritchie, D., *et al.* (2007). Smoking in the home after the smoke-free legislation in Scotland: Qualitative study. *British Medical Journal,* **335**, 553–7.

This is available at http://www.bmj.com/cgi/reprint/335/7619/553.

In some ways, a qualitative study is simpler to interpret (and therefore appraise) than a randomized trial, as more of the content may be easily understandable or intuitive. On the other hand, it may lend itself less readily to the checklist approach, as it may not be as obvious where to look for the answers to all of the questions. Also, the language of psychological or sociological research (often used in qualitative studies) can in itself be just as difficult to understand as medical or scientific terminology. Nonetheless, a checklist for appraising qualitative research is available at http://www.phru.nhs.uk/Doc_Links/Qualitative%20Appraisal%20Tool.pdf. Just as we found with the randomized controlled trial checklist, this one begins by asking two 'screening questions'.

Was there a clear statement of the aims of the research?

As with the randomized controlled trial example, the abstract of the paper clearly states the aims of the research. The primary aim is to establish the impact of the recent smoke-free legislation on smoking in the home or car. The secondary aim is to consider the implications on any future initiatives aimed at reducing children's exposure to passive smoking.

Why is it important? This is explained by the description of the secondary aim of the study – to inform future decision making or legislation for the protection of children's health by reducing their exposure to second-hand smoke. Its relevance? To help further the cause of providing smoke-free homes for children. The study passes the first screening question.

Is a qualitative methodology appropriate?

Smoking generally, but especially its effect on children exposed to passive smoking in the home or family car, is an emotive issue that provokes strong opinions on both sides. Issues separate from those directly to do with child health, which may be concerned with individual personal liberty, the perception of a 'Nanny State', frequently reinforce these opinions or beliefs concerning what constitutes responsible parenthood. A qualitative approach is the only research method that can adequately address such a range of opinion and subjective belief. The study, therefore, passes the second screening question and we can proceed to a full appraisal.

Was the research design appropriate to address the aims of the research?

Has the researcher justified the research design (e.g. have they discussed how they decided which method to use)? The study design was based around qualitative semi-structured interviews in the respondents' homes. Did the interviewers describe fully the method used? Did they, for example, use the same method as the Health Education Population Survey (HEPS) that the respondents' would have been familiar with already (Computer Aided Personal Interviewing [CAPI])? If not, why did they choose the method actually used?

Was the recruitment strategy appropriate to the aims of the research?

The study participants were recruited from wave 10 of HEPS and thus were already familiar with the interviewing approach used in the study.

> HEPS sought interviews with adults aged between 16 and 74 living in mainland Scotland (i.e. excluding all islands). For the second series of HEPS a sample of 1,540 addresses was drawn for each of waves one to six, and this was slightly increased to a sample of 1,584 for waves seven to 10 in order to maintain an achieved sample of around 900 interviews in each wave. The sample was drawn at random from the Postcode Address File; 22 addresses were selected from each of 70 postcode sectors for the first wave. In subsequent waves 35 postcode sectors that had been sampled for the previous wave were re-sampled, using a different starting point, so that although all the addresses were new for each wave there was a degree of overlap by common areas between adjacent waves. From wave seven onwards, the sample was increased to 72 postcode sectors with 36 overlapping. At each sampled address an interview was sought with the eligible adult whose birthday had fallen most recently before the interviewer's visit. (Health Education Population Survey (http://www.healthscotland.com/scotlands-health/population/HEPS.aspx))

The researchers sampled on three characteristics: composition of smokers in the household, socio-economic group and gender. They invited 106 people to take part, of which 54 were designated 'eligible' and 50 were actually interviewed. Did the researchers provide an adequate explanation of how they decided upon eligibility and why less than half of those invited to take part were actually interviewed?

Were the data collected in a way that addressed the research issue?

The researchers here have given quite a lot of detail that matches methods mentioned in this section of the checklist. A semi-structured interview format was used, as well as a topic guide tailored to each of the three different categories of participant: smoker living alone or with another smoker, smoker living with a non-smoker and non-smoker living with a smoker. The topic guide helps the interviewer to keep the interview on track and relevant to the research aim; otherwise, human nature would result in much digression and the value of the data would be diminished. The interviews were also tape recorded and analysed later by at least two researchers for each interview. Recording interviews provides an extra safeguard against possible misrepresentation on the part of the interviewers.

The term 'data saturation' mentioned in the checklist refers to a situation in which the interviewers are repeatedly encountering the same responses from successive interviewees. Did this occur in this study and, if it did, would it have constituted a problem?

Has the relationship between researcher and participants been adequately considered?

This question focuses on whether the researcher thinks their role has introduced bias or influenced the responses of the interviewees. It also asks if the researcher has been flexible enough to respond to changing emphasis or emerging themes (including unexpected ones) that might arise during the course of the study. Under 'Analysis', the statement is made that 'a modified grounded theory approach was taken whereby themes were revised iteratively as the fieldwork and analysis progressed'.

This means that a recognized sociological method (grounded theory, Chapter 8) was used in order to allow a theme to gradually emerge during the course of data analysis; that is, the researcher has no preconceived ideas about what might develop but allows a pattern to appear gradually. 'Iteratively' in this context means constantly going over previously visited data as a pattern emerges, to see how subsequent data may have suggested modification.

Apart from the fact that the interviews were conducted in the respondents' homes, where they were more likely to feel at ease, and that they were recruited from a sample of the population that had already taken part in the HEPS survey and would therefore be used to being interviewed, have the researchers given sufficient information about their role? Could they have influenced the data in any way?

Have ethical issues been taken into consideration?

Research studies generally have to be approved by local ethics committees before they can go ahead (Chapter 6). This is to protect the study population from any adverse effects that might arise from the research and also to protect the researchers from possible litigation if any harm was to be caused, or confidentiality compromised. One of the emerging themes suggested by this study is that smokers sometimes found themselves in a 'double bind' situation. This was because their sense of moral obligation not to damage the health of their children or grandchildren may have been in conflict with their self-image as hospitable (i.e. sharing cigarettes with smoking guests or allowing them to smoke indoors), non-judgmental and non-hypocritical individuals. Was any impact on the interviewees considered? Should it have been? Did the researchers divulge any information about whether or not they themselves were smokers?

Was the data analysis sufficiently rigorous?

The checklist asks us to consider if the process of data analysis has been described in depth. Is it made clear how categories/themes were derived from the data? Is a description given of how the data presented was selected from the total collected in the course of the interviews? If not, what do you think the reason for this might be?

Is there a clear statement of findings?

Some of the prompts given by the checklist for this question may not be applicable for this particular study. As the study was open-ended, with the researchers not starting out with a pre-conceived idea of what they thought the findings might be, the prompt 'If there is adequate discussion of the evidence both for and against the researcher's arguments' obviously does not apply. Again, as the findings consist mainly of the reported views of the interviewees on smoking in the home or car, the 'credibility' of the findings cannot very well be questioned. Although, as we agreed in the first screening question, the aim of the research was clear, there was no formal question to be answered, or hypothesis to be supported or denied. In the light of this, do you think that the findings of the study were well presented and clear?

How valuable is the research?

Research is often criticized on the grounds that it either tells us what we already 'know' or that it produces results for which no practical application can be found. What has this particular piece of research discovered? The smoke-free legislation passed in Scotland in 2006 was mainly aimed at protecting adults who work and/or socialize in environments, such as pubs and clubs, that were previously often heavily contaminated by second-hand tobacco smoke. It was already known that such second-hand smoke was harmful to children and that their main source of exposure to it was in their own homes and their family's cars. The logical next step of any future legislation would be to try to ensure that children's exposure to smoke was minimized in these environments. Short of introducing a total ban on smoking by the withdrawal of tobacco from legal sale, the only options would appear to be to step up media campaigns to increase awareness of the dangers of passive smoking and/or to offer 'tailored advice' to individuals to help them to develop strategies to avoid exposing children to second-hand smoke. Do you think that this study has found any 'new' information that was previously unknown? Do you think that such studies are useful in providing 'ammunition' for supporting future legislation? Do the findings of this study suggest any avenues for further research?

Conclusion

The process of critical appraisal need not be as daunting as it might first appear. Nobody is expecting you to acquire an in-depth knowledge of research design and statistical method before you attempt your first appraisal; '90% is pure common sense and 10% is jargon' (NHS Education for Scotland). http://www.nes.scot.nhs.uk/medicine/gpst/sho/information/critical_appraisal/default.asp).

A relatively recent development in online journal production can help you a great deal. A few journals, such as the BMJ and the Canadian Medical Association Journal (CMAJ), accept 'rapid responses' to papers published online. There is no limit on these responses, unlike those for print journals, which may vary between four and eight weeks following publication (Altman, 2002). Refer to these rapid responses alongside the original article when doing your appraisal – they can often suggest areas for discussion that you may otherwise have missed (and the contributors are frequently expert at spotting discrepancies in trial design and statistics). Finally, do try to do at least the first few appraisals that you attempt in company – the process becomes much easier when up to four or five people (especially if they have a variety of subject expertise and experience between them) are contributing ideas and suggestions.

 Action Point

Select a paper relevant to your area of practice using one of the methods listed in Box 5.1 – ideally choose a method different from the two examples you have already completed by working through this chapter. Use either a CASP checklist or other resource from the Resources list at the end of this chapter and conduct a critical appraisal of the paper.

References

Altman, D.G. (2002) Poor-quality medical research: What can journals do? *Journal of the American Medical Association*, **287**, 2765–2767.

Altman, D.G. (1994) The scandal of poor medical research. *British Medical Journal*, **308**, 283–284.

Hill, A. and Spittlehouse, C. (2001) *What is Critical Appraisal?* Hayward Medical Communications, London. http://www.evidence-based-medicine.co.uk/ebmfiles/WhatisCriticalAppraisal.pdf.

Jones, R., Scouller, J., Grainer, F. *et al.* (1994) The scandal of poor medical research: Sloppy use of literature often to blame. *British Medical Journal*, **308**, 591.

Land, M.H., Rouster-Stevens, K., Woods, C.R. *et al.* (2005) Lactobacillus sepsis associated with probiotic therapy. *Pediatrics*, **115**, 178–181.

MacCoun, R.J. (1998) Biases in the interpretation and use of research results. *Annual Review of Psychology*, **49**, 259–287.

NHS Education for Scotland. http://www.nes.scot.nhs.uk/medicine/gpst/sho/information/critical_appraisal/default.asp.

Resources for critical appraisal

Birmingham Critical Appraisal Skills Programme: provides training and appraisal resources. http://www.casp-birmingham.org/

CASP (Critical Appraisal Skills Programme) provides a series of checklists to help you ask the right questions in the right order when appraising a paper. http://www.phru.nhs.uk/pages/PHD/CASP.htm

CEBM (Centre for Evidence-Based Medicine) has, amongst many other resources, a searchable database of CATS (Critically Appraised Topics) and a free software program (CATMaker) to assist in calculating confidence intervals, NNT (numbers needed to treat) and other statistical components of critical appraisal. www.cebm.net/

ScHARR (Sheffield School of Health and Related Studies) offers a range of helpful resources and articles, including worked examples of critical appraisal. http://www.shef.ac.uk/scharr/ir/units/critapp/

Williams, K. (2009) *Getting Critical*, Palgrave Macmillan, Basingstoke.

Young, J. and Solomon, M. (2009) How to critically appraise an article. *Nature Clinical Practice*, **6** (2), 82–91.

6 Conducting Ethical Research in Healthcare

Helena Priest and Paula Roberts

Introduction

In this chapter, we explore the nature of ethics as applied to healthcare research, and discuss the reasons why any research that is conducted involving humans within a health or social care context must be conducted in an ethical manner. Structures and procedures that are current in the United Kingdom for ensuring that such research is indeed ethical are explained, including Codes of Ethical conduct, the Research Governance Framework, the peer review system, the National Research Ethics Service and the NHS Research and Development approvals required to conduct research in specific local NHS settings. Consideration is given to research that falls outside the UK National Health Service guidelines, such as that conducted in private organizations, charities or voluntary agencies. The chapter will also help you to read published research critically to judge how researchers have ensured that their research is ethical, and how to consider conflicts of interest or other ethical breaches.

Ethics

What do we mean when we talk about ethics? The word translated literally means 'moral philosophy', but that does not help us greatly. Dictionaries and thesauri suggest that ethics is to do with the principles, morals, beliefs or values of a person or group of people. It seems to be something to do with right and wrong in relation to human behaviour, and something that is normally shared amongst a group of people in the form of a custom or habit. For example, most people in the United Kingdom would consider it ethically wrong to cause deliberate distress or pain to another human being or to steal their possessions. However, a minority of people do cause harm to others, or steal possessions, thereby breaching not only generally accepted ethical principles but also breaking the law. In such cases, there is overlap between ethics and law; so, for example, not it is only ethically wrong to cause harm to other people but is also, in most cases, legally wrong and punishable by law. However, there are many ethical issues that are not so clear cut, such as deciding the age at which a child can understand information and consent to a medical procedure, or agree to participate in research.

Ethics in relation to healthcare research

Using these descriptions of ethics in relation to human behaviour, we can suppose that ethics in relation to research might have something to do with conducting research in a way that most people would consider appropriate and right, and in a way that does others no harm. There are a number of important documents available to guide people in conducting ethical research, and help ensure that these broad principles are upheld. These include:

- World Medical Association Declaration of Helsinki (2008), which is a statement of ethical principles to guide people involved in medical research involving human subjects;
- Data Protection Act (1998), which gives rights to individuals in relation to personal information that is held about them;
- Professional guidelines and codes, such as those produced by the UK Royal College of Nursing and the British Psychological Society;
- Department of Health Research Governance Framework (DH, 2005).

We will look at some of this guidance in detail later in the chapter.

Why must research be ethical?

People working within health and social care settings must ensure that their patients and clients receive safe and competent care, including when they are participating in health or social care research. Ethics lies at the heart of all research activity, particularly that involving humans and even more so research that includes people who may be considered vulnerable in some way, such as being an NHS patient, or a child, or a person with an intellectual disability or serious mental health problem. In most professional disciplines, conducting ethical research is a professional requirement not only for the practitioners of that discipline, but also in order to access research participants such as NHS patients. Furthermore, it is a requirement when applying to external agencies to obtain funding to conduct research.

When research is not ethical

A number of high profile cases in recent years have demonstrated to the public the importance of conducting research in accordance with the strictest of ethical principles.

 Action Point

Use the internet to find out about some research undertaken in North Staffordshire in the 1980s and 1990s in relation to covert videotaped surveillance of children admitted to hospital with their parents.

Hint: The research in question related to Munchausen's Syndrome by Proxy.

Reflection Point

Was this research justified? What, if any, do you think are the ethical issues inherent in this research?

This research has been hotly debated over many years. Some people argue that convert surveillance had positive outcomes, in that children may have been spared further harm. However, the actions of the researchers were criticized by some commentators as being unethical, because prior consent of the parents was not obtained. We will consider these ethical issues in greater detail later in this chapter.

 Action Point

Use the internet to find out about an enquiry in 2001 into the actions of a pathologist at Alder Hey Children's Hospital in the United Kingdom.

Hint: This concerned research into sudden infant death syndrome and other childhood illnesses.

 Reflection Point

What are the main ethical issues in retaining organs as in this case?

We could argue that it is only by carrying our research that important medical advancements can be made. Sudden infant death syndrome is unfortunately a common and extremely devastating occurrence, and any information gleaned that could help to prevent or reduce it would be very welcome. However, in the Alder Hay situation, most of the parents involved were unaware that their children's organs had been retained until much later, and were distressed to learn that in many cases they had buried or had cremated their children minus some of their organs or body parts.

Key ethical principles in relation to research

In both these case examples, some key ethical principles, such as provision of information and gaining consent, were ignored. Listed below are key ethical principles that, if observed, will help to ensure that research does not do any harm to participants or, indeed, researchers; that, where possible, it does some good; and that it ensures the rights, safety, privacy and dignity of those participating are protected:

- non-maleficence;
- beneficence;
- deception/debriefing;
- competence;
- confidentiality/anonymity;
- consent/capacity to consent;
- right to withdraw.

Non-maleficence

Non-maleficence means that research should do no harm to those participating in it. Hence, issues of risk and safety, not only to research participants but also to those conducting the research, must be considered before the research commences. However, it has been argued that all research may be potentially harmful to participants or researchers (Long and Johnson, 2007), and even the most rigorous research conducted to the highest ethical standards could sometimes be said to cause harm. For example, if a researcher is interviewing parents about their experiences of losing a child to Sudden Infant Death Syndrome, in the hope of providing better support services to such parents, it is likely that these parents will be upset and distressed at having to talk about a very difficult time in their lives. The good researcher will anticipate this and have in place a strategy to deal with it if it occurs, such as pausing or stopping the interview, and providing telephone numbers of appropriate support services for the parents to use. Any risk of harm or discomfort to participants must always be kept to a minimum and be balanced against the potential benefits of the research. Research participants should always be made aware if any proposed research activities are likely to cause distress, before they agree to participate in it. Following the activity, they should be offered a full debriefing (see below) and further explanation of the research aims and purpose.

Beneficence

This means that the research should aim to do good, if not directly to the participants themselves, then at least to others who may benefit from the research findings in the future. For example, a researcher may want to interview people who have accessed an NHS audiology service about their experiences of accessing that service; asking how they felt they were treated, whether they were able to communicate their wishes to the healthcare practitioner, and whether their needs were understood. The researcher may also wish to gather factual information, such as how long a patient had waited for an audiology clinic appointment. Clearly, these events and experiences have already taken place, so any changes made to service provision as a result of the research will not benefit these participants directly. Yet most people are happy to contribute their experiences and knowledge in the hope that people having the same problems or needs in the future will have a better experience and improved quality of care.

Deception/debriefing

Unless it is absolutely necessary, research should not be conducted if it involves deceiving the research participant in any way. There are exceptions to this ethical principle, such as testing a new drug, product or intervention against a 'placebo' or dummy product (Chapter 5). For the research to be effective, it would be important that neither the participants, nor the people administering the drugs, should know which patients were actually getting the real drug and which the placebo, for fear of hopes and expectations influencing their responses. Despite this, any patient agreeing to participate in a drug trial must be given as much information as possible about the research, and give consent to their participation in the knowledge that they may receive a product that will not help them. Indeed, they should be made aware that they may actually feel worse because of possible side effects if they receive the 'real' drug. Once the trial is over, it is important to inform the patients which of the two products they had received, and to provide full details of the findings of the study once available. This information and explanation after the event is known as debriefing, and is good practice in research even where deception has not been employed.

There are other situations where, although there is no attempt to deceive people, they may unwittingly be involved in research activities without being aware of it. For example, a researcher is conducting research into hand-washing practices of nurses in a hospital ward. The researcher is a non-participant observer; that is, he or she is not involved in the ward practices, but is simply observing and recording what is seen. Clearly, the nurses who are being observed will have given their full consent to participate in this research, and it is they who are being observed, not the patients that they are caring for. Nonetheless, it is unlikely that the researcher would be able to carry out a rigorous observation without observing some of the patients with whom the nurses are interacting as they go about their daily work. In a busy hospital ward with rapid patient turnover, it would be unrealistic to seek consent from every possible person that might enter the nurses' space, so it could be argued that these patients are being deceived and will not have access to debriefing. In such situations, creative ways of keeping people informed have to be found, such as displaying posters in the ward advising that research is being carried out, and making provision for people to 'opt out' if required.

Competence

It is important for a potential research participant to know that the people responsible for designing and conducting the research, collecting data and analysing it, possess the necessary skills and knowledge to do so. Clearly, some research is conducted as part of educational programmes, and is often intended to be 'research training'. The UK PhD system, for example, requires doctoral students to design and conduct empirical research that makes an original contribution to the knowledge base of their particular profession, but which at the same time equips them with the knowledge and skills to become independent researchers in the future. In such research, it is important that the student is well supervised and advised by someone with the necessary expertise and competence, and that potential research participants are made aware of the nature of the research and its purpose, the supervision arrangements, and who they can contact if they have a concern or query. It is also a requirement that research students undertake a programme of approved research training in the educational institution in which they are registered to do their PhDs. The same applies to people who are employed as contract researchers on a particular project, and to 'career young' researchers who are beginning to develop their research expertise. Students conducting NHS or social care research are not exempt from research governance and ethical approval procedures.

In all cases, research participants should be able to expect that the research in which they are participating has been subjected to a rigorous approval process that has judged the research to be scientifically and ethically sound, and conducted by competent or well supervised researchers.

Confidentiality and anonymity

The protection of participants' privacy and information is essential when conducting research, particularly personal and sensitive information. Researchers must undertake to keep all information confidential and secure, and to inform participants where and how it will be stored, who will have access to it and how it will be used. One way in which information can be kept confidential is to make it as anonymous as possible; that is, to disguise any information that could lead to a research participant being identifiable from any research output (such as reports and publications). Thus, participants' names can be replaced with code numbers or pseudonyms, with actual names and numbers or pseudonyms stored separately, and only the researcher able to put the two together. Sometimes it is not even necessary to have participants' names at all; for example, if you pick up a questionnaire in a library asking for comments about the services provided, and return it to a collection point in the library, no-one will ever know who you are. However, respecting confidentiality does not just apply to the use of people's names. For example, if research is being conducted with people suffering from a rare medical condition within a specialist unit in a particular part of the country, it would not take too much detective work by someone reading a report of this research to at least guess the identity of some of the likely participants. It is, therefore, important for researchers to make anonymous as far as possible any information that might lead to a breach of participants' privacy. The Data Protection Act (1998) outlines the law on information storage, use and disposal and should be adhered to at all times by researchers.

Storage of data

In the interests of maintaining confidentiality, attention must be paid to the storage of research data, whether this is completed questionnaires or recordings of interviews or scores on a test. All information should be handled and stored in a way that enables it to be accurately reported, interpreted, verified and reconstructed, while protecting participants' confidentiality. Data collected in the course of research must be retained securely for an appropriate period; organizations such as universities and research bodies give guidance on the time scale, but it is unlikely to be less that five years. The Data Protection Act (1998) also provides guidance. Data can be stored in any form as long as it is easily retrievable and in a format that will not go quickly out of date. It is important that electronic data is backed up regularly.

Consent

It is important that people considering participating in a research project have sufficient information about the project and exactly what their participation will entail, to enable them to give informed consent to participate. Normally, information about the proposed project, and about confidentiality and anonymity, is produced in the form of a written Participant Information

Sheet (Chapter 3), so that participants can keep and refer to it as they wish. Participant Information Sheets introduce the researcher, outline the study and its rationale, explain what data will be collected, and how and when; what will be done with the data; and potential benefits and potential harms or risks to taking part. A potential participant must be given adequate time to read and digest the information, and to seek independent advice, before making a decision whether to participate. Participant information sheet templates (together with sample consent forms) are available through the NHS Research Ethics Service (NRES, 2009) which should be closely followed where possible.

Research participants should be informed of all pertinent aspects of the research in a language understandable to them or their representative. Sometimes, adaptations to the information and consent procedures need to be made, such as when a potential participant cannot read. In this case, the participant information might be produced in video or DVD format so that the participant can keep and replay it as required. Alternatively, those with intellectual difficulties might have written information supplemented by pictures or symbols (see Chapter 14 for more information).

They will then be asked to read and sign a consent form, indicating that they have had the research explained to them and the opportunity to ask questions. They may also consent to additional activities, such as giving access to their medical records, or permission to inform their General Practitioner of their participation, or to the publication of data arising from their participation (made suitably anonymous) in an academic journal.

   Action Point

Find the online document entitled 'Information sheets and Consent Forms: Guidance for Researchers and Reviewers' by accessing NRES (www.nres.npsa.nhs.uk) and selecting 'Guidance'.

Draft a consent form for a project you are working on or interested in, using the template provided in this document.

A completed consent form based on the NRES template might look like the one in Box 6.1.

Process consent

Giving consent should not be a 'one-off' activity; rather, it should be considered as an ongoing process throughout the research project, and checks must be made with participants to ensure that they continue to consent to the activities initially proposed. This is known as process consent. For example, issues of confidentiality and anonymity must be explained and reiterated at the start of focus group or individual interviews, and at every subsequent stage of data collection. A participant may initially have consented to be interviewed, to have the interview content recorded and transcribed onto a computer, and for quotations from the interview to be used by the researcher in the written research report. However, after completing the interview, the participant decides that she is no longer happy to have her words quoted in a report. It would be important, therefore, that the researcher checks that all elements of consent remain in force and, if they do not, to respect the participants' rights to withdraw some of all of their initial consent without penalty.

Box 6.1   Consent Form

Title of Project: An exploration of the experiences of people with multiple sclerosis undergoing out-patient physiotherapy.
Name of Researcher: Dr Helena Priest
Please initial box
I confirm that I have read and understand the information sheet dated June 9th 2009, version
1, for the above study. I have had the opportunity to consider the information, ask questions
and have had these answered satisfactorily.   ☐

I understand that my participation is voluntary and that I am free to withdraw at any time
without giving any reason, without my medical care or legal rights being affected.   ☐

I understand that relevant sections of my medical notes and data collected during the study,
may be looked at by individuals from XX University, where it is relevant to my taking part
in this research. I give permission for these individuals to have access to my records.   ☐

I agree to my GP and physiotherapist being informed of my participation in the study.   ☐

I agree to take part in the above study.   ☐

Name of Patient   Date   Signature

Name of Person taking consent   Date   Signature

As far as possible, it is best to use an 'opt-in' rather than an 'opt-out' approach to the consent
process. So, for example, an invitation letter might be sent to potential research participants,
briefly outlining the proposed study and asking them to indicate (perhaps by returning a tear-off
slip in a self-addressed envelope) their interest and give permission for the researcher to contact
them.

There are, as mentioned in relation to deception, research situations where informed consent
from every participant is not possible. In situations like this, where it would not be possible or
practical to seek informed consent from everyone who may inadvertently enter the 'research
site', the researcher should ensure that any such observation takes place only where people
'would reasonably expect to be observed by strangers' (British Psychological Society, 2006).

Capacity to consent

There are particular issues to be considered when designing research to be undertaken by
children or vulnerable adults (e.g. people with intellectual disabilities or serious mental health
problems), as it is crucial to ascertain that they understand and consent to what is being asked
of them. In line with the law, the researcher has to be as sure as possible that the participant
is able to understand information about the nature, purpose and consequences of the research;
that they can retain that information and weigh it in balance to arrive at a decision; and can
communicate that decision.

The Mental Capacity Act (2005) considers these issues, and provides safeguards for people
who lack capacity to consent to research. For example, if a person cannot consent, researchers
must respect the person's previous wishes if these are known, and consult someone who can
give a view on the person's interests, wishes and feelings.

While it might be tempting to avoid conducting research where there are particular challenges to gaining consent, it is vitally important to include vulnerable or marginalized populations in research in order that their unique concerns, experiences and insights can be sought and gained. The case studies presented in Part 2 of this book provide specific examples.

Right to withdraw

Having consented to participate in a research project, all individuals must be offered the opportunity to withdraw from the project at any stage, without any adverse effects upon them or their care and treatment. This respects participants' autonomy and right to express personal choice. In most cases, they can also request that any data already collected from them should not be used in the research study.

Ensuring healthcare research is ethical

Having explored the ethical principles that should underpin all healthcare research, how can we be sure that they are put into practice when designing and conducting research? Indeed, how can we be sure that the research that we read about in published reports and journal articles has been conducted ethically? There are a number of guidelines and procedures available in the United Kingdom to help researchers in this respect. These include codes of ethical conduct relevant to specific professional groups; research governance, sponsorship and indemnity arrangements; review of scientific merit ('peer review') of the research proposal; and the work of National Research Ethics Services. We will explore these in more detail.

Ethical codes and guidelines

Most professional organizations have codes of ethical practice. For example, the UK Nursing and Midwifery Council (NMC) has its Code of Professional Conduct: Standards for Conduct, Performance and Ethics (Nursing and Midwifery Council, 2007); the British Association for Counselling and Psychotherapy has an Ethical Framework for Good Practice in Counselling and Psychotherapy (British Association for Counselling and Psychotherapy, 2009); the British Psychological Society has a Code of Ethics and Conduct (British Psychological Society, 2006). Equally, most professions whose members conduct healthcare research are expected to abide by a specific code of research ethics. For example:

- *Counselling*: British Association for Counselling and Psychotherapy, Ethical Guidelines for Researching Counselling and Psychotherapy, 2004;
- *Medicine*: Medical Research Council Good Research Practice, 2005; EU Clinical Trials Directive 2001/20/EC (2001);
- *Nursing*: Royal College of Nursing Research Society: Research Ethics, 2007;
- *Psychology*: British Psychological Society Good Practice Guidelines for the Conduct of Psychological Research within the NHS (2005).

If the relevant professional code is consulted at the outset, this will go a long way towards ensuring that all the key principles are considered when the research proposal is being prepared. Having consulted the relevant code, the health or social care researcher will need to turn to guidance from the relevant government Department. For example, in England, the Department of Health provides a Research Governance Framework (DH, 2005) to guide all researchers in health and social care, and those who may be in any way affected by such research.

Research governance

Partly driven by instances where research of dubious ethical standards had been conducted in the United Kingdom health service, in 2001 the English Department of Health produced a Research Government Framework for healthcare research (updated in 2005 to include social care settings; DH, 2005). Similar frameworks have been produced to guide research undertaken in other part of the United Kingdom, and are in operation in other countries. The English framework aims to provide a common standard to ensure respect for those who take part in research, and to ensure that no unreasonable or unsafe demands are made by researchers. It sets out a number of principles, requirements and standards, and explains how these should be delivered and monitored, in order to improve research and safeguard the public. Above all, it aims to ensure that the dignity, rights, safety and well-being of participants are the primary consideration in any research study.

The Research Governance Framework applies to research involving any of the following:

- research undertaken **in** or **by** the Department of Health, its non Departmental Public Bodies and the NHS;
- NHS or Social Care patients/ service users (including those in primary care, secondary care, tertiary care or social care);
- relatives of the above;
- NHS or social care professionals or volunteers;
- human organs or tissue;
- data from patients/relatives or care professionals, such as medical records or test results.

Is it research?

It is important to note that some forms of information generation that might be conducted in health and social care contexts are not, in fact, research. For example, healthcare professionals are likely to want to evaluate the services they provide in order to ensure that they are meeting the needs of their patients and clients. Indeed, such activities would be expected of most health and social care practitioners. In this sense, they may conduct a clinical audit or a service evaluation. Neither of these activities is deemed to carry much, if any, risk to service users, and they do not warrant ethical review in accordance with the Research Governance Framework. They should, however, always be conducted with advice from and under the auspices of relevant bodies, such as an NHS Trust's Clinical Audit Department.

Sometimes, however, it is difficult to judge whether an intended piece of work is in fact research; guidance is provided by the NHS Research Ethics Service (NRES, 2008), which defines clinical audit as an activity 'designed and conducted to produce information to inform delivery of best care'. Clinical audit was formally introduced into the NHS in 1993 and provides a method for systematically reflecting on and reviewing healthcare activity, particularly in relation to pre-set standards. Audits are undertaken to examine existing practices and to measure how care is routinely delivered. Clinical audit can be conducted as a 'one off' activity but is most often completed as part of an 'audit cycle' (Gould, 2008), where information is collected, improvements are made to address identified problems, and the audit is repeated at a later date. In this way, small but regular improvements to practices can be made.

As an example of how audits can be used to improve care practices, in 2001 the English Government introduced the Essence of Care strategy and toolkit (DH, 2003), using benchmarking to identify examples of best practice in care delivery, and using these examples as standards against which to compare actual practice. Thus, it is possible to identify when, and by how much, actual care delivered is falling short of the stated benchmark or standard, and to put action plans in place to ensure that the standard can be met. One of the areas included in Essence of Care is pressure ulcers, with an overall standard stating that 'The condition of the patients' skin will be maintained or improved'. This is then subdivided into separate factors that are individually audited. For example, the benchmark for best practice for Factor 4 is that there will be an 'Individualized documented plan agreed with multidisciplinary team in partnership with patients and/or carers, with evidence of ongoing reassessment'. This can easily be measured with reference to clinical documents and in discussion with patients and carers.

Clinical audits often form part of a service evaluation, which is 'designed and conducted solely to define or judge current care' (NRES, 2008). Service evaluation is similar to audit but is more likely to measure the delivery of a service against agreed standards, rather than simply providing a measure of clinical activity. For example, a service evaluation of a support service for parents of children with physical disabilities might include an audit of waiting times to access the service, plus a questionnaire to GPs to see whether they are aware of the service or how it might be improved, and an interview with parents to explore whether the service is meeting their needs.

In contrast, research is defined as 'the attempt to derive . . . new knowledge . . . which usually involves collecting data that are in addition to those for routine care' (NRES, 2008). In other words, in order to increase existing knowledge or produce new knowledge, activities need to be undertaken that would not normally be expected within the care environment. These activities are aimed at either testing out existing theories or ideas or at producing new theories or ideas.

Having established that the proposed piece of work is in fact research and not audit or service evaluation, the researcher must adhere to the relevant Research Governance Framework (DH, 2005) guidance and desirable standards to be achieved in five key areas:

1. Science;
2. Ethics;
3. Information;
4. Health, safety and employment;
5. Finance and intellectual property.

These standards are applicable to everyone involved as a researcher, research host or research participant. In this chapter, we will address the first three areas, which are particularly important in relation to ethics.

Standard 1: Science

It is a requirement of research governance that research proposals are reviewed for their scientific merit. This is sometimes known as the 'independent peer review' process, because committees of 'peers', that is people from similar professional or academic backgrounds as those likely to be making applications, but not connected with the applicants in any way, are formed specifically to receive and review research proposals. As a general principle, project proposals must be subjected to independent peer review in line with the scale of the study. This will sometimes mean that expert opinions are sought from outside the committee itself to supplement and enhance the review process. In some cases, where the research is commissioned and funded by a large organization or government body, the organization itself will conduct the peer review to decide which projects to fund and support.

Concerned mainly with the scientific elements of the proposed project, peer reviewers will consider a range of questions such as:

- Is the topic or problem worthwhile and, in particular, of value to health or social care?
- Is there adequate background information provided such that the reviewer can judge the rationale for and relevance of the proposed research?
- Are the proposed research design, methods of data collection and analysis appropriate for the topic and questions under study?
- Do the researchers have the required expertise and resources to conduct this study?

It is important for these questions to be answered early on, because research that is deemed unsound in any way, or that duplicates work that has already been done, or is not of sufficient quality to contribute something useful to existing knowledge, is unethical. If the study is a quantitative study, consultation with a statistician at an early stage of proposal development is recommended.

We have looked in detail at preparing a proposal for review, and the likely outcomes, in Chapter 3. Once the project proposal has received a favourable outcome from a peer review committee, application for sponsorship and ethical approval is permitted.

Sponsorship/indemnity arrangements

The role of a research sponsor is to be responsible for the science and conduct of the study. This role might be undertaken by a senior member of University staff, if the research is being conducted by academic researchers or students, or by a senior member of an NHS Trust if the researchers are NHS employees. Sponsorship can be joint, where, for example, a University and a NHS Trust share all the responsibilities; or there can be a co-sponsorship arrangement where the responsibilities are divided between sponsors.

The sponsor should be prepared to guarantee the quality of the research and the competence of the researcher (RCN, 2007), and hence will rely heavily on the judgement of the peer review committee. It is normal also for the sponsor to take responsibility for insuring/indemnifying the researcher against causing harm, whether through negligence or inadvertently.

Standard 2: Ethics

Once a researcher has obtained sponsorship and also satisfied a peer review committee that their research proposal is scientifically sound and that there is good reason for the research to be conducted, the next step is to apply for and gain ethical approval from a Research Ethics Committee (REC). RECs form part of the National Research Ethics Service (NRES) in the United Kingdom, which is in turn part of the NHS National Patient Safety Agency (NPSA). The function of the NRES is to 'maintain a UK-wide system of ethical review that protects the *safety*, *dignity* and *well-being* of research participants, whilst facilitating and promoting ethical research' (NPSA, 2008). In addition, the organization will ensure that the rights of participants are upheld, and that risks to researchers are kept to a minimum.

Research Ethics Committees (RECs) are groups of people who ensure the requirements of the NRES are met across the United Kingdom. They are convened in various locations to provide independent advice to research participants, researchers, funders and employers on the extent to which proposals for research studies comply with ethical standards. RECs comprise expert and lay members who generally carry out this role on a voluntary basis. They also seek to ensure that research is conducted that will benefit all groups in society, regardless of age, gender, ability, economic status, culture or ethnic background.

Detailed information about the application procedure is provided on-line by NRES (2009), and a standard application form is accessed online via an IRAS (Integrated Research Application System; see: www.myresearchproject.org.uk). For special cases, such as applications involving human tissue or issues to do with mental capacity, there are around 30 specialist RECs which are accessed via a central application system. Other applications are dealt with by more local RECs.

IRAS is 'a single system for applying for the permissions and approvals for health and social care/community care research in the UK'. It enables applicants to enter all the information that will be required by RECs and other NHS research bodies to approve the research. Furthermore, it 'uses filters to ensure that the data collected and collated is appropriate to the type of study, and consequently the permissions and approvals required'. Completion of the form and submission of required documentation will ensure that key ethical principles have been addressed, in particular:

- risks, benefits and safety;
- researcher competence/scientific merit;
- participant information;
- informed consent;
- capacity to consent by vulnerable groups;
- recruitment to a research study;
- involvement of the public in the design and conduct of the research;
- confidentiality;
- data storage;
- conflicts of interest.

Most of these key principles have already been discussed in this chapter; here we discuss some additional concerns of RECs and the wider NPSA.

Risks, benefits and safety

RECs will consider whether there are risks to participants, such as potential harm, distress or deception, and, if there are risks, whether the likely benefits of conducting the research outweigh these. The REC will also wish to know how any identified risks are being managed, including potential risks to researchers. In some cases, they will require evidence of risk assessment and some applications, such as those involving research with children, may require evidence of police clearance via the Criminal Records Bureau (CRB).

Researcher competence/scientific merit

Even though scientific merit has already been assessed via the peer review process, the ethics committee will also assure itself that the proposal is scientifically as well as ethically sound. It will consider whether the research is properly designed, that the researcher is competent or well supervised if appropriate, and whether any measures proposed are likely to demonstrate reliability and validity. They will also check whether any statistical analyses proposed are appropriate and justified, and whether the numbers of participants to be recruited are sufficient to demonstrate useful outcomes.

In some cases, they will ask whether the number of participants proposed is in fact too many. For example, if a statistical test indicated that 80 people were required to participate in order for the research to have adequate power and to demonstrate an appropriate effect size (Chapter 8), yet the researcher wishes to recruit 100, it could be argued that, as 20 people will be giving their time to participate when they are not needed, that this is unethical.

Recruitment of participants to a research study

The REC will consider the means of recruiting participants to the study; for example, if the researcher wishes to access a sample of participants to complete a questionnaire, it may be best in terms of anonymity if a neutral third party selects the participants from, say, a hospital caseload. Similarly, if a researcher attends a self-help group to explain the research and ask for volunteers to participate, this could be seen as coercion, and an invitation via a third party or letter may be preferable. RECs endorse the principle of 'opting in' to research, thus giving control over whether to participate to the potential participant.

Conflicts of interest/insider perspectives

RECs will need to check that the people conducting the research are not researching in their own organization or workplace in such a way that they might introduce bias into the design or outcomes of the study. For example, a senior nurse researching hand-washing practices within her own hospital may, albeit unwittingly, be seeing 'better' practices and ignoring bad practice when she is observing in her own ward, but the reverse when she is on another. In such an example, the REC might suggest that a different researcher conducts this part of the project.

This is an example of conflict of interest, which often arise when people are researching within their own organizations and thus taking an 'insider perspective'. However, more serious conflicts of interest can arise, and these must be disclosed at the outset and steps taken to ensure as far as possible objectivity and lack of bias in the research process. Conflicts of interest may be legal, ethical, moral, financial or academic, and these secondary influences might affect judgement and decision making about the primary focus of the research.

Equally, it is important for RECs to trust that the researcher will not plagiarize other researchers' ideas or data without permission or acknowledgement (Chapter 9), or engage in piracy (exploiting ideas with out permission or acknowledgement) or fraud (using deliberate deception such as inventing data or omitting inconvenient data from a project's findings and report (Medical Research Council, 2005)).

Involvement of the public

We have made the point in this chapter that it is vital for research participants to be fully informed about and consent to their participation. However, a further step can be taken, which is strongly advocated by RECs, to demonstrate that research is not simply being carried out 'on' people but, more ethically, 'with' people. Hence, service users and carers relevant to the project should be involved wherever possible in all aspects of the research. At a simple level, this might involve testing out a participant information sheet with representatives of the group that will be reading it in the research proper or, better still, involving them in the design and content of the information sheets. Increasingly, research funding bodies and ethics committees require evidence that relevant members of the public are involved at some level, and the organization INVOLVE (www.invo.org.uk) exists to promote public involvement in NHS, public health and social care research. We discuss user involvement in research further in Part 2 of this book.

Standard 3: Information

Extending the principle of public involvement, this standard refers to the ethical duty of researchers to disseminate: to make information about and findings from their projects accessible to the public. This might mean producing different types of information for different audiences, such as a summary report for a local community group, and an academic paper for publication in a journal. Within such reports, it is also ethically important that all contributors, including service users, are fully acknowledged. We discuss dissemination further in Chapter 10.

After REC approval

You might imagine, having gone through such a rigorous process and having received approval from a REC to proceed with the study, that this element of the research journey is over. However, we still need to obtain permission to carry out the research in the specific places or research sites we are interested in. Where these are NHS sites, then this approval must ultimately be gained from the local NHS Research and Development (R & D) office. Fortunately, most of the information that these offices need has already been collected for the Ethics application, and submitted via IRAS, so it is simply a matter of assembling what they require (such as the proposal, the information sheet, the consent forms, the researcher's CV, evidence of sponsorship, written permission from site managers and, most importantly, the letter giving ethical approval), and submitting it to the local office. Finally, once R & D approval has been received, you are ready to commence your research! Your responsibilities thereafter will be to remain in contact with the REC and R & D offices that approved the project, informing them of any adverse events or changes that you might need to make, and providing annual progress reports until the project is completed. At this point, the REC will ask for an 'end of project' report and your relationship with them will end . . . until your next project!

Timescales

This may all sound daunting and time consuming, but most of the approval bodies (peer review committees, ethics committees, R & D offices) observe strict timescales for reviewing projects and communicating the outcomes to applicants. RECs, for example, have a '60 day clock' in which a period of 60 calendar days is allowed for the issue of an ethical opinion on a new application. The clock may stop once, while the REC awaits a response from the applicant for further information or clarification.

Given that the whole business of seeking approval to conduct research is potentially time consuming and complex, it is tempting to try to design research that is uncontroversial and in no way risky to participants or researchers, such that the researcher will have a smooth ride through the approval processes. They might, for example, choose to conduct a survey of staff groups' understanding of recovery from mental health problems, rather than seeking the views and experiences of people who are recovering from mental health problems themselves. This would be unfortunate, because if no-one carried out research with vulnerable or hard to reach groups, then those groups would suffer a double jeopardy by not only being members of disadvantaged or marginalized groups, but also by not having their views sought or represented to inform policy or practice.

At the present, as part of a project to ensure that ethical review is commensurate with the nature and risks involved in projects, 'fast-track' routes for low risk projects through the ethical approval system are being piloted (NRES, 2008).

Ethics and non-NHS research

Health and social care research does not always take place under the auspices of the NHS. Much research is funded by charities or voluntary organizations, or other statutory organizations such as the Prison Service or Youth Offending Teams. You could be forgiven for thinking that as it is such a complex procedure to get to the point of being approved to conduct research in the NHS, it might be best to avoid the NHS and social care organizations altogether, and by-pass the arduous process. This would be wrong for two reasons. Firstly, if everyone took this approach, then the future development of knowledge in the NHS – including medical research – would end; clearly a most undesirable outcome.

The second reason that opting out of NHS/social care settings for research merely to avoid the ethical scrutiny involved is undesirable is because it remains vital that non-NHS research is also conducted ethically. So, at an early stage of proposal development, you should contact the organization in which you propose to carry out your research, to gain approval in principle and to ask for information about relevant ethical procedures. Some organizations such as the Prison Service have their own ethical approval systems; others such as patient support groups may not have formal arrangements but will discuss projects on a case-by-case basis with the researcher. In all cases, it is important to obtain and keep written evidence of all approvals requested and granted.

Internet Mediated Research (IMR) and ethical issues

It is becoming increasingly common to use the Internet as a means of gathering information and indeed recruiting research participants. Examples include 'observing' the conversations of people in chat rooms; accessing members of an online discussion group to complete an online survey; and administering certain experiments online. There are advantages to using IMR; for example, it might allow people who might not ordinarily do so to participate in research, such as people who are housebound or incapacitated in some way and who would not be able to attend an interview or focus group discussion. It might allow access to people who would not feel comfortable discussing sensitive topics face to face but are happy to do so given the relative anonymity of the Internet. Other advantages are that it is possible to access large numbers of participants, and relatively easy to ensure anonymity and confidentiality. There is emerging evidence to suggest that IMR is at least equivalent in effectiveness to more traditional methods of collecting data (Buchanan and Smith, 1999).

However, there are a number of issues inherent in IMR that must be considered over and above the core ethical principles that we have outlined in this chapter. One key factor is that as there is no physical contact between researcher and researched, there is no opportunity to intervene, support participants, or point them in the direction of support services, should they become distressed by any of the online material (British Psychological Society, 2007). Furthermore, it is impossible to ensure that participants are who they say they are, given the potential to change or invent identities online, and thus it is difficult to ensure that consent is valid. Furthermore, participants may believe that their communication with the researcher is private, when in fact the security of unencrypted e-mails, for example, is low (British Psychological Society, 2007). Other problems include self-selection resulting in sampling bias.

To overcome some of these difficulties, permissions to 'observe' chat groups and discussion boards should be sought where possible from the group's moderator. Potential research participants should be provided with as much information as possible about the security and use of their data, and, where it might be of a sensitive or distressing nature, provided information on relevant sources of support. You should avoid reporting direct quotes that could be traced back to their owner via search engines, unless the owner has expressly consented to their use. In sum, the key ethical principles of informed consent, right to withdraw, deception/debriefing and security of data are as applicable within IMR as in any other, but additional caution is required. The Association of Internet Researchers (www.aoir.org) can provide additional support and guidance.

Reading research reports for ethical issues

We have, thus far, outlined the key principles of ethical research and how to ensure that any research you conduct or are involved in is ethical. In the course of studying for qualifications or preparing to undertake a piece of research, you will read many published accounts of research that have been conducted in health and social care settings, and which should therefore have been bound by these same ethical principles. But how can we be certain? Often due to strict word limits, researchers cannot report every detail of their research in a written paper. So they may omit details of where and how they obtained peer review and ethical approval and local NHS support.

 Action Point

Imagine that you are scrutinizing a research paper for evidence that the research has been conducted ethically. What words/phrases/sentences in the paper would assure you that this was the case?

You might have identified words such as consent, confidentiality, anonymity, information, data security, sponsorship, REC, approval, involvement, service user, risk, safety, debriefing or feedback. Adequate information should be included within reports of published research to assure you that the research was conducted ethically.

 Action Point

Locate a copy of a research paper in a journal relevant to your discipline. Ensure that it **is** research using the guidance provided by the NHS Research Ethics Service (NRES, 2008).

Highlight all the points that would assure you that this was ethical research. Where you are not sure or cannot find evidence, note down what especially is the nature of your concern. You may wish to consider:

Who (if anyone) sponsored or funded the research?
What difference might this have made?
Does it appear that the rights of any individual were infringed in the carrying out of this research? If so, how?
What measures did the researcher take to ensure that the research was ethically sound and that individual rights were protected?

In future, when reading published research, always ask and try to answer the above questions.

Conclusion

In this chapter, we have followed the journey that a researcher might take in designing a research project ethically, and in ensuring that all ethical principles have been considered and met before the research commences. While these procedures may appear daunting and lengthy, they are necessary to ensure the integrity of the project, and above all the safety and well-being of the intended research participants. Recently, procedures have been introduced to streamline the process of applying for NHS approvals and these procedures are constantly evolving and improving to ensure that there are no undue barriers or delays to conducting worthwhile health and social care research.

References

British Psychological Society (2005) *Good Practice Guidelines for the Conduct of Psychological Research within the NHS*, British Psychological Society, Leicester.
British Psychological Society (2006) *Code of Ethics and Conduct*, British Psychological Society, Leicester.
British Psychological Society (2007) *Report of the Working Party on Conducting Research on the Internet. Guidelines for Ethical Practice in Psychological Research Online*, British Psychological Society, Leicester.
British Association for Counselling and Psychotherapy (2004) *Ethical guidelines for researching counselling and Psychotherapy*. Retrieved from: http://ethics.iit.edu/codes/coe/british.assoc.counselling.psychotherapy.2004.html.

British Association for Counselling and Psychotherapy (BACUP) (2009) *Ethical Framework for Good Practice in Counselling & Psychotherapy*, BACAP, Lutterworth.

Buchanan, T. and Smith, J.L. (1999) Using the Internet for psychological research: Personality testing on the World-Wide Web. *British Journal of Psychology*, **90**, 125–144.

Data Protection Act (1998) Retrieved from: http://www.opsi.gov.uk/Acts/Acts1998/ukpga_19980029_en_1.

Department of Health (DH) (2003) Essence of Care; Patient-focused benchmarks for clinical governance. Retrieved from: http://www.dh.gov.uk/PublicationsAndStatistics/Publications/PublicationsPolicyAndGuidance/PublicationsPolicyAndGuidanceArticle/fs/en?CONTENT_ID=4005475&chk=A0A4iz.

Department of Health (DH) (2005) *Research Governance Framework for Health and Social Care*, 2nd edn, DH, London.

Gould, D. (2008) Audit and research: similarities and differences. *Nursing Standard*, **22** (37), 51–56.

Long, T. and Johnson, M. (2007) *Research Ethics in the Real World*, Churchill Livingstone, Edinburgh.

Medical Research Council (MRC) (2001) *EU Clinical Trials Directive (2001/20/EC) [Online]*. Retrieved from: http://www.wctn.org.uk/downloads/EU_Directive/Directive.pdf.

Medical Research Council (MRC) (2005) *Good Research Practice*, MRC, London.

Mental Capacity Act (2005) Retrieved from: http://www.opsi.gov.uk/acts/acts2005/ukpga_20050009_en_1.

NRES (2008) Defining research. Retrieved from: http://www.nres.npsa.nhs.uk/news-and-publications/publications/general-publications/.

NRES (2009) Information sheets & consent forms. Guidance for researchers & reviewers. Retrieved from: http://www.nres.npsa.nhs.uk/rec-community/guidance/#PIS.

National Patient Safety Agency (NPSA) (2008) Retrieved from: http://www.nres.npsa.nhs.uk/applicants/apply/research-in-the-nhs/.

Nursing and Midwifery Council (NMC) (2007) *Code of professional conduct: Standards for Conduct, Performance and Ethics*, NMC, London.

Royal College of Nursing (RCN) Research Society (2007) *Research Ethics*, RCN, London.

World Medical Association Declaration of Helsinki (2008) Retrieved from: http://www.wma.net/e/policy/b3.htm.

Resources

Association of Internet Researchers: Retrieved from: http://www.aoir.org.

The Good Clinical Practice Directive (Directive 2005/28/EC of 8 April 2005 of the European Parliament and of the Council). Retrieved from: http://eur-lex.europa.eu/LexUriServ/LexUriServ.do?uri=OJ:L:2005:091:0013:0019:EN:PDF.

Integrated Research Application Service (IRAS) (2008). Retrieved from: www.myresearchproject.org.uk.

National Research Ethics Service (NRES) (2008). Retrieved from: www.nres.npsa.nhs.uk.

National Research Ethics Service (NRES) (2008). Developing commensurate review: a report of the National Research Ethics Service 'fast track' project. Retrieved from: http://www.nres.npsa.nhs.uk/aboutus/developing-nres.

Royal College of Nursing (RCN) (2005) *Informed Consent in Health and Social Care Research*, RCN, London.

7 Quantitative Research Methods: Gathering and Making Sense of Numbers

David Clark-Carter

Introduction

In this chapter, we explore the quantitative approach to research methodology. Unlike in other chapters, we have not included specific action points or exercises, as we cannot assume that all readers have access to the necessary statistical software. However, for readers who wish to explore and practise quantitative techniques, we provide some suggested references and resources at the end of the chapter.

The term quantitative research can be used to describe a large number of research techniques. These can range from carefully controlled experiments to unstructured interviews. What all the techniques share is that numbers are in some way being applied to the results of the research. However, those numbers could be as seemingly straightforward as the number of people who practice some behaviour, such as smoking, or the number of times behaviour of a particular type is shown, such as smiling. I say 'seemingly straightforward', because the researcher may have to make a judgement about how to classify a piece of behaviour; this is an issue that will be returned to later.

Whatever the method we use, it should employ the appropriate design to address our research questions. Typically, research questions can be classified into two types: either *'are there differences between people in different groups?'* Or *'is there a relationship between two variables?'* For an example of the first type, imagine that you split a sample of smokers into two equal-sized groups. One group will receive standard leaflets designed to stop them smoking (the usual care group), while the other group receives usual care plus a new intervention (the intervention group). Our research question could be: after the intervention do fewer people smoke in the intervention group than in the usual care group?

For an example of the second type of research question, imagine that you are studying people with Type 2 diabetes and you wish to see whether there is a relationship between the amount of daily exercise they take and their level of cholesterol.

Unless we are taking a census – in other words, taking data from an entire population – we will have based our research on a sample of people. What constitutes the population of interest depends on the nature of our research. Thus, in the first design above, it could be all smokers, and in the second, all people with Type 2 diabetes. Usually, we are not just interested in the results from our sample but want to know whether the results can be generalized to the wider population; in other words, we are likely to want the design to have external validity. To try to ensure that the results can be generalized we need to design the research carefully, including how we choose our sample. An additional issue is over whether we want to identify a causal link within the research; in other words, do we want the design to have internal validity?

In addition to choosing a design, we need to choose what we are going to measure. In the smoking example, we are interested in whether the intervention is having an effect. However, although we may not have affected smoking behaviour we may have had an effect on a precursor to this: attitudes to smoking. Thus, we could assess effectiveness in more than one way. Before we take a measure we want to be sure that it has certain properties which mean that we are measuring what we think we are measuring, that is that the measure is valid, and that, where appropriate, we would get the same result on another occasion, that is that the measure is reliable.

Once we have the results of a research study we have a number of decisions to make. The two most important decisions are over what the results are telling us and how to present the results in the clearest possible way. The presentation of the results usually has two elements. The first involves what are termed descriptive statistics, such as an average, while the second involves what are termed inferential statistics, which are designed to give an objective answer to our research question. This chapter cannot be treated as a complete manual on how to conduct quantitative analysis; whole books are required to do that. However, it will explain the essentials and give you a clear idea of the issues that you need to consider when designing, analysing and reporting your own research or when critically evaluating someone else's research.

The validity of designs

External validity of designs

A study that has external validity is one from which the results can be generalized beyond the very specific conditions which pertained to the study. The two main aspects that a researcher may want to generalize are the nature of the participants and the nature of the setting in which the research occurred. For, while it may be of interest to have demonstrated that a particular phenomenon can occur, such as an intervention appearing to reduce smoking, the research was probably conducted to test the usefulness of an intervention which is more widely applicable. A distinction which is sometimes made when referring to an intervention is between efficacy – does it work – and effectiveness – does it work in the more usual settings where it is likely to be applied. Although we cannot guarantee that the phenomenon demonstrated in a given piece of research is generalizable, we can at least take steps to make it more likely that it is. To do this we need to think about the nature of our sample and the nature of the setting.

The sample

To be able to generalize to our population we want to have a representative sample. The safest way to do this is by random sampling. However, this can also be very expensive in terms of time and money. A quicker and cheaper method can be a convenience sampling.

Random sampling

There seems to be a misconception about what random means in this context; it doesn't mean arbitrary. Rather, it means that every person in the population has an equal likelihood of being selected. To take a true random sample you need to identify everyone in the population and give them some code, such as a unique number. You need to have chosen what size of sample you want. You then use a method to choose random numbers, such as a computer package or a table of random numbers, and select the required number of participants. What has been described is sometimes called a simple random sample (some use the term simple probability sample to describe it). There are ways to make the sampling less expensive, particularly if you are having to interview each participant or otherwise work with them in person, such as in an experiment. Such methods can involve cluster sampling. Here, instead of identifying every person in the population you could treat groupings (or clusters) as your initial basis for selection. As an example, you might identify every hospital in the area you are interested in and randomly select from them. Once the hospitals have been selected you could then select randomly from the patients involved with each hospital that has been selected. While this method has advantages, the data collected may need more complex analysis than would be the case for a simple random sample.

Convenience sampling

Alternative terms for convenience sampling are accidental or opportunistic sampling. In such methods you treat anyone who you can get as a participant. Thus, you might stand outside a supermarket entrance and approach everyone as they attempt to enter it. Unless your notional population is very restricted, such a method is likely to be very unrepresentative. You will only be sampling people who shop at that branch of that supermarket at that time. Accordingly, if you want to make the sample more representative you will have to sample from a wider range of places and times.

Quota sampling and snowballing

One technique that is employed when you want to include people with specific characteristics is quota sampling. Here you might want to make sure that you have a reasonable proportion of each sex or of particular age ranges. To do this you would initially approach everyone but once you had sufficient people with a required characteristic you could stop approaching others with that characteristic. An alternative sampling technique when you are looking for particular characteristic, particularly if it is unusual, is snowballing. Imagine that you wish to identify people with a particular interest, such as music, in order to see whether it can have an effect on a therapeutic technique that you have devised. Having found some people with an interest in music you could ask them for details of people they know who share that interest.

Dealing with refusals

Whichever sampling method you use, it is likely that you will get some people refusing to take part in the research. In the case of random sampling, you should select a potential sample that is larger than you actually require and then go to the next person in that potential sample if a person refuses. In both cases, it is a good idea to make a note of details about those who are refusing so that you can see whether you have ended up with a biased sample.

The setting

If you want the phenomenon you are testing to occur in places other than the one in which you conducted the study, then you need to think carefully about whether you are making the setting too unique. Accordingly, if you have devised a therapy which patients are meant to implement at home, it might be wise to test whether it works in people's homes and not just in a consulting room; you would be checking its effectiveness as well as its efficacy.

Other aspects of external validity

There may be other factors which influence whether a phenomenon occurs. These could include the nature of the researcher or the time when the study was conducted. Thus, if only one researcher conducted the research we don't know whether another person would get the same result. Equally, there may be phenomena which are affected by diurnal rhythms and so only conducting the research at the same time of day would not pick this up.

Internal validity of designs

This is only an issue if you are trying to establish causal relations between aspects of a study. Thus, you might want to know whether particular dietary practices are better for people with Type 2 diabetes. The safest method of establishing such a causal link is via an experiment where you have allocated people to different groups and you have manipulated what people in a given group eat. If you simply observe people who already have different diets from each other then all you can do is establish whether a relationship exists, not that one element influences another. Thus, in trying to establish internal validity for a study you need to allow for other variables which could explain the result; in the previous example, it may be that other factors such as amount of exercise are related to the diet as well.

The design that is often treated as the gold standard for having internal validity is the RCT or randomized control trial. In this you have a control group, members of which are not given the intervention, and participants are randomly assigned to the groups. By having a control group you can gauge whether any changes between before and after the intervention would have happened spontaneously without experiencing the intervention. By randomly allocating people to the groups you make it less likely that people in the different groups will differ on other aspects which are relevant to the study, such as motivation to change or amount of exercise they take. Such variables can be called confounding variables, as they can vary with the phenomenon you are investigating and either create the false impression of effectiveness of an intervention or even mask its effectiveness. Some studies employ a within-subjects design, where rather than have different people in each group (or condition) each participant does each of the conditions. As an example, you might be investigating a breast milk substitute to see how it compared with breastfeeding. You might weigh infants prior to and after feeding either with a bottle or when breastfed. In using such a design, you need to guard against order effects. In other words, you don't want your result to be an artefact of the order in which your participants carried out the different conditions. In this example, you would assign some infants to the bottle feeding condition first and some to the breastfeeding condition first.

There are many other threats to internal validity (see Clark-Carter, 2010; Cook and Campbell, 1979; or Pedhazur and Schmelkin, 1991 for a fuller list). Three worth noting when looking for changes over time are measurement, history and attrition. If you are trying to assess change over time then you need to use the same measure, as you will not be able to distinguish differences produced over time from those that are simply a consequence of the change in measurement. History is where there has been a change over the time of the study which is not part of your study but which could affect your results. An example could be where you are testing an intervention designed to improve amount of exercise taken, but while the study was being conducted the price of petrol rose and people started walking or cycling to work as a consequence. Attrition (sometimes called mortality) is where people have dropped out of a study. If this happens in a non-random way it could affect the conclusions drawn from the research. An example would be if less motivated people dropped out of an intervention to improve diet, while there was no drop out from the control group. Those who completed the intervention might show an improvement in diet but this wouldn't mean that the intervention worked; the more motivated people in the control group might also have improved their diets.

Another distinction that is made between designs is cross-sectional and longitudinal. In the former, we might be comparing people of different ages but we would have different people in the different age groups. In a longitudinal study, we would study a group of people over time. It is not a good idea to use a cross-sectional design to study the effects of ageing. You might find differences in a cross-sectional study between older and younger participants. However, this may be due to the different experiences which the older people had at the age which the younger sample are now; for example in nutrition or type of exercise, rather than due to a change which inevitably occurs with age. A longitudinal study would follow the same participants over time and thus could observe changes which are a consequence of ageing.

The dilemma of trying to establish both types of validity

In order to establish greater internal validity for a piece of research there can be a danger of lessening the external validity. More control of extraneous variables can make a study lack ecological validity. In other words, the conditions under which the study has been conducted are less like the real world. Therefore, to establish both the causal link and the generalizability of the findings it may be necessary to conduct a series of studies. Initially, highly controlled but more artificial studies to establish a causal link may be conducted. These could be followed by studies conducted under conditions that are less restrictive. Such a series of studies would address the efficacy and the effectiveness of an intervention.

The properties of measures

Validity of measures

Validity of a measure refers to what it is testing. There are various forms of validity. Face validity refers to how the measure is perceived. When conducting a study you want the measurement you take from participants to reflect what you are trying to measure. This can be a problem particularly with measures such as questionnaires, which involve some element of interpretation on the part of participants. If you have told participants that you are measuring their quality of life, then for them to take the measure seriously and answer it truthfully they need to perceive it as a measure of quality of life. Face validity extends to the people administering the measure, who may not always be the person who designed the research. If the person taking the measure does not perceive it as a useful measure of what it is purporting to measure then they can affect the results. An example of a measure that would have poor face validity could be one conducted to test young children's hearing. The conditions under which the test is conducted may not be ideal and so there may be a tendency for children who have perfectly normal hearing to fail the test. Those using the test know this and so don't refer those who fail on for further checks but wait to see what happens next time parents bring the child for a check.

Other forms of validity of measures include construct validity, content validity and criterion-related validity. Construct validity refers to the measure measuring the theoretical construct. An example would be of trying to measure health related locus of control (Rotter, 1954), which is the extent to which individuals believe that they can control events (in this case, their health). The person devising the measure has to have a theory about what constitutes locus of control and will try to address aspects of that construct. One way to check this form of validity is to see how the measure is related to other measures. Thus, you would want such a measure to show a good relationship with any other existing measure of health locus of control; it should have convergent construct validity. On the other hand, you do not want the measure to be strongly related to measures of a different construct, such as depression; it should have good divergent construct validity, otherwise you might simply have devised another measure of depression. Content validity refers to the measure addressing all the aspects of the construct. Criterion-related validity refers to the measure's ability to do what you require of it. To check this you would again check the measure against some existing criteria. A typical example would be where you have devised a screening questionnaire to be completed by patients, which is designed to replace more time-consuming and expensive interviews with consultants. During the creation of the questionnaire you would have participants complete the questionnaire and be interviewed by a consultant. You would then check whether your measure came to the same conclusions as a consultant.

Reliability of measures

The basic idea of reliability of a measure is that it should be measuring the person's true score. That is impossible to establish. However, attempts can be made to establish whether it is likely. We could give the same test on two occasions and see whether the results are the same. A problem with this approach, particularly when applied to measures of psychological phenomena, such as an ability or an attitude, is that there may be an artificially high similarity between the two occasions because participants have remembered what they did on the first occasion. This method is called test–retest and it is worth checking, but there needs to be a reasonable gap between the two occasions; Kline (2000) recommends a minimum of a three-month gap between test and retest. However, often when we are trying to establish the reliability of a measure we want to create the measure and apply it without having to wait for an appropriate period to have elapsed to conduct a retest.

To solve the problem with testing and retesting using the same version of the measure, we could produce two versions of the same measure and then see whether a person achieves the same score from both versions. Unfortunately, this approach, known as alternate form (or parallel form), introduces its own problems. We now have two attempts to measure what we want to measure and the source of any lack of agreement between them cannot be identified as being in one particular version. In addition, when we wish to look for change, say between before and after an intervention, we will not know whether a change in score is due to a change in the phenomenon we are measuring or the fact that we have used a slightly different measure. A solution to the above problems is to treat different parts within the same version of the test as though they were producing a measure of the phenomenon. At its simplest we could compare the result on half the test with the result on the other half; what is termed split-half reliability. Many tests of ability involve the questions becoming increasingly more difficult as the test progresses. Therefore, it would not be sensible to compare the first and second halves of the test. A commonly accepted solution to many of the above problems is provided by Cronbach's alpha (a statistical formula; Cronbach, 1951). This produces the equivalent of the mean of the reliabilities from all possible split halves. Kline (2000) notes that an alpha of greater than 0.7 is usually seen as a sufficiently reliable test. We can interpret this as telling us how closely the current version of the measure would be related to an alternate test of the same length. It can also be interpreted as the square of the correlation between the measured score and the true score.

Inter-rater reliability

When scoring a phenomenon involves subjective judgement we need to be reassured that the score given would be the same regardless of the person providing the score. As an example, we may wish to rate communication between a health worker and a patient. As part of our scoring system, we may want to note aspects of the interaction such as listening, giving information or giving reassurance. To check that our method of scoring was reliable we would start by operationalizing what we meant by our terms and producing examples of the specific type of behaviour. We could produce a scoring manual that included definitions. We would then train raters in the method and then get two or more to rate the same interaction separately, but obviously a different one from the one on which they were trained. We would then look to see how well the raters agree. A common statistic that is calculated to assess inter-rater reliability is Cohen's Kappa (Cohen, 1988). This produces a figure that can be interpreted as the degree of agreement between raters, with the agreements that could occur by chance having been removed. When inter-rater reliability is poor, the scoring system will need to be refined until an acceptable level of agreement is achieved. Even when the level of agreement is good, you need to have a system to resolve disagreements and you need to report what it was.

Choosing a measure

When we wish to take measurements, we should look to see what already exists before creating our own. Part of the evidence we should use to decide whether an existing measure could be used is to look at the psychometric properties of the measure. A manual for a measure should report details of the checks which have been made on aspects of validity and reliability. In addition, they will report the norms for the test. These are the descriptive statistics for the samples that were used in the checks of psychometric properties.

Exploring and describing data

In order to give a context for the following section it is worth looking at an aspect of data: the nature of the scale on which it is measured. Often data is split into four types: nominal, ordinal, interval and ratio.

Nominal data

Nominal (or categorical) data exists when all we know is the categories into which the data fall. Thus, eye colour or gender would be examples of nominal data. We could use numbers to code the different categories in order to enter data into a computer statistical package, such as *PASW* (Predictive Analytics Software), but those numbers would be arbitrary. If we coded blue eyes as 1 and brown eyes as 2 we wouldn't be dealing with a scale on which we are saying those with brown eyes have a higher score; we could just as easily coded blue as 2 and brown as 1.

Ordinal data

As its name suggests, the numbers used to code ordinal data give information about the order in which the data should be ranked and so are not arbitrary. However, they may give us no more information than the rank. As an example, if we know the order of people arriving at a clinic we do not know how far apart they were in time. The first person could have arrived at 10.00 a.m., the second person at 10.01 a.m. and the third person at 11.00 a.m. Therefore, the gaps between the arrival times don't have to be regular. There is another form of data that is considered ordinal, but may be treated as though it were reflecting a more continuous scale. An example of this would be the frequently used Likert scale. Here a person with a long-term condition could be asked to respond to the statement: 'My condition prevents me from having a normal life' by endorsing one of the following: 'strongly disagree', disagree', 'undecided', 'agree' or 'strongly agree'. We can see that there is an order for these responses but we might argue that they are indications of points on a more continuous scale and so we might treat them as though they have more equal distances between them than would be the case for the order of people arriving at the clinic.

Interval data

The classic example of interval data is temperature, for example in degrees Celsius. Here gaps between data points of the same size have the same meaning. Thus, the increases in temperature between 0 and 5 degrees and 5 and 10 degrees are both 5 degrees. However, one restriction of interval data is that it does not have a true zero, in the sense of an absence of the quality being measured; 0 degrees Celsius is still a measurable temperature as emphasized by the fact that when you convert it to Fahrenheit it is 32 degrees. Without a true zero, it becomes meaningless to talk of ratios within the scale. Thus, if you suggested that 100 degrees Celsius is double 50 degrees Celsius, by converting the figures to Fahrenheit we see that the equivalent figures do not have the same ratio: 212 degrees is not double 122 degrees.

Ratio scales

Ratio scales have all the properties of interval scales plus a true zero. This does allow statements about ratios to be made; 50 centimetres is twice as long as 25 centimetres, and when we convert this to imperial measure the same ratio is maintained: 19.68 inches is twice as long as 9.84 inches.

Where possible it is best to try to preserve our measures in their most detailed form. For, as you move from ratio to nominal data you lose information. Hence it is usually better to know a participant's age than that they were in a given age range if your analysis is going to include age. On the other hand, if you are asking about age in order to be able to describe your sample then an age range would be adequate.

Descriptive statistics

To get an impression of what the results of a study tell us, we need to be able to summarize those results because simply visually scanning a set of numbers could create a false impression. The problem is increased when we want to know whether two sets of figures differ, such as between a control and an intervention group, or whether there is a relationship between two sets of numbers. To describe or summarize data from a sample, statisticians have developed descriptive statistics. The most frequently quoted statistics are measures of central tendency (Box 7.1), such as the mean, median and mode, all of which are sometimes referred to as averages.

Each of the above measures of central tendency has advantages and disadvantages. The mean takes all the data into its calculation but by so doing can be affected by extreme high or low values (often termed outliers) in the set. Accordingly, if a group of five people has a mean age of 25 years, adding a person who is 50 will change the mean to just over 29 years. This leads to another feature of the mean, that it may not be a value that is shared by any of the data points. In this example, there may be nobody of 29 in the sample. In addition, for some data a mean can produce a value that can't exist for that scale. An example of this would be if we were told that the average family had 2.4 children.

The median is virtually unaffected by outliers as each new data point is simply placed in its rank order, and so a 50-year-old added to a set of ages with a median of 25 would have no more effect on the median than if a 29-year-old were added instead. The median doesn't use all the values of the data in its calculation.

The mode may not exist, may not be unique or may be very unrepresentative of the set of data. Thus, if every score in the set is different there is no mode. You could group data into ranges and then you might find a modal range, that is the range of scores that occurs most frequently. There may be more than one value in the data that has the same high frequency; for example if the number of both 21-year-olds and 23-year-olds was the same and both were

---

Box 7.1 Measures of Central Tendency

Mean

The mean, which is usually quoted, should be more correctly described as the arithmetic mean, as it is only one of many versions of the mean. To calculate it, add all the numbers in the set together and then divide by the number of numbers.

Median

The median is the central figure in the sense that the data are placed in numerical order and then the middle number is the median.

Mode

The mode is the most frequently occurring number in the set.

higher than the number of any other age. This is described as a bimodal distribution. When there are more than two figures with the highest frequency then it is sometimes described as multimodal. The unrepresentativeness of the mode could occur when a value near one end of the range of scores has the mode and the frequency of that value is not that much higher than for other values in the range. An example would be if you had a set of people whose ages ranged from 25 to 75 and if every age in the range was represented once except for the 74-year-olds, of which there were two, then the mode would be 74-years, while the median and mean might be closer to 50.

The mean is usually the measure of central tendency which is quoted. This is partly because it is used in certain types of inferential test (see below). However, if the median is markedly different from the mean then it should also be quoted.

One thing that the discussion of measures of central tendency should have alerted you to is that when you are told that the average is a particular value, your first question should be about which version of the average is being quoted. Typically in the media, figures are quoted without that information. Thus, you might learn that the average wage is a particular figure but if there are a few very highly paid people in the calculation then the mean and median may differ by quite a lot. A second point is that it isn't sensible to quote such statistics for data on certain scales. Given that the coding of gender is arbitrary, say 1 for male and 2 for female, then quoting a mean is merely going to tell whether there were an equal number of males and females: if the mean for the sample is 1.5 then there is a balance of males and females. However, this seems an unnecessarily circuitous route to finding that information. It would be better to quote frequencies or percentages when data are on a nominal scale.

A problem with all the measures of central tendency is that they don't give any context for the number. Thus, two samples may have the same mean age of 25 years. However, in one sample everyone may be exactly 25 whereas in the other the youngest might be 16 and the oldest 55. To give a context, statisticians have devised what are called measures of spread (or dispersion).

Measures of dispersion

Minimum and maximum

The minimum and the maximum are the lowest and highest values in the set of data. In the previous example, the minimum would be 16 years and the maximum would be 55 years.

Range

The range has a formal meaning which is the difference between the maximum and the minimum. Therefore, the range in the previous example would be 39 years.

Variance

To calculate variance it is necessary to introduce another statistical notion, that of deviation. Deviation, in this context, refers to the difference between a given person's score and the mean for the sample. Accordingly, if the mean age for a group were 25, a person who was 29 would have a deviation of $+4$ and a person aged 21 would have a deviation of -4. Having found each deviation, we want a method to summarize them. If we added them together, we would have the problem that they would cancel each other out and the total would be zero. A way to get around this problem is to square each deviation and then add them; the square of −4 is 16, as is the square of +4. Clearly, if we simply add them then the larger the number of people the larger the variance. Therefore, we could adjust for the sample size by finding the mean of the squared deviations: now you have the variance. There is a further complication. What has been described is the variance for the sample. Frequently statisticians want an estimate of the equivalent value in the population (what is sometimes called a parameter, in this case the variance in the population). They have found that dividing the sum of the squared deviations by one fewer than the sample size produces a better estimate of the population variance. This version is the one that is usually quoted by computer software and is reported in journal articles.

Variance has its uses but there is a drawback to it in that it is not in the original units; in the age example, it is the square of age. A solution to this problem is to quote the standard deviation.

Standard deviation

A standard deviation (SD) is found by taking the square root of the variance. As SDs are in the original units they can be quoted in the following form: *the sample had a mean age of 25 ± 3 years*. In other words, the standard deviation was three years. As well as being in the original units, SDs have an additional useful property when the data are distributed in a particular way. You have probably come across the idea of a normal distribution. This is where if you plotted the data in a graph (a histogram) showing the number of people who had a particular score, then you would produce a curve which is often referred to as bell shaped. If the data in the population are normally distributed then approximately 34% of the population will have a score between the mean and 1 SD above the mean, while approximately 34% will have a score which is between the mean and 1 SD below the mean. Therefore, if our sample has a mean age of 25 with an SD of three and age forms a normal distribution, then approximately 68% of the population will be aged between 22 and 28.

Interquartile range

If data are placed in numerical order then the first quartile is one quarter of the way along the sample, the second quartile (the median) is half way along the data and the third quartile is three quarters of the way along the sample. The interquartile range is the range between the first and third quartiles.

Semi-interquartile range

The semi-interquartile range (sometimes known as the quartile deviation) is the interquartile range divided by 2.

Descriptive statistics looking at relationships between variables

As well as wanting to describe or summarize a single variable we often want a way to look at how two variables are related, such as amount of daily exercise and cholesterol level in people with Type 2 diabetes. Two such statistics are covariance and correlation.

Measures of degree of relationship

Covariance

Here we return to the notion of deviation: the difference between the mean for a sample and a participant's score. We find the deviation for a person on one variable – for example amount of exercise – and the deviation for the same person on the other variable – for example level of cholesterol. We then multiply these two deviations; in other words, we find their product (termed a cross product). As usual, we want to summarize these cross products and so we can add them and, as usual because the sum will be larger the greater the number of participants, we can find their mean: the covariance. However, as with variance, this will be a less accurate estimate of the population parameter than if we divide the sum of cross products by one fewer than the sample size.

As a measure of the relationship between two variables, covariance has a drawback because it will be affected by the variability of the individual variables. The larger the variability, for the same degree of closeness of the relationship between the variables, the bigger the covariance. Therefore, you cannot use covariance to compare degrees of relationship between different variables. Accordingly, it would not be useful to ask whether exercise and cholesterol were more related than exercise and HbA1C (a chemical formed when red blood cells combine with glucose). We need a way of standardizing the statistic so that such comparisons can be made. A correlation coefficient is a solution to that problem.

Correlation coefficient

Pearson's product moment correlation coefficient (r) is a measure of correlation. It can be found by multiplying the standard deviations of the two variables and then dividing the covariance of the two variables by the product of the standard deviations. If two variables are perfectly positively correlated (that is, as one goes up so does the other, in a completely predictable way), then r will be $+1$. If the two variables are perfectly inversely correlated (as one goes up the other goes down), then r will equal -1. If there is absolutely no relationship between the variables then r will equal 0. We now have a way to evaluate Cronbach's alpha, which is described above as an indication of a measure's reliability. 0.7 was given as a minimal level for Cronbach's alpha. It was explained that the square root of this figure (0.84) can be interpreted as the correlation between true score and score on the measure.

Graphs

Graphical representation of data can be useful for at least two reasons. It can help you to explore your data and it can help to explain them to others. Using graphs you can look at the distribution of the data via histograms, stem-and-leaf plots or box plots, including looking at extreme scores. To look at the relationship between two variables you can use scatter plots. To get an impression of differences between groups you can use line charts or bar charts and you can even show measures of dispersion around the means to see how much overlap there is likely to be between the distributions of the different groups. Graphs and tables perform different functions. A good graph can give an overall impression of the data, while a table gives more exact figures, but with complex data it can take some work to get the same impression from a table of figures. Nonetheless, mainly for reasons of space, journal editors tend to ask for only one form of data presentation. For more detail on graphical representation see Chambers *et al.* (1983), Clark-Carter (2010) or Cleveland (1985).

Inferential statistics

As mentioned above, researchers often want to go beyond what they have found to be the case within the sample of people they have been studying to asking whether this could be a more generalizable phenomenon. For example, if a relationship was found between exercise and cholesterol in my sample, I would want to know whether this is just a fluke or whether it is likely to occur in other samples. The conventional way to test this is what follows. Formally, a null hypothesis is created; for example: *there is no relationship between exercise and cholesterol level*. It may seem odd that we need a statement that is actually *not* what we are looking to find. The reason is that we can never prove that something is the case simply by accumulating examples of it. In fact, we need to get away from the notion that we can prove anything. What we can do is demonstrate that the result we have found in our study would be unlikely to have occurred if the null hypothesis were true. We would take this as support for our hypothesis (often called the alternative hypothesis), which could be that there is an inverse relationship between exercise and level of cholesterol; the more exercise a person takes the lower his or her cholesterol. It is this inability to *prove* that makes it difficult to communicate the results of research to those who are not trained in this approach. We cannot prove that smoking is linked to various forms of cancer but we can say that the relationships that we have found in studies are very unlikely to be present if there weren't such links.

Typically, researchers accept a result which is only likely to have occurred with a probability of one in twenty or less if the null hypothesis were true, as being evidence for the alternative hypothesis. Other ways of expressing one in twenty is as a probability of 5% or 0.05. In this context, 0.05 is often described as the alpha level or even the rejection region; the level of probability at or below which we are willing to reject the null hypothesis. When the probability is at or below the alpha level (and therefore in the rejection region) we say that the result is statistically significant.

Directional hypotheses

Sometimes we are conducting exploratory research where we are uncertain of the outcome. For example, we might be exploring binge drinking in teenagers to see whether more males or females indulge in it. We might not have a prediction as to which direction the results will go. The null hypothesis in this case will be unaffected by that uncertainty and will be something like: *male and female teenagers are equally likely to indulge in binge drinking*. However, the alternative hypothesis will reflect the uncertainty and will be of the form *male and female teenagers will differ in the likelihood of indulging in binge drinking*. Such a hypothesis is described as non-directional or bidirectional. On the other hand, if we predicted that females would be more likely to binge drink then we would propose a directional or unidirectional hypothesis.

Parametric tests

Statistical tests are often split into two types: those that make assumptions about aspects of the population from which the sample has come – the parameters – called parametric tests, and those that do not make such assumptions, called non-parametric tests. Another distinction is between tests which use a particular distribution to find their probability and tests which do not use such distributions. The latter are called distribution-free tests. Although the two ways of characterizing the tests are not exactly the same, distribution-free tests are usually non-parametric tests. An example of a parametric test is the *t*-test. This can be used when two conditions are being compared with a dependant variable that is more continuous. An example would be if we were comparing depression scores in a control group with those in an intervention group.

Degrees of freedom

One attribute which some tests rely on for their probability on a particular distribution is degrees of freedom. Formally, degrees of freedom (df) are based on the data used to calculate the statistic and the number of parameters which are being estimated. It is the df which determine the shape of the distribution from which the probability is derived. In the case of *r*, the df is the sample size minus two. In most cases, the way to work out the df involves a similarly straightforward calculation. However, usually statistical computer packages will report the df and the probability for a test routinely. It is standard practice to report the df when giving the results of a statistical test.

Tails of statistical tests

The probability of a result for many statistical tests is affected by the nature of the alternative hypothesis. If the alternative hypothesis is non-directional then the probability is described as two-tailed. A way to understand this term is to think of the distribution of possible values for *r* when the null hypothesis is that *r* will be zero. The possible values will look like a normal distribution with values ranging from -1 to $+1$. When we make a non-directional hypothesis, we are saying that we don't know in which 'tail' of the distribution our result will be; the result could be in either of the two tails. However, when we make a directional hypothesis then we are predicting the one tail in which the result will be. The consequence for the probability of our result of having a one- or a two-tailed test is that in the case of a two-tailed test half of our rejection region is in each tail of the distribution, whereas in a one-tailed test the rejection region is only in one tail. Thus, the value of the statistic has to be larger (further along the distribution) to reach the rejection region when you have a two-tailed test than when you have a one-tailed test. In tests based on such distributions, the probability of a one-tailed test is half that for a two tailed test. However, this is only true if the result has gone in the direction we predicted. Accordingly, if we predict that amount of exercise and cholesterol level will be negatively correlated, then we can use a one-tailed probability only if the correlation is negative, as that is the tail in which we predicted the result would occur (Box 7.2). In one approach to probability, if the correlation were positive when we predicted a negative correlation, then we should subtract the one-tailed probability from one to get the true probability.

Reporting the results of a statistical test

You will see many approaches to reporting results in journal articles. My advice is to report thoroughly. Sometimes, for example in meta-analyses (reviews of several studies), others may

---

Box 7.2   An Example of Running a Statistical Test

Imagine that we have conducted a study to look at the relationship between exercise and cholesterol level. Our null hypothesis is: *there is no relation between amount of exercise taken and cholesterol level.* Based on previous research we make a directional hypothesis and our alternative hypothesis is: *there is a negative relation between amount of exercise taken and cholesterol level.* We have surveyed 20 people, measured their cholesterol level, and asked them about how much time they spent in at least moderate exercise in the previous week. We calculate r and find that it is -0.3. The computer reports that the one-tailed probability is $p = 0.099$. As this is greater than 0.05, the result is not statistically significant and we do not have sufficient evidence to reject the null hypothesis.

---

need that information, and even if they do not it allows readers to make more informed comparisons across studies. There are three elements to reporting the results of a statistical test:

- what you did and on what;
- what you conclude;
- the statistical evidence for that conclusion.

The detail entailed in the appropriate statistical evidence varies from test to test. In the above example, I would write: A Pearson's Product Moment correlation coefficient was calculated for the relationship between amount of exercise and level of cholesterol. The relationship was not statistically significant ($r_{(18)} = -0.3$, $p = 0.099$, one-tailed test). The 18 in parentheses is following a common convention for presenting the df. An additional element that is useful when reporting the results of a study is the effect size; this is discussed later.

When we make a decision about whether to reject the null hypothesis we don't know whether we are correct; we could be making an error. If we reject the null hypothesis when the null hypothesis is true, then we are committing what is called a Type I error. However, when we fail to reject the null hypothesis we also do not know whether the decision is correct. If we do not reject the null hypothesis when it is false we are committing a Type II error. The probability of committing a Type II error is usually described as beta. Clearly, we want to minimize this probability. Statisticians use the term statistical power to refer to the likelihood of avoiding a Type II error. Therefore, we want to maximize the power of our statistical test. Typically, power of 0.8 is considered a minimum below which you would not want to go. Power and beta are related in that power = 1 − beta and so beta = 1 − power. This means that the maximum beta you would not want to go above is 0.2; by convention we are willing to accept a probability of 0.05 of making a Type I error but a probability of 0.2 of making a Type II error. In fact this convention can be circumvented depending on the importance of avoiding the two types of error. Having said that, it is likely that your research will be viewed as unusual if you set alpha as larger than 0.05 or your beta as larger than 0.2. It should be noted that alpha and beta are linked so that lessening alpha increases beta; in other words, by decreasing the likelihood of making a Type I error you increase the likelihood of making a Type II error, if everything else is held constant.

Many aspects of a study have an effect on statistical power. Once all aspects of the design of a study have been decided, including the nature of the hypotheses, then two important determinants of power are the sample size and the size of the effect: the effect size. If we want to compare the results of different studies, we cannot use the statistic which is derived from many inferential statistical tests or the probability, as both are affected by the sample size. Therefore, if two studies had used different sample sizes then they may lead to different decisions simply because the sample sizes differed. Effect sizes are designed to give a result of a study that is not dependent on the sample size.

Effect sizes

There are numerous examples of effect sizes, including variants devised by statisticians to improve their estimation of what the value would be in the population. From the detail introduced so far, two can be mentioned at this stage. Cohen's d is an appropriate effect size when you are comparing the means of two groups. It is calculated by finding the difference between the two means and dividing that result by the standard deviation. Thus, the result has been converted into numbers of standard deviations that the two means differ by. By dividing by the standard deviation, the result has been standardized. In other words, the variability of the scale has been taken into account. This allows comparison across studies that have used different scales to measure the same phenomena. Therefore, if two studies had used different measures of depression when comparing an intervention to reduce depression with a control group, if we know Cohen's d for each study then we can see which has shown a larger effect. Just comparing the differences between the means for the control and intervention groups would not be sensible, as it would ignore the inherent variability of the different measures of depression.

A second effect size is r. It is relatively unusual in that it is used as an inferential test but it has been standardized so that it can be used to compare studies which have used different measures.

Putting an effect size in context

Presented with an effect size, the reader might ask about how to judge its importance. This can be done in a number of ways. Cohen (1988) evaluated published research in the behavioural sciences and drew up three categories for each effect size, what constituted a small, a medium and a large effect size. In the case of Cohen's d the figures are: 0.2 or below (just under a $\frac{1}{4}$ of a standard deviation) is a small effect; around 0.5 ($\frac{1}{2}$ an SD) is a medium effect; and 0.8 or above (just above $\frac{3}{4}$ of an SD) is a large effect. That puts the effect size in a very general context. However, what constitutes an important effect depends on the situation. In the case of a study that was looking at an intervention designed to save life, even a small effect would be considered important.

Determining statistical power

If you are going to use statistical significance as your basis for judging the result of your research, then it makes little sense to conduct a study which means that you would have difficulty in achieving a statistically significant result. If you did run such a study then you are wasting your participants' time. This is why ethics committees want to know that you are going to conduct a study that has sufficient statistical power. Therefore, during the design stage you should work out what sample size would be necessary to achieve an adequate level of statistical power. Statistical power is inextricably linked with effect size and sample size. Therefore, to work out what sample size we need in order to achieve our desired level of power we need to know the effect size. However, if we knew the effect size it is unlikely that we would be conducting the study. Therefore, we need an estimate of what effect size we are likely to get or a minimum effect size below which we are not interested.

Estimating effect size prior to conducting the study

There are a number of sources for an effect size to use in a power calculation. Firstly, we should have read reports of relevant research. If they have reported effect sizes, in line with current advice, then it is straightforward. However, if they have given sufficient detail we should be able to calculate an effect size, for example if means and SDs are reported. Secondly, you should always conduct a pilot study to check how your research design works. The data you collect from this could give you an indication of a possible effect size. However, it is worth noting that as with any descriptive statistic, the smaller the sample on which it is based the less accurate it is likely to be as an estimate of the population value. In the absence of any other indication as to the possible effect size, we can decide what would constitute the minimum effect which would be of clinical interest. Thus, in a study involving an intervention to lessen depression, we could look at the size of change we want in terms of the scale we are using and divide that by the test's SD from the norms for the test. A final way to estimate effect size, in the absence of any other indication of what would be the likely size, would be to use Cohen's guidelines as to what constitutes a small, medium or large effect. Thus, you might decide that the area of research was sufficiently important that you would want to detect a small effect size.

Once you have an effect size there are simple sources for working out statistical power. These range from power tables (Clark-Carter, 2010; Cohen, 1988) to statistical packages such as *SamplePower* (Borenstein, Rothstein and Cohen, 1997) or G*Power (Faul *et al.*, 2007).

Retrospective power analysis

When a result is not statistically significant, as we have seen above this could be for one of two reasons: either the null hypothesis is correct or the effect was sufficiently large to be of interest but we had insufficient statistical power to find a statistically significant result. Routinely, we should be calculating and reporting effect sizes from our studies. However, now that we know the effect size we can conduct another power analysis to find out what sample size would give us a reasonable level of power for that effect size. This can help us make recommendations for future research. If the necessary sample size is unrealistically large then the design needs modifying; for example an intervention might need to be applied for a longer period. On the other hand, if the sample size is within reasonable bounds then we could recommend a replication of the study but with this recommended sample size.

In the case of the relationship between exercise and cholesterol, the result was not significant. Power analysis shows that for a one-tailed test, with alpha set at 0.05, for that effect size ($r = 0.3$) you would need a sample of 68 people to have power of the recommended minimum of 0.8. As this isn't an unreasonable sample, particularly as the area of research is an important one, then we would recommend attempting to replicate the study but with the increased sample size.

Confidence intervals

One way to put a result in context is to find a confidence interval (CI) for it. The calculation of a CI follows the same principles as inferential tests. However, the result is interpreted in a slightly different way. At an intuitive level a CI can be interpreted as a range of values in which the population parameter is likely to lie. Thus, a CI for the mean of a sample is likely to contain the mean for the population. Confidence intervals are calculated with a certain level of confidence. The most common level is 95%, which is the equivalent of applying our usual alpha level of 0.05 (or 5%). Put more formally, we can interpret a CI in the following way. Imagine that we took a sample of a given size from a population and calculated a mean and a 95% CI for the mean. We then took another sample of the same size and again calculated the 95% CI and kept repeating this process. On 95% of occasions the CIs would contain the population parameter.

When you interpret a CI there is often an important value which you are looking to see whether the CI contains, and that would demonstrate no effect; for example if we are comparing the depression scores for an intervention and a control group. A statistic of interest will be the difference between the mean depression scores. If we calculate a CI for the difference then we should look to see whether it contains zero, and if it does then even if we find that the mean difference in the sample favours the intervention group, the CI is suggesting that this may not be true in the population. In fact, if the CI contains negative as well as positive values then the value in the population could even favour the control group.

Non-parametric tests

As was stated earlier, a defining characteristic of a non-parametric test is that it doesn't entail assumptions about the population from which the sample comes. However, the probability found from running a non-parametric test can be made inaccurate if the data do not conform to certain guidelines. An example is the Mann–Whitney U test, which is a non-parametric equivalent of the between-subjects t-test, and which needs the variance of the two groups to be sufficiently similar.

A second issue to be aware of is that the probability quoted by statistical packages for non-parametric tests can be inaccurate if the sample size is small. This is because they often rely on what is termed a z-approximation. In other words, they are using the information from the data to produce an equivalent of a parametric test that finds its probability from the normal distribution. You will sometimes see the probability referred to as *asymp* (or asymptotic). The probabilities given by such tests only become accurate when the sample size is sufficiently large, and what constitutes sufficiently large depends on the specific test. In the case of the Mann–Whitney U test, as long as you have at least 20 in each group then the approximation can be considered accurate, whereas in the case of Spearman's rho, a non-parametric equivalent of Pearson's Product Moment Correlation Coefficient, you need at least 100 participants for the approximation to be accurate.

When the sample sizes are below the necessary size then there are two possible ways to find a more accurate probability. If the software you are using has the facility to ask for exact probabilities (as some versions of *PASW* will), then you can choose that option. However, it does rely on your computer having sufficient processing power to cope. An alternative way to find the exact probability, or at least to find whether your result achieves statistical significance, is to use tables provided in books (e.g. Clark-Carter, 2010; Neave and Worthington, 1988). If your computer can't work out exact probabilities it may have the facility to find what is sometimes called a Monte-Carlo version (as in *PASW*). This can be an accurate estimate of the exact probability and will be more accurate than the one based on the z-approximation.

A misunderstanding has developed over non-parametric tests, which is probably due to the way in which many of them are calculated. You may come across the statement that they are only for ordinal or ranked data and not for interval or ratio data. This isn't true. However, some of them, such as the Mann–Whitney U test, convert the data into ranks. This has two possible benefits. If there are outliers in the data they will just be given the next rank along. In addition, if the data in two groups have different variances then the effect of ranking can lessen this problem.

A final point to make about non-parametric tests is to do with statistical power. If all the assumptions of a parametric test are fulfilled but you run the non-parametric equivalent then your test will have less power. This can be calculated by what is termed power efficiency. As an example, if you ran a Mann–Whitney U test when all the assumptions of a between-subjects t-test are fulfilled, then to get the same level of statistical power in the two tests you would need 27 per group for the Mann–Whitney U and 25 per group for the t-test. However, if assumptions of the parametric test are not fulfilled, then the non-parametric test can have more power than the parametric test.

Contingency tables or cross tabulation

When you are examining a variable which forms different categories and another variable which also forms categories, for example, comparing males and females to see whether different proportions smoke, then the data can be placed in a contingency table. As long as the data are independent, in the sense that no participant could be placed in more than one combination of the two variables, then a useful inferential test is Pearson's chi-square. Taking two categories from each variable, one can calculate a useful statistic which can be used as an effect size: the odds ratio.

Odds ratios

To explain an odds ratio requires two related ideas to be introduced: probability and odds. A probability, in this context, is the proportion of participants who fall into one category, for example the proportion of males who smoke. The related probability, for example the proportion of males who do not smoke, can be found by subtracting the original probability from one. Odds can be found by dividing one probability by the other. In this way, we could find the odds of being a smoker (relative to being a non-smoker) amongst the males. The odds for the other category, for example women who smoke (relative to those who do not smoke), can then be calculated. The odds ratio is found by dividing one odds by the other. Odds ratios can be expressed in two ways. In the current example, we could divide the odds for males by the odds for females or we could divide the odds for females by the odds for males. It is perhaps easier to interpret an odds ratio by finding which of the two ways produces a figure greater than one. To convert from one version of the odds ratio to the other, simply divide one version into one. Thus an odds ratio of 0.2 converts to an odds ratio of 5. If the odds ratio is exactly one then clearly the two odds are the same and there is no difference between the two groups. In the above example, when the odds of being a smoker for males was divided by the odds of being a smoker for females, we found that the odds ratio was greater than one. This can be interpreted as showing that the odds of being a smoker for males is greater than it is for females.

Once again, a confidence interval can tell us useful additional information. If the confidence interval contains one, then this suggests that whatever the sample is showing there may be no difference in the odds of the two categories in the population.

Conclusion

In this chapter, the need to consider issues such as the internal and external validity of your designs has been emphasized. The importance of your measures having validity and reliability has been shown. The ways in which you should explore data and present it to others has been discussed. It has been shown what form hypotheses take and how they are tested. The distinction between parametric and non-parametric tests and how to decide which is the more appropriate has been explained. It has been shown how to choose an appropriate sample size for a study. Finally, the argument has been made for the importance of reporting effect sizes and confidence intervals in order to put a research finding in a wider context.

References

Borenstein, M., Rothstein, H. and Cohen, J. (1997) *SamplePower 1.0*, PASW Inc., Chicago.

Chambers, J.M., Cleveland, W.S., Kleiner, B. and Tukey, J. (1983) *Graphical Methods for Data Analysis*, Wadsworth International Group, Belmont.

Clark-Carter, D. (2010) *Quantitative Psychological Research: The Complete Student's Companion*, Psychology Press, Hove.

Cleveland, W.S. (1985) *The Elements of Graphing Data*, Wadsworth, Monterey, CA.

Cohen, J. (1988) *Statistical Power Analysis for the Behavioral Sciences*, 2nd edn, Lawrence Erlbaum Associates, Hillsdale, NJ.

Cook, T.D. and Campbell, D.T. (1979) *Quasi-experimentation: Design & Analysis Issues for Field Settings*, Houghton Mifflin Company, Boston, MA.

Cronbach, L.J. (1951) Coefficient alpha and the internal structure of tests. *Psychometrika*, **16**, 297–334.

Faul, F., Erdfelder, E., Lang, A.-G. and Buchner, A. (2007) G*Power 3: A flexible statistical power analysis for the social, behavioral, and biomedical sciences. *Behavior Research Methods*, **39**, 175–191.

Kline, P. (2000) *The Handbook of Psychological Testing*, 2nd edn, Routledge, London.

Neave, H.R. and Worthington, P.L. (1988) *Distribution-free Tests*, Routledge, London.

Pedhazur, E. J. and Schmelkin, L.P. (1991) *Measurement, Design, and Analysis: An Integrated Approach*, Lawrence Erlbaum Associates, Hillsdale, NJ.

Rotter, J.B. (1954). *Social learning and clinical psychology*, Prentice-Hall, NJ.

Further resources

Coolican, H. (2009) *Research Methods and Statistics in Psychology*, 5th edn, Hodder Education, London.

Field, A. (2009) *Discovering Statistics: Using SPSS*, 3rd edn, Sage, London.

Pallant, J. (2007) *SPSS Survival Manual*, 3rd edn, Open University Press, Maidenhead.

8   Qualitative Research Methods: Gathering and Making Sense of Words

Helena Priest and Paula Roberts

Introduction

This chapter describes qualitative research: what it is, how it is done, the kinds of topics, data and people that are amenable to qualitative research; and, in this way, helps the reader to assess the merit of published qualitative research as well as to consider using qualitative research to answer their own clinical or academic questions. The chapter introduces common approaches to generating qualitative data, such as interviews and observations, before outlining a number of specific approaches to qualitative research, such as phenomenology and grounded theory. Strengths, weaknesses and rigour in qualitative research are addressed, considering the extent to which measures such as validity and reliability are applicable to qualitative research, and how to ensure the accuracy, trustworthiness and transferability of procedures used. Finally, the chapter discusses the role of the researcher in qualitative research, and considers the concept of reflexivity.

What is qualitative research?

In Chapter 7, we looked at the kinds of research that can be done which produce information in the form of numbers. We turn our attention now to a different kind of research, one which produces data in the form of words. Famously, the 'Whiskas' cat food company once produced a TV advert claiming that this brand of cat food was the brand of choice for most cat owners. However, people who conduct qualitative research are more interested in exploring people's unique personal experiences and understanding of the world, rather than finding out that '8 out of 10 cat owners say their cats prefer it', a claim made about 'Whiskas' at the time. What we can't tell from such numbers or statistics is what made an individual cat owner choose the particular product, how they evaluated it as a suitable cat food, how they felt when their cat devoured the lot or left it untouched, and so on. Qualitative research allows us some access to people's experiences, views, opinions, beliefs, feelings and judgments by asking them to tell us, in spoken word or in writing, about these. In turn, we as researchers make our own interpretations of these words and arrive at some conclusions.

The use of qualitative methods in research supports the notion that there is no external reality or truth. Rather, humans make sense of, or construct, their individual world, and qualitative research tries to 'tap into' this world – taking an emic or internal perspective rather than using an external frame of reference (an etic perspective), as used in quantitative research.

There have been many attempts to define the common and essential features of qualitative research. Bryman (1988), in the early years of qualitative research, considered the key features to be 'seeing through the eyes of another person'; 'describing the other person's perspective'; 'understanding actions and meanings in their social context'; 'favouring open and relatively unstructured research designs'; and 'avoiding concepts and theories at an early stage'. More recently, Willig (2001, p. 8) has described qualitative researchers as being interested in 'how people make sense of the world and how they experience events. They aim to understand what it is like to experience particular conditions . . . and how people manage certain situations . . .'

The key principles of qualitative research can be summarized as:

- **Naturalistic:** because human behaviour is best understood within its natural context, qualitative researchers do not alter aspects of human behaviour, but rather observe, describe and make sense of naturally occurring situations;
- **Subjective:** the researcher does not try to be an objective outsider. Rather, the researcher tries to 'tap into' the experience of the research participant;
- **Interpretive:** because human beings actively strive to make sense of (interpret) their social world and the world of others, researchers therefore try to interpret the world of the people they are studying;
- **Unique:** because of the uniqueness of the individual, there are thus multiple possible interpretations of the social world. Researchers try to discover these unique interpretations but may also seek to draw out commonalities from different people's experiences;
- **Holistic:** the researcher tries to take into account the 'big picture' as well as looking at specific detail within it;
- **Flexible:** the detail of the research is not always totally specified at the outset, allowing some flexibility in questions and methods as the research progresses;
- **Inductive, hypothesis generating:** conclusions are drawn from information and premises, which may lead to the generation of new hypotheses or theories.

In summary, then, qualitative research is a means of exploring an area of human experience, in order to try to understand how humans make sense of their world. It allows us to identify and describe topics or phenomena about which little is known, and explore and explain the scope and meaning of such phenomena.

What can we study using qualitative research?

The main subjects of qualitative research are any or all of:

- people;
- human phenomena;
- the process and experience of carrying out the research itself (more about this under 'reflexivity').

 Action Point

Reflecting on your own area of practice, which people or which aspects of human phenomena could be explored using a qualitative approach?

You may have identified particular groups of people that you meet in your daily practice, such as patients undergoing heart surgery; or nurses undertaking higher education courses. You might want to work with such groups of people to explore aspects of human phenomena that are particularly relevant to those groups. These might include, for example, pain, fear of death or reassurance for the people undergoing heart surgery, or motivation and determination in nurses choosing to undertake further study. These complex yet nebulous topics lend themselves well to exploration using qualitative methods, as we shall see.

History of qualitative research

As we learnt in Chapter 2, qualitative research initially developed as an alternative to the dominant scientific/quantitative paradigm. It has gone through many phases of development since the 1940s, during which time several seminal texts have been published, such as 'The Discovery of Grounded Theory' (Glaser and Strauss, 1967), which aimed to explain how to 'do' qualitative research. Many of these remain influential today. Such approaches were an attempt to demonstrate that qualitative research could be as systematic and rigorous as the dominant quantitative methods of the time (McLeod, 2001).

Today, there is a wide range of different types of qualitative research, some of which will answer some questions better than others. Qualitative research is becoming increasingly accepted and influential within social science, education and healthcare research. It is particularly appropriate for exploring healthcare practices as it shares many of healthcare's key activities: listening, observing, questioning, recording, hearing people's stories and building and checking understanding. The kind of knowledge generated from these activities aims, therefore, to be holistic, personal and relevant within its natural setting.

Some myths and misconceptions

Despite it having become acceptable and legitimate as an approach to information gathering and research, there remain some myths and misconceptions about precisely what qualitative research is and does. There is a view in some quarters that 'quantitative research is quantitative research without numbers'; this is a misconception. It is not a 'version' of quantitative research, it is a completely different type of research designed to answer different types of questions in different ways. Others believe that it is in some way easier to do than quantitative research because the researcher does not have to trouble themselves with numbers, statistical tests, calculations and complex computer programs such as SPSS. Alternatively, there is a belief that it is harder to conduct than quantitative research, precisely because there are no set 'rules' that determine which statistical test will produce what kind of information, nor computer programs that, provided the right information is inputted, will produce the answer to the question. This too is a misconception, as even when analysing quantitative data, despite the availability of 'rules', you still have to decide what data to select, how to screen and diagnose its properties, how to enter it into the relevant spreadsheet, which test to use, what analysis to perform, and what sense can be made of the data output (Chapter 7).

Another common myth is that qualitative research, because it is not 'scientific' and we cannot 'prove' anything from it, is somehow less rigorous and, therefore, of less value than quantitative research. This idea arose and has persisted since the early days of qualitative research development and use. Qualitative research can indeed be conducted rigorously and faithfully; we explore some of the ways in this can be done and discuss issues of reliability and validity under the section headed 'rigour'.

Finally, some people have argued that, as each human being is unique, and will therefore have a unique understanding of the world, any qualitative research designed to explore people's experiences will result in as many different answers and interpretations as there are people! The conclusion from this is that we cannot draw any meaningful or generalizable answers from such diverse personal experiences. We return to this debate, too, in the section on rigour.

Asking qualitative questions

Qualitative research usually starts with a question or series of questions. It is these questions that determine the precise method, the type of data that will be gathered, the people that will be involved (referred to as 'participants' or co-researchers) and the way that data will be handled.

 Action Point

Imagine that you want to find out what people who had just been discharged from hospital thought about their hospital stay. What sort of questions might you ask?

You might ask whether there were things about their stay they were unhappy with and anything that could have been done to improve their experience. You might ask what they thought of the food and facilities. Of course, you could do this by constructing a questionnaire with 'tick boxes', but patients' experiences are unique, and you might miss some important and detailed information that could not be captured by ticking a five point scale. We return to 'qualitative questions' later in this chapter.

Methods of sampling in qualitative studies

The key aim, in most qualitative research, is to gather information from participants who are most likely to be able to answer our questions. Seeking such participants is referred to as purposive or theoretical sampling; we select a sub-population from the target population who are willing and able to contribute their views on our topic of interest, rather than recruit participants with little interest in or insight into the phenomenon.

 Action Point

Can you think of any disadvantages of seeking out and selecting participants in this focused and purposive manner?

One possible risk is that we will only seek out those people who are articulate, informed and willing to share their views. This is sometimes described as 'elite bias'. We may unwittingly or even deliberately exclude people who seem difficult to engage in the research process, such as people in prison, or those who may find it difficult to communicate with us, such as people with sensory impairments or those with intellectual disabilities. To avoid this possibility, researchers must work hard to include at all stages of the research process those groups of people whose lives might be affected by the findings of the research undertaken.

Homogeneity

It follows from the purposive sampling argument that in qualitative research there is no particular aim to recruit groups who are representative of a larger population. Instead, the aim is normally to recruit participants who share similar characteristics, for example people with intellectual disabilities who have been physically abused, or people who have recently undergone a kidney transplant. The aim is, therefore, to obtain a homogenous sample, homogenous meaning 'similar'.

How many people do we need in our sample?

There are no hard and fast rules; decisions are based on the methods, the topic of interest; how many people are likely to fall into the category; and how easy it will be to recruit them. Some types of qualitative research provide guidance on numbers of people; for example, Interpretative Phenomenological Analysis (see below) generally recommends between six and ten participants, while grounded theory (see below) suggests that sampling should continue until saturation is reached, which is when new participants do not add any new information or insights to those already identified. It is possible for qualitative research to be undertaken using just one participant or many more than that in a single study; multisite studies can increase numbers considerably. However, it is not all about numbers – more is not necessarily better! It is more important to consider the quality and richness of the data that you wish to obtain. It is important also to consider the resources available for analysing the data. Consider that it takes about four hours to transcribe a one hour taped interview using a transcribing machine, and the amount of time needed simply to manage the data can quickly mount up.

Finding participants

Action Point

Imagine that you want to conduct a study on people's experiences of being in hospital. List all the possible methods you could use to identify people who might become part of your study.

You might have thought of advertising in hospital Out Patient clinics or General Practitioners' surgeries, or contacting 'gatekeepers' to relevant organizations (such as hospital managers). When there are a relatively small number of potential participants, it is likely that most will be included in your sample. In this case you can use snowball sampling, whereby participants suggest other potential participants you could approach to make up your sample. If participants are to be recruited from a large organization, however, it is often helpful to prepare materials and offer to visit the team and outline your research; in this way staff are more likely to be supportive and 'sell' involvement in your project to potential participants.

Data for qualitative research

Qualitative research draws upon many different types and sources of data that are amenable to its methods, and draws upon a diverse range of approaches for analysing data.

 Action Point

Given that qualitative data is generally in the form of words, what sources might a qualitative researcher use to obtain words to analyse?

Perhaps the most obvious source is the written word, such as is available in books, newspapers, journals, diaries, and so on. Indeed, a form of research devotes itself to analysing such sources, which can be referred to as documentary analysis. Other sources, though, are more frequently used, in particular the spoken words of someone who has been interviewed about a topic, or has written down their thoughts and ideas in an open-ended questionnaire, journal or diary. Alternative sources of qualitative data are observations, where researchers note down what is happening around them, or record observations on audiotape or video camera and later analyse the words spoken and interactions observed. We will now look in more depth at four common sources of qualitative data: interviews, focus groups, observations and questionnaires, and consider their uses and limitations.

Interviews

Interviews are a popular means of exploring and capturing an individual's thoughts, opinions, feelings and experience of a topic that is particularly significant to him/her. However, interviews are not the same as informal conversations between friends. They need to be well prepared. An appropriate venue that is accessible to participants needs to be identified and booked, if necessary; it needs to be a place that is warm and comfortable and where there will be no distractions, such as from a ringing telephone. If interviews are to take place in a participant's own home, then special considerations might be needed, such as following local organization lone worker policies.

Refreshments should be available (at the very least drinking water) and tissues. Other equipment needed includes a clock, tape recorder or digital recorder, a list of topics or interview schedule, and a 'do not disturb' sign for the door if the interview is in a public location. Although the interview participant will already have consented to being interviewed, it is important to check this before the interview starts (this is known as process consent, indicating that consent is not a 'one-off' activity) and to ensure that they are still happy for the interview to be recorded. The opening of the interview should include some 'settling' questions to help the participant feel at ease. Thereafter, they should be encouraged to talk freely, but the interviewer should decide when to allow them to deviate from the key topic areas and when to bring them 'back on track'. Sometimes the most important and relevant information comes out naturally when people are allowed to tell their stories freely, so it may be important to be flexible. At the end of the interview, you should thank participants for their contribution and arrange to send a transcript of the interview for checking, if this has previously been agreed.

Interview structure

Normally conducted on a one-to-one basis, the researcher/interviewer has to decide from the outset on the level of structure required for the interview. This can be unstructured, where the interviewer draws on previous experience to explore the topic of interest, allowing the interviewee to talk freely around the topic. An advantage of unstructured interviews is that there is considerable scope for the interviewee to develop their ideas without being constrained by pre-set questions. However, this type of interview requires great skill on the part of the interviewer to ensure that key topic areas are being addressed and, if not, to guide the interview back on track.

At the other end of the spectrum, structured interviews have a pre-prepared list of questions that will be posed in the same order and using the same words to all participants. Too highly structured (almost like an oral version of a paper questionnaire), and the interview participant will be restricted to direct answers to questions posed, with little opportunity to expand or elaborate, or take the conversation in a different direction. Too loosely structured, and the participant may be struggling to focus ideas and wonder what the researcher is looking for. Hence, the most common type of interview in qualitative research is the semi-structured interview (Willig, 2001).

Semi-structured interviews allow the researcher to dictate to some extent the topics and content of the interview, but also allow the participant to add, elaborate, deviate, provide examples and tell illustrative stories, as they feel appropriate. To this end, researchers normally draw up an interview schedule to facilitate the general areas of discussion, with some broad question areas and some accompanying prompt questions, should the participant not be forthcoming or need more explanation on a topic. The areas of focus should be viewed as broad objectives, rather than specific questions requiring specific answers. Participants should also be given the opportunity to add further contributions, if they wish, to a more general discussion at the end of the interview. Often important data is yielded in this spontaneous discussion time.

Whatever the level of structure in the interview, as a general rule all questions other than those designed to collect essential factual information, are open ended. This means that they cannot usually be answered with a simple 'yes' or 'no' or single category answer, but instead steer the interviewee to respond more extensively. So, for example, if we want to find out about someone's experience of caring for a relative who has had a stroke, we might want to ask 'what was it like for you when your relative first came home from hospital?' Useful words to start open-ended questions are what, when, where, who, why and how (5w + h).

Did you find any difficulty with wording these questions? Sometimes, questions prefixed with 'why' are difficult to answer and can appear challenging or confrontational; for example, 'why did you do that?' Wherever possible, try to avoid too many questions beginning with why, as this can lead to your respondent having to justify their response.

Other types of questions to avoid are leading questions, such as 'how severe is your pain?', as this leads the respondent to think of their pain in terms of severity, when in fact it may be quite mild. Instead, they may respond with 'quite severe', a different meaning altogether. Equally, double-barrelled questions, where two things are asked at once, are difficult to answer, especially if the respondent would like to answer each part of the question in a different way. For example if you ask 'would you like a cup of tea and then go and have your bath?' the respondent may feel pressure to say yes to both, even though it is only the tea they want!

 Action Point

Using the 5 w + h method, devise some open ended questions to help you interview someone about caring for their relative after a stroke:

What . . .
When . . .
Where. . .
Who. . .
Why. . .
How . . .

Recording interview data

Typically, interviews are recorded using digital recording equipment that can later be transcribed onto computer, producing a semi-permanent record of the entire interview. It is a good idea, though, to take some written notes as a precaution against equipment failure, unless this would seem to interfere with the spontaneity and flow of the interview itself. It goes without saying that equipment should be checked at the outset, and backup systems put in place in case equipment fails. Carefully label your data with the date of the interview and participant number for later verification and cross-referencing.

Strengths and weaknesses of interviews

Interviews are useful in that they generate immediate responses and produce much detailed data that would otherwise be difficult to capture, such as people's emotional responses. They also allow both the interviewer and interviewee to clarify ideas at the time. It is perhaps less likely for interviewees to evade questions, lie or mislead, as they might do in completing a questionnaire, as they have agreed to be there and are 'face-to-face' in a human interaction. However, interviewing is time consuming, both in terms of preparing for and conducting the interview, as well as in transcribing and analysing the interview data. In this way, it can be an expensive option in terms of interviewer time and resources. Equally, interviewing is a highly skilled activity and the unskilled or unprepared interviewer may not make the most of the interview situation if they do not practice good questioning and listening skills.

Focus groups

Alternatives to the face-to-face interview include telephone interviewing and group interviews, often known as focus groups. For several decades, focus groups have been used in marketing research to generate ideas, attitudes and opinions on various topics (Fern, 2001). Focus groups comprise small gatherings of people (usually between six and ten, together with a moderator) brought together to participate in a group discussion. The importance of focus groups lies in their capacity to generate interactive discussion. Consequently, the right balance of participants, in terms of manageability and potential contribution, needs prior consideration. Smaller groups may detract from the advantages of collectivism whilst large numbers of participants may be difficult to facilitate. In larger groups, some participants may feel excluded or sense that they are a source of unintended or undesirable effects on group dynamics (Fern, 2001).

Advantages of focus groups include: speed and expediency (in that several people are seen and data is gathered from several people simultaneously); snowballing (triggering responses from group members); spontaneity of responses; synergism (the group's combined efforts comprising more than the sum of individual contributions); stimulation from other group members; and the security of group settings. Indeed 'many focus groups gather a momentum and spontaneity which provide invaluable data for future analysis' (Roberts, 1997, p. 81). Focus group discussion can yield sufficiently rich data to use alone, or be compared with the everyday experience of other people, or to facilitate further data collection such as individual interviews or the development of questionnaires.

Focus groups must be carefully planned to maximize the opportunity for data gathering. The assistance of a host coordinator (an identified contact in your host organization who will assist in booking rooms and facilitating contact with participants) is invaluable. Focus groups can be undertaken in informal or formal settings, but it is important that the group can see and hear each other and the moderator. A large conference table is often useful, around which participants can sit facing each other, with space for copies of the interview schedules. An appropriate and reliable recording device is necessary to ensure all voices are heard for subsequent review and reproduction.

Participants should be sent invitation letters in advance, outlining the aims and purpose of the research, issues of anonymity and confidentiality, requesting that the discussion be recorded, and enclosing an interview schedule. This information will give participants time to consider the issues involved and to appreciate what the discussions are to accomplish, thus enabling the available time to be used more effectively.

When planning a focus group, incentives can greatly improve participation rates. For example offer refreshments or payment and expenses if the budget permits. You will need to allow half an hour before each interview commences to set up recording equipment and work through the key issues, such as explaining the purpose of research and the interview process, gaining consent, making introductions, giving the opportunity to ask questions and explaining issues of confidentiality and data storage.

The role of the moderator in such exploratory investigations is that of facilitator, and it is important to be an attentive and active listener, using non-verbal communication skills to encourage participants to speak freely. To facilitate the process, the counselling skills of reflection (putting 'back' to participants not just the content of what they have said but also what is understood by it) and summarizing (focusing participants' scattered thoughts and feelings, or closing a particular theme) are useful (Tschudin, 1995).

Strengths and weaknesses of focus groups

Most of the principles that apply to individual interviews (such as consent, anonymity, process and data storage) apply to focus groups, except that normally one would only conduct one interview and perhaps a follow up with the same person, whereas multiple focus groups are often conducted. They share similar strengths and weaknesses to individual interviews, with the additional strength that the collective responses generated from group discussion often provide insights that would not have been gained from individual interviews.

Observation

Useful qualitative data can be obtained from observing the behaviour and interactions of people and recording it in ways that can later be translated into verbal data for analysis. The researcher can adopt a number of different roles in observational research ranging from complete participation, where the researcher becomes part of the group under study, to complete observation, where the researcher is 'on the sidelines' and takes no part in the activities of the people being observed. Various other positions along this continuum can also be adopted. Whichever style of observation is chosen, it involves producing detailed descriptions of people's behaviour within its natural context.

Before conducting an observational study, it will be necessary to gain permissions to enter the 'field', taking into account that some people may be incidentally observed that are not the focus of your study (see Chapter 6 for more information). You must then decide how to record what is occurring in the setting; do you take notes, or rely on your memory, or use a digital recorder? If the former, how much will you actually remember? Will the fact that you are writing everything down mean that you will miss seeing what's going on? Will you distract people around you if it appears that you are writing about them? The latter will require consent from key people whose words and actions will be recorded. How will you ensure that you record events faithfully, and do not just concentrate on those things that you find particularly interesting, thus introducing bias into your study? How will people take to being recorded? These questions all need to be answered and justified before embarking on an observational study.

Strengths and weaknesses of observation

 Action Point

Can you think of any disadvantages of being:

(a) a participant observer;
(b) a non participant observer?

As a participant observer, one of the difficulties is in capturing the full extent of what is going on. If you are trying to observe everything around you at the same time as being part of the context that you are observing (say, practising as a nurse while at the same time observing the way in which senior nurses are managing the ward), it is inevitable that you will be caught up in fulfilling your role and will miss important elements of the behaviour you are observing. Equally, you may experience role conflict, whereby your 'researcher' duties are set aside because of competing priorities of your 'nurse' role. A further difficulty is that you may need to spend considerable time in the research setting, and may also need to spend time getting to know people and develop relationships before actually commencing observations.

On the other hand, spending this time to build relationships as a participant observer does help those being observed to relax, behave naturally and speak openly to the researcher, allowing the researcher to get a good understanding of activities and their possible meanings in the chosen setting.

A disadvantage of non-participant observation, on the other hand, is that if people know they are being observed, their behaviour may change subtly in response, thus the researcher is unable to gather naturally occurring data. In some cases, a degree of 'covertness' is adopted to avoid this (but see Chapter 6 on the ethical issues involved, and the importance of debriefing). In addition, conducting a thorough observational study requires extensive time for data collection, something that is not often available to the busy clinician.

Questionnaires

Questionnaires may not immediately be thought of as providing qualitative data, but depending on the structure of the questionnaire, they can provide textual data that lends itself to qualitative analysis. For example, it is common in questionnaires, after asking the respondent to rank something on a five point scale, to ask for 'comments' and to provide a free text box in which these comments can be written. This textual data can then be analysed using methods such as qualitative thematic analysis (see below), which can support and enhance the data provided from statistical analysis of the numerical data.

Strengths and weaknesses of questionnaires

One of the key advantages is that, apart from postage or other distribution costs, questionnaires are a relatively quick and cheap form of data collection. Once the content has been designed and agreed, it is quick and easy to duplicate multiple copies and distribute these widely, and this costs little in terms of researcher time. Once competed questionnaires have been returned, the researcher has direct access to the respondents' words on paper (or, as is becoming popular, on a computer file). There is no need to spend time listening to or transcribing recordings before analysis can take place.

On the other hand, once a questionnaire has been posted or made available for completion, and even when the researcher has included a self addressed envelope, the 'control' of the process is out of the researcher's hands, and it is entirely up to the recipient whether or not to complete and return the questionnaire. An acceptable response rate is often judged to be around 33%; this begs the question of what the remaining 67% of recipients thought, and whether there is something unique about those that chose to respond that means responses cannot be generalized to the wider population. Other disadvantages are that it is not possible to guarantee that respondents will fill in a 'further comments' box or open-ended question section, or, where they do so, to probe meanings further or to ask for examples.

Approaches to qualitative research

As with the range of data sources, qualitative research is characterized by its 'immense diversity', in which each different approach has 'quite different traditions and procedures' (Yardley, 2000, pp. 216–217). Such traditions include sociology, social interactionism, linguistics, history, psychology and philosophy, or a mixture of these. The topic, as well as your own theoretical interests and leanings, will influence choice of method and this choice will, in turn, influence the research design, questions, data collected and the way the data is analysed. We will introduce four research methods (phenomenology, ethnography, grounded theory and narrative analysis) that are used frequently in health care research, and outline data collection and analysis procedures according to these different methods.

Phenomenology

The word 'phenomenology' has its origins in the Greek *phainein*, which means 'to appear'. Its origins are attributed to Husserl (1859–1938), a mathematician and philosopher, who sought to identify the true content of human consciousness; that is, to make explicit, or make 'appear', those things that humans are consciously aware of or experience. He described phenomenology as 'the scientific study of the essential structures of consciousness'; his proposed method is eidetic or descriptive, in which individuals are the vehicle through which the essential structure or 'essence' of the phenomenon may be accessed and described (Priest, 2002). Husserl's method suggests four fundamental processes: intentionality, reduction, description and essence, which are applied by individuals to their personal experience.

Intentionality is the process whereby, in consciousness, the mind focuses its thoughts on an object or idea. Phenomenological reduction (sometimes referred to as 'bracketing' or 'epoché') is the process that facilitates transcendence from our natural attitude (the common sense assumptions we use to make sense of the everyday world) to a phenomenological standpoint, in which we focus not on natural objects but on conscious ideas of those objects. Phenomenological reduction is, then, the deliberate suspension of judgement, commonly held beliefs and presuppositions about a particular phenomenon, in order to investigate it from a new perspective (Priest, 2002). A further strategy required to achieve this transcendence is imaginative variation, which involves asking questions of the phenomenon in order to remove non-essential features and to test its limits. Imaginative variation continues until a common understanding about the phenomenon has been achieved. Then, a description of the phenomenon can be produced and its essential structure or 'essence' uncovered.

Later manifestations of phenomenology have taken issue with the search for 'essence', arguing that each human will bring their own experience and interpretations to bear on phenomena and that there are likely to be as many unique descriptions of a phenomenon as there are people! Therefore, a branch of 'interpretative phenomenology' or hermeneutics (the science of interpretation) developed, based originally on the ideas of Heidegger (1889–1976). Hermeneutics produces an interpretation of the meaning of an experience or phenomenon. In carrying out the hermeneutic cycle, the researcher builds up an interpretation of a text, moving backwards and forwards through the text and between parts of it and the whole, carrying out micro analyses of small sections, and using these to challenge and reinterpret the overall sense of the whole text. The aim is to achieve a comprehensive and coherent interpretation.

Phenomenology's most recent manifestation, designed initially for use with within psychology, is Interpretive Phenomenological Analysis or IPA (Smith, Larkin and Flowers, 2009; Smith and Osborn, 2003). IPA draws on both phenomenology and symbolic interactionism (a belief that the meaning of objects, events and behaviours comes from the interpretation we give to them). Its aim is to explore how participants experience and make sense of their world, while at the same time acknowledging that the researcher is also trying to 'make sense of the participants making sense' of their world (Smith and Osborn, 2003, p. 51). The following steps can be taken to analyse qualitative interview data using an IPA approach (adapted from Smith and Osborn, 2003):

- Read the interview transcript a number of times;
- Use the left hand margin to annotate what is interesting or significant about what the respondent has said;
- Use the right hand margin to document emerging theme titles – concise phrases that capture the essential quality of what was found in the text. This moves the response to a higher level of abstraction;
- List emergent themes on a sheet of paper and look for connections between them – a more analytical or theoretical ordering;
- Cluster themes together into super-ordinate themes where possible and give a name to these;
- Check clusters with the transcript (iterative analysis);
- Produce a table of super-ordinate themes with their constituent themes, ordered coherently;
- Illustrate themes with verbatim quotations from the transcript;
- Drop any themes which do not fit well with the emerging structure or are not very rich in evidence in the transcript;
- Write up as a case study;
- Repeat with interviews from other participants, either starting from scratch or using themes from first participant as a starting point.

Ethnography

Ethnography is designed to understand the shared lives and experiences of cultural groups, from the perspective of the people within those groups. It has its origins in social anthropology and requires the researcher to spend considerable time in the field, sharing and observing the routine, normal aspects of life of those studied. In this way, it produces a detailed study of the 'way of life' of small groups in their social and cultural context. There are many forms of ethnography, including life history and visual ethnography (using photography or video) (Creswell, 2007). Creswell notes that the most traditional approach is realist ethnography, which produces an objective account of the situation, reporting on what is observed and overheard in the field, and written in the third person to demonstrate lack of personal bias on the part of the researcher. A more recent alternative is critical ethnography, in which the researcher aims to advocate on behalf of the group (often a marginalized group) being studied, and in this way empower the group to challenge their marginalized status. The broad steps required to conduct an ethnographic study are:

- Identify and locate a culture-sharing group to study;
- Select cultural themes or issues of relevance to this group;
- Carry out fieldwork (gather information of many types from where the group works and lives);
- From the data, produce a description of the group;
- Identify the rules, patterns and themes that emerge from the group that indicate how the group works and lives;
- Produce a cultural portrait of the group that incorporates the group's views as well as the views of the researcher. This may be in the form of words, pictures, plays or poems (adapted from Creswell, 2007).

Language based approaches

Given that language is the medium through which much social interaction takes place, a study of language and its use is a legitimate qualitative research approach. Language based research approaches include Discourse analysis (DA), introduced by Potter and Wetherell (1987), and Narrative analysis. We will explore narrative analysis in this chapter.

Narrative analysis

The basic assumption of a narrative approach to generating and analysing research data is that story telling is the primary means by which people make sense of and communicate human experience (McLeod, 2001). We live in a 'storied world' (Murray, 2003). Ask anyone to tell you about something and they will often naturally tell you a story – 'well. I remember once when I ...' Narrative analysis aims to uncover how people construct their world through language and stories It seeks to understand the meaning of an experience by exploring the stories that the person tells about that experience, and the way in which those stories are told.

The most common method of narrative data collection is the interview, and the interview style is likely to be unstructured or only lightly structured. Within the interview, we have two options – we can ask people specifically to tell a story, for example 'can you think of a time when that happened to you', or we can simply encourage people to talk freely and look for the presence, structure and function of stories within our interview transcripts afterwards. Or we might do both; we might begin, for example, with a broad question such as 'I'm interested in finding out about your recent experience of being in hospital. Can you start by telling me about how you came to be there...?' While many people are very willing to provide lengthy and detailed accounts of their experiences to a willing listener, it may be that specific prompts are needed to encourage more reticent participants towards 'story telling'.

In terms of data analysis, whereas other qualitative approaches tend to 'carve up' the data into themes, codes, categories or meaning units, narrative analysis aims for a more holistic approach to the data (Crossley, 2007), retaining the social context in which the stories are based and told (Murray, 2003). Riessman (1993) suggests that sections of text can be identified as stories if they have a beginning, a middle and an end, as well as a logical temporal sequence. Emden (1998) provides a step-by-step guide to conducting a narrative analysis:

- Read the text several times;
- Delete interviewer questions;
- Delete words that detract from the key idea of each sentence or group of sentences;
- Read the remaining text for sense;
- Repeat the last two steps several times;
- Identify fragments of themes (subplots);
- Move fragments of themes together to create a coherent core story.

However, it is worth noting that there are many other approaches. Labov and Waletzky's (1967) approach, for example enables us to identify the defining features of a story, which are orientation, complicating action, evaluation, resolution and coda; there are also many different ways of producing the 'core story', such as in stanza (poetic) form (Gee, 1986, 1991; McLeod and Balamoutsou, 2000).

Grounded theory

First developed in 1967 by Glaser and Strauss, the aim of grounded theory is to discover the underlying social forces that shape human behaviour and, from this, to generate new theory. This theory is developed from ('grounded in') the research data and is represented as a core category with related categories and concepts. In addition to generating theory, existing theories can be modified or developed further (McCann and Clark, 2009). There are two key processes:

Constant comparative analysis: data collection and analysis take place simultaneously; teasing out the categories and their related properties until saturation is reached, and a theory with sufficient detail and abstraction is generated. Saturation occurs when the researcher is seeing repeated examples of categories in the data similar to those already identified, and is confident that no further development of the category can be achieved (Glaser and Strauss, 1967).

Theoretical sampling: new data is collected specifically to compare with emerging categories and to establish conceptual boundaries that are related to the evolving theory. An outline for common grounded theory procedures that are used to help break down the original data, conceptualize it, and re-arrange it in new ways is:

- **Immersion in the data:** Reading and re-reading transcripts;
- **Open coding:** identifying and labelling meaningful units (words, phrases or sentences) in the text. By looking for similarities and asking questions, units or **categories** that are in essence very similar can eventually be labelled with the same name. The same data may be attributed to more than one category;
- **Writing definitions:** once categories appear to be saturated, definitions of the properties of each category are written;
- **Axial coding:** categories are refined and reduced, and new connections are made between them;
- **Selective coding:** one or two core categories are identified to which all other categories relate;
- **Emergent theory:** linking to existing theory and building a conceptual framework from which to develop a new (grounded) theory. The grounded theory offers a coherent account that explains the topic of interest;
- **Constant comparison** of new theory against existing data;
- **Theoretical sampling:** selecting more participants who it is believed will further illuminate or test the emergent theory.

A unique feature of grounded theory is that the literature review normally takes place after the data has been generated and analysed. There are two reasons for this. Firstly, it means that the researcher is not prejudiced by other theories and ideas and comes to the data 'fresh'; a similar concept to the 'bracketing' of descriptive phenomenology. Secondly, it is then possible to link existing research and theory with the concepts, constructs and properties identified within the grounded theory.

Since the inception of Grounded Theory, alternative approaches have been developed, notably that of Charmaz (2000), which takes the view that a definitive theory does not simply emerge from the data; rather, theory is constructed by the researcher through interaction with the data. In this way, the theory is only one of many possible interpretations of the data (Willig, 2001).

Generic qualitative approaches

What all these qualitative approaches to analysis have in common is that they all involve immersion in the data, identifying meanings, labelling or coding sections of the text, clustering them and testing them out. So why, you might ask, is there not simply a 'common' method for analysing all kinds of qualitative data? In fact, several authors have developed and described generic approaches to qualitative. These might broadly be described as qualitative content analysis. Content analysis originated in the 1950s as an approach to analysing text in the publishing industry, whereby text was broken down into quantifiable units (Berelson, 1952). The method was quickly challenged by Kracauer (1953) who argued that text lost its meaning through such reduction, and advocated a qualitative approach to content analysis whereby meanings and insights are elicited from the text more holistically within the context from which they are derived. Qualitative content analysis helps the researcher to create meanings in the text, through the construction of emergent themes. Codes or labels are assigned to sections of the data. This helps to reduce, organize and retrieve the data and supports the generation of ideas.

One approach to thematic content *analysis* is proposed by Newell and Burnard (2006) as a pragmatic approach and a way of analysing qualitative interview data without the need to be wedded to any particular tradition:

- **Stage 1:** Make notes or 'memos' after each interview on the topics talked about – thoughts, feelings and ideas that have occurred to the researcher;
- **Stage 2:** Read through transcripts and make notes on general themes;
- **Stage 3:** Re-read transcripts, writing down in the transcript margins as many headings as are needed to summarize/categorize/describe all aspects of the content (similar to 'open coding' in grounded theory);
- **Stage 4:** Look for similar or overlapping categories and combine them where possible. Aim for no more than 12 final category codes;
- **Stage 5:** Return to the transcripts with the final category codes, marking up the parts of the text where the category codes occur using a different coloured marker or highlighter pen. Draw one vertical line down the transcript from the first participant, two for the second, and so on (This is to identify from which interview each section came, once pages are cut up). Cut up the separately coloured sections and file separately;
- **Stage 6:** Write up findings based on the organized data. Illustrate with quotations from the text.

 Action Point

Select a piece of written text (part of a journal article, a page of a book, etc.), and type it into your computer. It should occupy no more than 30 lines on the page. Having been introduced to several different approaches to qualitative data analysis in this chapter, select two of the approaches and follow the analytical steps outlined with your own data. Compare the outcome of your analyses using the two methods.

Qualitative data analysis software

In today's computer age, it may seem that using highlighter pens, scissors and glue, as advocated by Newell and Burnard (2006), is a somewhat antiquated and cumbersome approach, particularly if there is a considerable amount of data to be worked through. An alternative is to use simple word processing packages to facilitate the highlighting, moving, cutting and pasting aspects of the process. Alternatively, it is possible to use qualitative data management packages such as NVivo or Ethnograph. Advantages include speed of coding and retrieval, the facility to attach notes and memos, and the production of index trees or other graphic mapping systems, all of which are time/date-stamped on print-outs so that the progress of a project is evident.

It is important to note, however, that such packages do not do the analysis for you. They simply aid in the management and organization of qualitative data. Decisions about codes, categories and themes are still left to you as the researcher, and it is still up to you to justify your analytic decisions.

Criticisms of qualitative research

Qualitative research is sometimes criticized as being unscientific and, therefore, of little value. Critics point out that as there is no real consensus on methods of data collection and analysis, and that it is a personal and subjective style of research, that it is difficult to demonstrate the reliability and validity of studies. (As we have seen in this chapter, methods and approaches are many and varied but there are, nevertheless, a number of common and key characteristics that define and justify the approach).

Other criticisms are that studies generally involve small numbers of participants and, therefore, findings cannot be generalized to the broader population; equally, that participants are not representative, as they may have been purposively selected for their specific knowledge or experience of a topic.

Overcoming criticisms: Rigour in qualitative research

We are not suggesting for one minute that qualitative research should not be subjected to critique and scrutiny, nor that it should not be evaluated in terms of its validity, reliability and generalizability. Nevertheless, demonstrating rigour is by no means straightforward. Cutcliffe and McKenna (1999) suggest that there are four possible ways of dealing with the difficulties:

- We can decide that it is impossible for *any* criteria to be used to judge qualitative studies;
- Qualitative studies should be judged using the same criteria and terminology as quantitative studies;
- Qualitative studies should be judged using criteria that are specifically developed for the qualitative paradigm;
- The credibility of qualitative research findings can be established by testing them with a deductive quantitative study.

We suggest that the traditional tests of rigour as applied within quantitative research need different emphases, given the essential subjectivity of qualitative studies, but that there is no major difficulty in using the same language (e.g. validity, reliability and generalizability), provided that its meaning in the qualitative context is explained and its use justified. Some approaches and suggestions for dealing with these tests of rigour are discussed below, as is an alternative approach to judging the quality of qualitative research.

Validity

Validity, in the qualitative context, is the extent to which the research is plausible, credible, trustworthy and defensible. A major challenge to achieving validity in qualitative research is researcher bias, whereby the research might selectively collect and record data, or base interpretations, on personal perspectives.

There are several ways in which validity can be increased and demonstrated. Firstly, the researcher should make explicit his or her presuppositions and subjective judgements about the research topic, so that the reader can judge to what extent the findings arise from the data presented. Using more than one data source (data triangulation; Chapters 2 and 11) can help to cross-check findings and, therefore, demonstrate validity. Using 'low inference descriptors', such as participants' verbatim quotations or stories, can help the reader to judge the credibility of the analyses made. Finally, validity can also be assessed in terms of how well the data represents the phenomena under scrutiny, so it is common to return analyses to research participants, to ask how well the findings resonate with their own experience and reflect their perspectives (respondent validation). However, there are counter arguments to returning analyses to participants for checking; for example, Newell and Burnard (2006) point out that such checking can never be accurate, as interviews happened in the past, and the analysis has involved separating out sections of the interview from the whole. Rather, it is argued, the researcher should have confidence in his or her own interpretation and acknowledge its inherent subjectivity.

Reliability

Reliability is the extent to which the results of a study are dependable and repeatable in different circumstances (such as with a different researcher or at a different time). Clearly, no two researchers would produce exactly the same analyses of a given piece of data, and this would not necessarily be desirable, as it would remove the essential subjectivity of qualitative research. However, steps can be taken to ensure that analyses are as reliable as possible. These include ensuring technical accuracy in recording and transcribing intensive engagement with the data and frequent moving between data and interpretation.

Generalizability

This refers to the extent to which research findings are transferable to other situations. Qualitative research is often thought to be weak in its generalizability, particularly as participants are often selected purposively in order to fulfil the needs of a particular study. However, findings from qualitative studies can be used to develop, test, refine and challenge theoretical propositions (Priest, 2002).

It is always important, in written accounts of qualitative studies, to provide detailed information about all aspects of the study, such as participants, recruitment methods, the research setting, and the data generation and analysis methods, in order for readers to decide how the findings may be applied.

Judging the quality of qualitative research

As an alternative to retaining the 'traditional' tests of rigour, Yardley (2000) suggests four flexible measures that may be used to judge the quality of qualitative research, while pointing out that these measures are in themselves open to interpretation by the person judging its quality:

Sensitivity to Context: Has the researcher demonstrated awareness of the theoretical context, the socio-cultural setting of the research, and the relationship between the researcher and participants?

Commitment and Rigour: Has the researcher reported sufficient detail to judge the thoroughness of data collection, analysis and reporting, and is there evidence that the researcher has had prolonged engagement with the topic?

Transparency and Coherence: Are the arguments and supporting evidence presented clear and persuasive? Has the researcher made honest disclosures about assumptions made and decisions taken? Such disclosure is often described as reflexivity, which is discussed later in this Chapter.

Impact and Importance: Are the findings presented likely to be useful in relation to the objectives set? Will they add to theory/knowledge or practice?

As Yardley indicates, the research process should be made transparent and communicated coherently within any written report, such that readers can trace the decision processes relating to theory, methodology and analysis throughout the life of the study. An audit trail or methodological log (Finlay and Gough, 2003) should be maintained for the duration of the study and used to inform the written report; this is commonly achieved through the maintenance of a research diary in which ideas, decisions, and reasons for them are recorded.

The role of the researcher in qualitative research

It is important to be aware that complete objectivity or detachment on the part of the researcher is impossible within qualitative research. The researcher is always subjectively involved to some degree. In some qualitative approaches, such as phenomenology, researchers attempt to retain objectivity through 'bracketing' or setting aside their own assumptions and knowledge, and trying to see the phenomenon through fresh eyes. In other approaches, such as grounded theory, they aim to remain sensitive to the data by delaying any exploration of the relevant literature until all data has been gathered.

As an alternative approach, given that objectivity is not possible or even desirable, many qualitative researchers acknowledge their own interpretive viewpoint and its influence on the research through the process of reflexivity. Reflexivity is considered by some to be a defining feature of qualitative research (Finlay and Gough, 2003), in recognition of the fact that research is co-constructed between researcher, participant and their relationship. Finlay and Gough outline different types of reflexivity including introspection and mutual collaboration, and suggest how it may be achieved within research projects. It is common, as part of being reflexive, for researchers to write a first person account of their own orientation and position within the research.

Action Point

Find a journal article that reports a qualitative study. What evidence is there within the paper that the author is being reflexive?

Conclusion

In summary, qualitative research is neither 'better' nor 'worse'; 'easier' or 'harder' than quantitative research – it is just different. The guiding principle is to select the most appropriate approach with which to answer the research question(s) you have identified. In some cases, this means using a combination of approaches and methods, such as when you need some in-depth information to add to the information provided by statistical analysis of data. This notion is illustrated in Chapters 11 and 16.

Action Point

Comparing Qualitative and Quantitative Research

Now that you have read chapters on both quantitative and qualitative methods, try to complete the boxes in Table 8.1.

Table 8.1   Key Features of Qualitative and Quantitative Research

	Qualitative Research	Quantitative Research
Objective/Purpose		
Participants		
Data Collection methods/tools		
Data Analysis methods		
Outcomes of research		
Advantages		
Disadvantages		

References

Berelson, B. (1952) *Content Analysis in Communication Research*, Free Press, Glencoe, IL.

Bryman, A. (1988) *Quantity and Quality in Social Research (Contemporary Social Research)*, Routledge, London.

Charmaz, K. (2000) *Constructing Grounded Theory: A Practical Guide Through Qualitative Analysis (Introducing Qualitative Methods series)*, Sage, Thousand Oaks.

Creswell, J.W. (2007) *Qualitative Inquiry and Research Design. Choosing among Five Approaches*, 2nd edn, Sage, Thousand Oaks.

Crossley, M. (2007) Narrative analysis, in *Analysing Qualitative Data in Psychology* (eds E. Lyons and A. Coyle), Sage, London, pp. 131–157.

Cutcliffe, J. and McKenna, H. (1999) Establishing the credibility of qualitative research findings: the plot thickens. *Journal of Advanced Nursing*, **30** (2), 374–380.

Emden C. (1998) Conducting a narrative analysis. *Collegian*, **5** (3), 34–39.

Fern, E.F. (2001) *Advanced Focus Group Research*, Sage, London.

Finlay, L. and Gough, B. (2003) *Reflexivity. A Practical Guide for Researchers in Health and Social Sciences*, Blackwell, Oxford.

Gee, J.P. (1986) Units in the production of narrative discourse. *Discourse Processes*, **9**, 391–422.

Gee, J.P. (1991) A linguistic approach to narrative. *Journal of Narrative and Life History*, **1** (1), 15–39.

Glaser, B. and Strauss, A. (1967) *The Discovery of Grounded Theory*, Aldine, Chicago.

Hawker, S. and Kerr, C. (2007) Doing grounded theory, in *Analysing Qualitative Data in Psychology* (eds E. Lyons and A. Coyle), Sage, London, pp. 87–97.

Kracauer, S. (1953) The challenge to qualitative content analysis. *Public Opinion Quarterly*, **16**, 631–642

Labov, W. and Waletzky, J. (1967) Narrative analysis: Oral versions of personal experience, in *Essays on the Verbal and Visual Arts* (ed. J. Helm), University of Washington Press, Seattle.

McLeod, J. and Balamoutsou, S. (2000) A method for qualitative narrative analysis of psychotherapy transcripts, in *Qualitative Psychotherapy Research: Methods and Methodology* (eds J. Frommer and D.L. Rennie), Pabst, Berlin.

McLeod, J. (2001) *Qualitative Research in Counselling and Psychotherapy*, Sage, London.

Murray, M. (2003) Narrative psychology, in *Qualitative Psychology. A Practical Guide to Research Methods* (ed. J.A. Smith), Sage, London, pp. 111–132.

Newell, R. and Burnard, P. (2006) *Vital Notes for Nursing Research: Research for Evidence-based Practice*, Blackwell, Oxford.

Payne, S. (2007) Grounded theory, in *Analysing Qualitative Data in Psychology* (eds E. Lyons and A. Coyle), Sage, London, pp. 65–86.

Potter, J. and Wetherell, M. (1987) *Discourse and Social Psychology: Beyond Attitudes and Behaviour*, Sage, London.

Priest, H. (2002) An approach to the phenomenological analysis of data. *Nurse Researcher*, **10** (2), 50–63.

Riessman, C. (1993) *Narrative Analysis*, Sage, Newbury Park.

Roberts, P.M. (1997) Planning and running a focus group. *Nurse Researcher*, **4** (4), 78–82.

Smith, J.A., Larkin, M. and Flowers, P. (2009) *Interpretative Phenomenological Analysis: Theory, Method and Research. Understanding Method and Application*, Sage, London.

Smith, J.A. and Osborn, M. (2003) Interpretative qualitative analysis, in (ed. J.A. Smith), *Qualitative Psychology. A Practical Guide to Research Methods*, Sage, London, pp. 51–80.

Tschudin, V. (1995) *Counselling Skills for Nurses*, 4th edn, Ballière Tindall, London.

Willig, C. (2001) *Introducing Qualitative Research in Psychology*, Open University Press, Maidenhead.

Yardley, L. (2000) Dilemmas in qualitative health research. *Psychology and Health*, **15**, 215–228.

Further reading

Greenbaum, T.L. (1998) *The Handbook for Focus Group Research*, 2nd edn, Sage, London.

Krueger, R.A. and Casey, M.A. (2009) *Focus Groups: a Practical Guide for Applied Research*, 4th edn, Sage, London.

Litosseliti, L. (2003) *Using Focus Groups in Research*, Continuum International Publishing Group, London.

McCann, T.V. and Clark, E. (2003) Grounded theory in nursing research: Part 1. methodology (grounded theory). *Nurse Researcher*, **11** (2), 7–18.

Redmond, R. and Curtis, E. (2009) Focus groups: Principles and process. *Nurse Researcher*, **16** (3), 57–69.

Schiffrin, D., Tannen, D. and Hamilton, H. (eds) (2003) *The Handbook of Discourse Analysis*, Blackwell, Oxford.

Stewart, D.W., Shamdasani, P.N. and Rook, D.W. (2006) *Focus Groups: Theory and Practice*, Sage, London.

Wolcott, H.F. (2009) *Writing up Qualitative Research*, 3rd edn, Sage, London.

Resources

Ethnograph 6: http://www.qualisresearch.com/.
Interpretative Phenomenological Analysis: http://www.ipa.bbk.ac.uk/.
NVivo 8: http://www.qsrinternational.com/.

9 Making Your Case: Writing for Your Audience

Mike Brough, Susan Smith, Paula Roberts and Helena Priest

Introduction

Writing was developed for record keeping and then communication only about 6000 years ago. Even 500 years ago, the majority of people in Europe could not read or write. Thus, reading and writing are clearly *learnt*. Your writing style is something that will constantly develop, and that you will adapt to the audience you wish to address. This chapter, therefore, focuses on academic writing. It considers the different contexts in which you might need to write, and the different approaches you might use in those contexts. We consider how you might use the work of others within your work, and explain the terms 'plagiarism' and 'copyright'. The chapter includes examples of good academic practice, including referencing in texts and the construction of reference lists.

 Action Point

Look at a piece of work you have written in the past for a project or assignment. In what way (if any) has your writing style altered since then? Who was the target audience, what was the purpose of the work and how has it affected your writing style?

 Action point

To help you to appreciate different writing styles, stop reading this chapter (temporarily!) and summarize the writing differences in: a textbook, a research journal, a leaflet on healthy eating, a diary, and a newspaper. List the main similarities and differences, such as sentence length, vocabulary, typeface, format and audience.

You may have commented on differences in structure, presentation, layout, style and language use. We will begin by focusing on language and consider issues of structure and style later in the chapter.

Writing and research

Linguistics, grammar and psychology

If you want to follow up some of the points made in this chapter, you might find yourself picking up books on linguistics. You will find the accepted view of writing is that it is one of the ways language can be expressed; speech is another type of language expression. Speech and written communication are two very different ways of expressing language. Language is best thought of as an intermediate between ideas and their manifestation as speech or written communication.

You may believe that there is a 'correct' way to use language with correct grammar, spelling and punctuation. There are conventional uses of language, grammar, spelling and punctuation, and, if you stick to the conventions, your writing will probably be accepted by your peers; or, at least, judged on the merits of its content. If you break the conventions, invent new words, use unusual spellings, or punctuate in arbitrary personal ways, you may alienate readers; they may stop reading your work. Great literary writers such as Shakespeare and Lewis Carroll felt empowered to break these rules, to make their own rules. If you want to compete with them, fine, but you are reading the wrong book!

Although we no longer have a simple prescriptive view of grammar, it is still believed that language uses some basic categories of structure, for example nouns (proper nouns for specific identifiable things, and common nouns for categories of thing or abstractions of things), as verbs, and so on.

You should also note that punctuation is now regarded as a way of breaking up the sentence structure (syntax) so that it is easier to see. Linguists do not think of punctuation as being a technique for explaining how sentences should be read or spoken (a comma is a short pause, the voice should go up when you get to a question mark . . .), although this was formerly a common description of punctuation (short pause/break, long pause/breaks, full stop, etc.). Box 9.1 summarizes some common stylistic, grammatical and punctuation issues, with tips on how to avoid errors in your writing.

Box 9.1   Tips on Academic Writing

Simplicity

There is no particular merit in using long or obscure words where simple ones will do. Similarly, excessively long sentences serve only to confuse the reader and obscure your message. Of course, it will be necessary to include technical terms relating to your discipline, which is acceptable, provided that they are initially defined and explained.

Abbreviations

It is acceptable to use abbreviations, provided that the full version is given the first time that the term is used. For example:

> Patients in the High Dependency Unit (HDU) expect to receive high quality care from experienced staff. It is therefore HDU policy to provide training courses for all clinical staff.

Person

The use of the first person singular – I/me – should generally be avoided in academic writing, as should the substitution of 'the student' or 'the author' for 'I'. However, there are some instances where writing in the first person is acceptable or even encouraged, such as in reflective writing or professional development diaries.

Spelling, grammar and punctuation

These *are* important and should always be checked either manually or by using checking facilities on a word-processing package. Remember, though, that spell-checking facilities will not pick up words correctly spelled but used in the wrong context; for example, it would accept all the following sentences:

Students should make an appointment to discuss **their** progress (CORRECT)
Students should make an appointment to discuss **there** progress (INCORRECT)
Students should make an appointment to discuss **they're** progress (INCORRECT)

A grammar check on your word-processor should, however, pick up the incorrect uses.
The use of apostrophes often causes difficulties. It is not uncommon to see signs advertising goods for sale such as:
APPLE'S 50p, PEAR'S 45p.
Apostrophes are never necessary to denote a plural. They are used either to denote the omission of a letter or letters from a word or phrase, such as **haven't**, or **can't** (and are best avoided in academic writing), or to denote possession, such as **the patient's temperature** (singular) or **the nurses' home** (plural). Care must be taken with words which become plural without the addition of an 's' such as **women** or **children.** To denote possession, the following would be used: **the women's group** or **the Children's Charter**.
An exception is the possessive form of the word **it.** If instead of saying **the cat's basket,** we wanted to use the word **it** instead of **the cat,** the correct phrase would be **its basket** and not **it's basket.** The apostrophe version (**it's**) is used only for the abbreviation of 'it is'.
Grammar-checking facilities available within most word-processing packages are useful, but usually make alternative suggestions rather than offer definitive alterations, so do not place too much reliance upon these unless you are confident in your ability to accept or reject suggestions.
Lynn Truss's (2003) best-selling book 'Eats, shoots and leaves' makes many punctuation difficulties very clear, in a humorous and accessible way.

Gender neutral language

Unless the gender of a person is known, do not make assumptions in your writing; for example, do not refer to nurses as 'she' and doctors as 'he'. Where the gender is unknown, some writers suggest using 'he or she'; 'she or he','s/he' or alternating between 'she' and 'he'. Writers who feel such usages are clumsy suggest the singular use of 'they', 'their' and 'them', and although strictly speaking grammatically incorrect, these terms are now widely accepted in academic writing. Take care, also, with the use of phrases such as 'the best man for the job' and use non-gender specific alternatives where possible.

In the last few years, electronic sources have been available to carry out research on what people actually do in writing. There are even some studies of the relationship between the way people write and the effectiveness of that writing. This is particularly true in pedagogic (teaching) literature, but there are also some studies on the visibility of materials and how this is affected by their language, keywords and abstracts. See Chapter 10 for further discussion on writing abstracts and selecting keywords.

The context of writing

There are many different contexts in which you might need to write. Some examples are:

1. A university essay on the relationship between a healthcare professional and a patient.
2. A proposal for some healthcare research (Chapter 3) to be considered by an ethics committee (Chapter 6).
3. A paper for a conference, describing ongoing progress in a research project; a joint paper written by yourself and others involved in a large project, and intended for publication in an authoritative journal; or a report of a meta-analysis of all studies of factors affecting incidence of late-onset diabetes (see Chapter 10 for more on disseminating research evidence).
4. A report to the management of an NHS Hospital Trust, summarizing findings on ongoing work to reduce the risk of infections acquired during hospital stays.
5. A document laying out hospital sterilization protocols, to minimize risk of infection; a leaflet for gout sufferers, explaining which foods and drinks to avoid; or an online help page, to provide guidance on lifestyle for those suffering from gout.
6. A chapter for a textbook on the kidney (in an undergraduate textbook); a textbook, describing the history of epidemiology and disease control.
7. A personal letter to a much-loved relative who has just been diagnosed with a serious illness.
8. A newspaper article on why a greater proportion of people seem to be dying of cancer in the early twenty first century than a hundred years ago, or why men living in some parts of the United Kingdom have lower life expectancies than those living in other areas.
9. A script for a television drama set in a hospital.

They all have a vaguely healthcare slant, but are quite different. Some might need to be produced as a professional task in a health or medical career. By contrast, writing a university essay is contrived; it is not ideal practice for any of the other tasks. However, university teachers may help students acquire writing skills by getting them to practice writing in hypothetical situations related to some or all of these different writing contexts.

We deliberately included one example of creative writing in the above list (the last), and we should also note that genres such as plays, novels and poetry also have their own distinctive style and relevance in healthcare. However, the rest of this chapter focuses on the other types of writing.

Writing styles should be chosen bearing in mind the following factors:

- **target audience:** who is expected to read the text; for example a medical researcher/ practitioner (in the same or different field), health manager, politician or the general public;
- **intent of the communication:** to present facts/observations, interpret facts or propose a course of action, for example.

These factors will determine the nature of the communication and its content. Depending on the audience, different assumptions about prior knowledge and understanding of the subject will be appropriate. It should also be obvious that documents with different intents will marshal different material to achieve that purpose.

The writing style will also depend on the aim of the communication. For example, research papers should not contain extraneous, redundant information. On the other hand, a textbook might include illustrative examples and worked discussions of the theory of common situations. Less obviously, perhaps, the writing style should be one that is acceptable to the target audience.

In the context of professional writing, there are a number of assumptions that probably always apply, even in quite different contexts. One is that the writing should be honest and not intended to deceive. We will assume that the intention will always be to present facts and arguments in the clearest way. This means that writing styles should be precise and be aimed at conveying intended information in the best way to avoid alternative interpretations from the one intended.

Different layers of the communication

The final document will contain elements relating to many different aspects of the communication. The ideas and concepts under discussion are a very important aspect of the communication, but they may not be very visible in the document. These are deep aspects of the communication. By contrast, punctuation (used to help clarify sentence structure) is a shallow aspect of communication. Table 9.1 outlines a more complete list of issues in the communication, roughly organized from deep to shallow issues.

Table 9.1 Levels of communication.

Level	Concerned with
Semantics, conceptual	Concepts and ideas in the subject domain; what they mean and how they are related
Organizational	The way a complex subject domain is broken into simpler inter-related chunks
Argumentation	How facts, interpretation and arguments are organized to advance an explanation or conclusion
Vocabulary	Choice of words to represent concepts under discussion
Rhetoric	Choice of mood, voice, style, for the writer–reader relationship and the aim of the communication
Grammar	How words, phrases and clauses are put together
Punctuation	Use of conventional marks to clarify grammatical structure
Typeface	Choice of typeface for readability and legibility and to distinguish different document elements
Typographic	Page layout, paragraph and line spacing, indentation

The table mostly goes from the 'large' aspects of a communication down to the detail, but this is not absolute. For example, organization is an issue at the most abstract level of communication. It is also important at lower levels: in choice of sentence and paragraph length.

Relating your writing to that of others

It is rare that your work will stand in isolation. You may want to compare your findings or conclusions with those of others, to confirm/extend their findings, or advance an alternative assumption. We should explicitly recognize and explain this dependency, as far as is possible. It is, of course, unlikely that you will know what all the influences on your thinking were. For this reason, it is suggested that you keep a note of what you read (and when), and even your own notes summarizing your reading, together with your reaction to what you read. You may find that something out of your current area of research might influence your thinking in a different area many years later.

It is also interesting to note that new ideas evolve and develop, with many people contributing to the ideas. The concept, approach or framework develops and evolves, with many people contributing a small, maybe even imperceptible amount to it, so it is often hard to trace your ideas back to their origins, but you should try. There are two main reasons why any dependency on the work of others should be acknowledged explicitly. The first is that it is part of the scholarly ethos. The second is that if your argument depends on the ideas or research results of others, someone reading your writing critically may need to review those sources if they wish to validate your conclusion. If you claim observational data supports your case, you must explain how the data was obtained, so that that research might be repeated. If you refer to arguments advanced by others to support your conclusion, you must give the critical reader sufficient information for them to review all the supporting arguments you have used in claiming your conclusions. This is a requirement for reproducibility and traceability of any arguments you put forward to support rational, objective conclusions.

Note an implicit paradigm of how we convince others of the truth of observations, validity of a particular point of view, or efficacy of treatments in particular situations. It should be done by clearly formulating an argument, backed up by verifiable evidence, and reviewed within an explicitly stated framework. This is the 'evidence based approach' (Chapters 1 and 2). It is the application of the modern scientific paradigm to situations where we are considering interventions to achieve explicit goals, set by ethical or sociological considerations. In such a paradigm, traceability of evidence and observations is essential.

Academic writing may be defined as writing with a wish to be objective, honest and scholarly in presenting our views, observations and conclusions with our peers in a given discipline. Those peers constitute a scholarly community; an 'academy'. The examples in the section 'The context of writing' were deliberately picked so that some could be described as academic writing and some as professional (but not academic) writing.

The document lifecycle

Books describing how to write a university essay often explain that you should research sources (discovering which are authoritative and which are derivative or secondary), make notes on the subject, plan the structure of your essay, draft the essay, review the essay and then hand in the essay. The essay is a personal creation, written in a short time frame, on a well-defined topic. It gives practice in researching a topic, critical review of ideas, organization of complex material and writing skills, including referencing. It is usually constrained by students being told that they should write in a particular style, for example an 'academic writing' style.

As mentioned earlier, however, writing essays is rare outside the school and university environment. Few will earn their living by writing essays. The nearest profession we can think of is that of journalism, although the writing style is quite different from what one might learn in writing essays at university. We have already met some of the very different types of document that might need to be written, and remarked on how the vocabulary, writing style, organization and so on might differ in those different types of document. What is perhaps less obvious is that the writing life cycle will differ.

Sources

Let us consider how we might plan the writing of a research report. Whilst at university or college, we are often asked to carry out research and then write it up. But this would be a very poor model for carrying out and writing up research, whether it involved controlled experiments, epidemiological surveys, or other approaches. The most obvious difference is that the researching of the literature would occur before and during the research. We do not do the research, then carry out a literature search so the report could be written.

The information that we need to write something may have been collated specifically for that writing task. This is typical in a university essay; indeed, it is good practice to ask students to list their sources in a bibliography (Box 9.4) and maybe even hand in their notes on those sources. However, real-life writing situations have a wider range of sources for our ideas used in that writing; indeed, we may not always be aware of where we got those ideas from. A responsible academic would, therefore, keep a notebook of what they had read in their subject, many shelves of books, a database of papers, maybe even filed print versions of the documents with notes about the subject. Nowadays, of course, digital copies of articles can be far easier to search than their print equivalent.

Since the early 1990s, an increasing amount of information has been disseminated via the World Wide Web. Many sources will be of this type. This brings some advantages. For example, the material is in electronic form, it can be saved compactly and quickly retrieved, but there are also downsides. One problem is that a web page may often change after you have read it; it may even disappear. By contrast, if you read and photocopied a journal article, you can be confident it won't have changed after you read it. Some web sites may offer a permalink option, which will link to that particular version of the page you were viewing. The permalink can then be included in writing reference details, along with the original date you accessed the page.

A more insidious danger of material being available in electronic form is that is easy to slip into misusing it. A quick cut and paste, and a bit of rewording, and we have a new document, but this is plagiarism (see below). Cutting and pasting can be used as a more efficient way of quoting someone else; quotation marks are then obligatory (or the equivalent block quotation), but cutting and pasting should never be used if the intention is to paraphrase the original source – as mentioned, rewording is plagiarism. The discipline is thus:

1. Take a read-only copy of an electronic source and record when you made the copy (read only, just in case you accidentally modify the other author's text).

2. If you subsequently access the web page and find it has changed, take a new copy of it; retain the first copy, too, in case you have referred to it in anything you wrote after your first access, but before you found it had changed.
3. If you need to refer to ideas from the archived text, give the source, and when you made the copy of it.
4. If you wish to quote something from the web page, copy (exactly) text from it, and enclose the copied text in quotes in your writing.
5. Never modify the text you copied; it should be regarded as read-only.

What about your own previous writing? Isn't it fair to cut and paste your own work? Not really. It's just lazy, and an abuse of your readers. If you want to summarize your own ideas, then you could write a book, or set up a web page, and update it from time to time and identify updates or revisions by using version numbers. Once you have published a document in a journal, you should refer to it, not reuse it. It can no longer be regarded as free content for future writing. Summarize your previous findings/opinions and give references.

After you have written your document

Once a student has written an essay, there is an immense sense of relief. The student may be keen to see the mark they have been awarded, and the more thoughtful will look forward to getting comments back on how they could have improved the logic, conceptual organization and argumentation of their work; and critical remarks about use of English, and punctuation, too, perhaps. Once out of the learning situation, however, completing the first version of the document is unlikely to be the end of the story. There are three parts of the lifecycle that do not occur in most student essays, but do occur in real-life situations:

1. *Editing:*
   a. *Technical editing:* reviews the intellectual content of a written work for accuracy, coherency, originality, and so on.
   b. *Copy-editing:* reviews grammar, punctuation and spelling in a written work; it may include advice on simplifying language to improve communication.
2. *Placement and advertising:* finding ways to make the work visible to a wider audience; for example, by providing a good title and abstract, maybe choosing keywords for web and electronic papers.
3. *Content management:* the provision of controlled access to authorized readers over the time the document has currency, management of revisions (version management) and final destruction or archiving of the document.

Technical editing may be carried out by the original author, taking into account the comments of reviewers. The reviewers may be course team members (for course work), research team members (for a research report), or external, often anonymous reviewers (for a journal paper). Technical editing may involve deletion of large sections of the original and/or additions of new sections. Most commonly, technical editing leads to some restructuring of the report and reformulation of detailed arguments and conclusions.

Copy-editing is usually carried out in a similar way to technical editing, but on the advice of someone with experience in publication, and a good knowledge of writing styles, grammar, punctuation and, to a lesser extent, typography and typesetting. Any author can learn a lot from the input of a good copy editor.

Most universities allow students to get others to help them with copy-editing in their essays (remember to check your own organisation's regulations and guidelines first). Technical editing is not generally allowed in university-assessed essays, as it would compromise their nature as personal work. A good university programme will include opportunities for a wide range of written reports, some of which would use technical editing. Once you move on from university, you will find the various types of editing process are a very important part of the document life-cycle. It is no good writing a brilliant exposition if no-one reads it. So you should think about where you are going to place it (this is further discussed in Chapter 10) for maximum effect.

Scoping your document

If you are asked to write an essay, you know what the scope of it is. At least, you will have a rough idea of what it is meant to cover. One of the first things you have to do is decide what to put in and what to leave out. If you miss out important points or include extraneous, unnecessary material, you will lose marks, but at least you will have a rough idea of what it should cover.

When it comes to writing up research, you have a much more open-ended situation. Should you just write one report when you have finished your research? Logical, but impractical; when will you know your research is finished? In fact, you are likely to find the decision is driven by political constraints. Maybe you should write a research report each year, or maybe there is an annual conference or special issue of a journal that you need to meet the deadline for. If you have been funded by a funding body, then there will be a time by which you will need to write a final report.

It should be clear that sometimes you will be writing several documents describing the research. This is unavoidable, particularly if the reports have different audiences and objectives: an end of funding report should show you met the original research plans, while a journal paper should show how (if at all) your research has contributed to the knowledge in that area. You need to spend some time planning which reports you will write, when you will write them, and the style in which you will write them.

It is tempting to write many papers, each covering a small part of your research, and getting each accepted in a reputable journal or conference. That way, you have more papers, and each is smaller and may thus have more chance of being accepted for publication. You should be careful not to abuse this just to push up the count of your publications (particularly if each of your papers cites the others). This is sometimes called the salami approach (slice the results up thin ...) and should be avoided. Your publications should be judged on the merit of their contribution to knowledge, not just 'counted'. You should include related results and ideas together, in one publication. That way, it will be a positive contribution to knowledge in the field.

What you choose not to put in is very important. You should not include irrelevant material, but you should always report negative findings from your research. If you only report what you consider positive findings, you can considerably distort the information. For example (a hypothetical case), suppose you looked at 20 different factors influencing whether mothers opting for home births needed to be referred to hospital for delivery. You might have a sample of 100 such births to look at, and (suppose) 30 of the 100 had to be referred to the hospital. As you looked at 20 factors, just by chance, some will have a very high correlation with those 30 deliveries. If you entitle your paper 'A study of the two main factors influencing referral of home deliveries to hospital' and then discuss two factors, the reader might think: 'This is significant'. You should really have described the study as originally designed, with all twenty factors. Statisticians can then point out the fact that the use of '5% levels' is somewhat misleading, given that you started with 20 factors. If you make it look as though there were only ever two factors under consideration, then your report will be misleading (see Chapter 7 for more information).

Similarly, if you were working for a pharmaceutical company and you are reporting a drug trial and a totally unexpected side effect occurred in a small number of the study patients, you have a moral and ethical obligation to report it.

Readability

Having completed your paper or essay, you may wonder how it would read to someone else. You can check your use of punctuation in the humorous 'Eats, shoots and leaves (Truss, 2003). You can check your writing and use of correct English grammar, syntax, style and choice of words in the latest edition of 'Fowler' (1998) or the Oxford Style Guide (Ritter, 2003), or you can ask someone else to read what you have written. If another person can make sense of what you have written, especially if that person is unfamiliar with the content, then that is a good measure of its readability. However, if you want a more objective measure, you can use a readability index such as the Flesh Reading Ease Score or the Flesh-Kinkaid Grade Level Score. These scores can be requested on word programming programs such as Microsoft Word, after a spelling and grammar check has been carried out. Readability scores are calculated from the numbers of syllables used per word and number of words used in a sentence. The logic is that if you use long words (where short ones would do) or too many long sentences, you may confuse your reader and reduce the readability of your work. However, do not assume that 'good' scores are necessarily a good thing; as Hart (2000) has noted: 'There's almost no correlation between the main readability indexes and actual readability, and there won't be . . . until someone develops a tool that can parse the content of text in the specific context of a well-defined audience'. So perhaps a long-suffering friend or colleague may be able to do as good a job!

Using others' ideas in writing

The first principle is that it should always be possible to distinguish your work from that of others. If you do not make this distinction, then it will appear that it is your work, when it is actually someone else's. Failure to declare that an element of what you have presented as your work is actually not your work is plagiarism. You should note that plagiarism is an absolute offence. Even if you do not plagiarize someone else's work deliberately, if it is their work, not yours, but you present it in a way that implies it is your work, then your work is plagiaristic.

The analogy often used is that of speeding. If you exceed the speed limit, then you are guilty. 'I didn't know I was doing 65 mph', or 'My speedometer is faulty', or 'I didn't know it was a 50 mph limit' are not defences. Knowing your speed, maintaining your vehicle and watching for road signs are legal responsibilities when you engage in a critical task such as driving a road vehicle. Proper attribution of ideas and work is a similar responsibility if you claim to be a scholar. The ultimate sanction may be quite draconian (e.g. losing your job). As honest scholarship is an important principle in all academic disciplines, plagiarism is an anathema to all scholars and academics. Today, most universities will request at least a sample of assignments to be submitted electronically; this is so they can by checked using software such as 'Tunitin' (http://turnitin.com/static_jisc/ac_uk_index.html; Turnitin allows students' work to be checked for 'improper citation or potential plagiarism by comparing it against continuously updated databases' (Turnitin, 2009). In fact, the whole manuscript of this textbook has been checked for plagiarism using Turnint!)

Reasons for referencing

Apart from avoiding plagiarism, Cottrell (2008) identifies other reasons why we should reference.

It is courteous to the author of the document referenced to acknowledge their work

As authors, we certainly want to know where and how our work has been used. In the modern world, referencing also drives the visibility of research in search engines, leading to improved prominence of both the authors and the article. Thompson Scientific uses the number of times an article from a particular journal has been cited as part of a calculation to determine the journal's impact in practice (Garfield, 2005). This impact factor is a measure of the esteem of a journal within its field, calculated annually by total number of citations received by that journal in that year to articles published over the previous two years, divided by the total number of citable items published by the journal in that two year period. Journal Citation Reports (JCR, http://thomsonreuters.com/content/press_room/sci/448197) indicate this impact factor; most journal home pages give their own impact factor. They are used as a proxy for the importance of a journal to its field and are hugely influential in helping authors to determine which publications to submit their research to, and help libraries determine which journals to stock.

It helps the reader locate the original source

A good reference list from an appropriate article is still one of the quickest and most favoured ways of locating further information on a specific topic. A bad reference list often gives a poor impression of a piece of work, and has the knock on effect of undermining the work to which it is attached. Reviewing the references is an important part of the critical evaluation of a paper. Poor referencing can affect the overall assessment of the quality of your research. This can be very important for researchers planning a follow-up article, a systematic review, or providing an evidence based summary for use in practice.

It enables double checking

Referencing improves your workflow and saves time when you want to go back and double check your work.

It instils confidence in the writing

Thorough research and good referencing can add credibility to your article. Good evidence based practice is essential in the workplace. The ability to justify decisions can help improve both local and national practice and, therefore, patient care. More importantly, it also helps to support decisions when things may go wrong and legal action is taken.

Although these are the main reasons why good referencing skills are required, it also helps the experienced reader locate the information they require with greater ease. When presented with a paper, we expect a certain format. As someone looking for specific information, we know where to go to examine the methodology of an experiment or to get a summary of conclusions. We also have set expectations of where to find references to highlight arguments or for further information. To make this easier for the author, not only do we display an acceptable layout of any report or article, but we have devised standards to determine how and when we use referencing.

A further principle of referencing is that you should distinguish between when you use or refer to other people's ideas and when you use their material. If you wish to summarize, review, or criticize someone else's ideas or findings originally reported in a paper or book, then you can either refer to that original publication or summarize the ideas given there, together with a reference to that publication. If you wish to quote an extract from the other scholar's work, that is acceptable, but you must make it clear that you are using their words, not their ideas. Conventionally, the quoted extract is shown between quotation marks, but longer sections could be shown as an indented paragraph, with the source reference below. The original source of the quotation must always be given; otherwise, it is plagiarism. Drawings and photographs should similarly be shown as having been taken from an earlier work (copyright permission is generally required, see below). If a diagram is a modification of a previously published diagram, it should be labelled, '*derived from that in* . . .' (and the reference given).

If you quote someone else, you must quote *exactly* what they said, even if you don't like their choice of words. You cannot alter them. You either summarize their ideas or quote their words. Rewording what they said is plagiarism, as discussed below. If you feel you really want to make editorial comments on their words, this is possible.

Example

Jones explains that 'one of the most critical factors in setting up a good relationship [rapport] with the patient is . . .' (Jones, 2003).

What is in the square brackets is an insertion that was not in the original material. Here it has been used to suggest an alternative word. It may also add additional information to help the reader to place the quote in its proper context.

One subtlety that many students find difficult is the difference between paraphrasing (which is allowed, providing the original source is referenced) and rewording. Rewording is never allowed. It is plagiarism. Box 9.2 illustrates this distinction.

In summary, you can quote original words. If you do, you should give the exact original words, and clearly indicate this, and where they were taken from. Alternatively, you can summarize someone else's ideas in your own words. To do that, you must understand the original and summarize those ideas from scratch. In short, the summarizing of the other person's ideas must involve your brain in understanding the ideas and the use of your own

Box 9.2 Distinguishing Between Paraphrasing and Rewording

Imagine that you have read the following:

> When organising a discussion of concepts in a complex subject domain, it is best to carry out some explicit modelling of those concepts. If no explicit modelling is carried out, the implicit ontology may be ill-defined, contradictory or confused. There are a range of approaches that can be used to model the semantics or ontology of a subject-domain, including the use of semantic nets (Brough, 2008).

If you read this (possibly with the aid of a dictionary) you might summarize it as:

> Brough (2008) suggests that it is best to carry out some explicit modelling of the subject domain's concepts or ontology, whenever the subject domain is complex.

That is fine. It is in your own words, summarizing the ideas in Brough's text, and you also indicated where you saw the ideas expounded. This is paraphrasing. As here, paraphrased text is usually shorter than the original. By contrast, consider:

> It is best to carry out explicit modelling of concepts when you organize a discussion of concepts in a complex subject domain. The implicit metaphysics may be confused, ill-defined or contradictory. There are several approaches for modelling the ontology of a subject domain, including semantic nets (Brough, 2008).

This is not acceptable. The words are different. The three sentences in the reworded text each have differences from the original text, but it is a rather mechanical rewording that shows no evidence of understanding the original. It is significant that there is a one-to-one correspondence between the sentences in the original text and the plagiaristic rewording of it. In the first sentence, there has been a mechanical transformation of the text. You should see how this has largely preserved the original meaning, even if you do not understand the sentence. The second sentence has had some words taken out, but omission of the first phrase has changed the meaning of what was said entirely, as the original implied the confusion was likely to arise *if no explicit concept modelling was carried out*. This qualification is no longer present.

The word 'ontology' has been replaced by 'metaphysics' in the second sentence, perhaps because the writer has consulted the 'thesaurus' facility available in most word processing packages in search of an alternative word. However, these words do not have the same meaning and are not equivalent concepts. Even if 'ontology' had been replaced with a precise synonym, the rewording would be mechanical, with no understanding of the original sentence required. The third sentence retained 'ontology' but has deleted some words, which results in making it appear as though 'semantic nets' is an 'approach'. It isn't; *using* semantics nets is an approach.

So detailed review of the reworded text shows it does not convey the same meaning as the original. It is a shuffling around of words and random deletion of some words. We might call this rewriting plagiarism. The reworded text has also chosen to replace one word with another thought to have the same meaning. It did not have the same meaning and the result was nonsense. Even if words are replaced with words that are equivalent, it would still be plagiarism (sometimes referred to as thesaurus plagiarism). The above can be characterized as an attempt to change the words of the original text by someone with knowledge of English grammar, but no understanding of the material being reworded.

Table 9.2   When to reference.

When to reference (from Cottrell, 2008)	When not to reference (from Neville, 2007)
To cite source of theory, argument or view	Historical overview with points taken from numerous sources
With specific information for example data	Your own experience or observation (unless published elsewhere)
When quoting (reproducing text exactly; sometimes knows as 'verbatim')	When drawing up summaries and conclusions
When paraphrasing (putting others' ideas in your own words)	Accepted common knowledge, for example the world is round
When directly inspired or influenced by others' work/ideas	

original words in conveying your understanding. It is worth noting that your finished work is likely to contain several phrases that also appear in the original text. In paraphrasing, this is coincidental. In plagiaristic rewording, this is a consequence of the transformation process. A competent scholar who is paraphrasing other work (i.e. summarizing ideas) has no concept of changing the text. If you only exercise grammatical and lexical (vocabulary) skills you have just reworded the text and the work is plagiaristic.

In summary, Table 9.2 is based on the work of Cottrell (2008) and Neville (2007). It provides a quick overview of the general principles to be applied when judging when work needs to be cited and referenced.

Copyright, intellectual property rights and fair use

Many people confuse the need to observe propriety in distinguishing your work from that of others with the issue of copyright. These are quite different issues. When someone develops an invention or an artistic work, within certain legal constraints they have the exclusive right to its commercial exploitation. Unless they have purposefully declared the work copyright free (where no commercial advantage can be gained) or give explicit permission to other individuals, they retain this commercial ownership. This is copyright. For published works, the copyright may reside with the author, publisher or organizer of a conference at which that paper was presented. In the case of teaching material prepared for a university course by an employee of that university, the copyright will almost always reside with the university. That is because the teaching material would have been prepared under the primary contract that the university has with its employee. They therefore 'own' what they produce in the course of that contract. Universities generally waive this ownership when academics write academic papers, textbooks, and so on.

You have to be careful not to breach copyright when you use other people's work. For example, if you wished to discuss two papers by other authors, you cannot reprint the whole of those papers. It would be a breach of copyright – commercial theft – and you might well end up in court. You are only allowed fair use of it for scholarly, non-commercial purposes. Quoting a short section is generally accepted as fair use. If you plan to quote more than a sentence or two, you should think carefully about getting permission to use the material in the way you propose. Be sensible: if you only plan to quote one sentence, the copyright owner may think your request for permission to use the material is frivolous.

In a similar respect, not all works need to be cited. Some ideas can be taken for granted, they are common knowledge in that subject domain. The basic fundamentals of the circulation of the blood can be taken as read in any medical treatment. We do not need to provide evidence in order to support the facts that veins bring blood back to the heart and that (except for the pulmonary vein) they are low in oxygen content. Any reader of an academic medical or health text is likely to know that. On the other hand, if we were writing a paper on gout, it might be helpful to provide a reference to papers discussing the relationship between blood parameters (e.g. blood pressure) and the likelihood of developing gout.

What is 'common knowledge' in a discipline will vary, depending on the audience. It will also depend on the date the text is being written. Today, if we were writing a report on the incidence of smoking in different social groups, education and family income, we would not have to provide references to the fact that long-term smoking habits increase the likelihood of developing lung cancer. Fifty years ago, we could not have assumed that everyone knew that. Indeed, there might have been many who thought there was no evidence of such a causal connection. Perhaps papers written thirty years ago would have merited references to sources supporting the premise that 'smoking increases the likelihood of incidence of lung cancer', but we don't need to do this now. Things have moved on. Now we are concerned with what causes people to smoke, how we can encourage them to stop, and how other factors predispose people to develop lung cancer. Work on these issues by other authorities would merit references. Sir Richard Doll's pioneering work on the relationship between smoking and lung cancer would of course still merit reference in a discussion of the development of epidemiology and the nature of health and the environment (Doll and Hill, 1950).

Primary and secondary sources

Students often include references to textbooks (or lecture notes) in their essays. Whilst their wish to be honest about where they got their ideas from is reasonable, it is rare that a textbook merits such a reference and, even rarer, lecture notes. This is because textbooks and lectures are (with very rare exceptions) secondary sources of knowledge. They usually describe original work by others: the primary sources. Thus, for example, if a student reads about a statistical study in a textbook, and then wants to discuss that study, they might feel tempted to refer to the textbook. It is much better to go back to the primary source in which the study was originally described.

Going back to primary sources is required in professional academic writing. That is not to say that you might never give references to sources that themselves describe other people's work. If Jones (for example) compared two different studies of risk factors for coronary heart disease (by Smith and Jenson), and those sources contained important information relevant to a paper you were writing, you would be likely to refer to those papers. We should obtain the original papers and read them ourselves, possibly using Jones's comments as a guide. You might then add your own view, maybe comparing it to the others, as shown in the fictitious example in Box 9.3, for example:

Sometimes the same research is described in several published works. If that is the case, then the first complete write up by the research's main scientists should be referred to. If there was a preliminary report, describing intermediate results, then the later fuller complete summary of the results should be referred to. This principle of referring to the first definitive statement of the facts holds in most cases. There is one exception to this, however. If an authority develops a theory, treatment or procedure that they are generally accepted to be responsible for, then the last (and most accessible) statement of that might be referred to.

Box 9.3   Using Secondary Sources

> Smith (1992) reported that . . . and in a similar study, Jenson (1993), reviewed the effects of . . . and concluded . . . However, as Jones commented 'In two previous studies . . .' (Jones 1998). We thus see there are alternative explanations of . . . .

The first sentence summarizes the findings of Smith and Jenson. The second sentence quotes a comment made by Jones in his 1998 paper about the two earlier pieces of research; there is also a paraphrased summary of Jones's conclusion. The third sentence is the author's own opinions, formed in the context of the earlier scholars' work.

There is a tempting trap here for the author who is pressed for time. Suppose you had access to Jones's work, but neither Jenson's nor Smith's work. You might be tempted to take what Jones said about the two other authors on trust. You should not do that; if you wrote the sample text above, that would be at best disingenuous. You have not read Smith and Jenson, so you cannot refer to them. We can call this kind of writing 'citation stealing': you have cited works as though you have seen them, when, in fact, you haven't. As this is being dishonest about how you have used other authors' work, it is a form of plagiarism. Even if you found Jones's work first, you had a duty to consult the originals of any work that you wish to cite. If you have not read Jenson or Smith, you cannot say anything about what they said. You certainly cannot quote something they said, if you haven't read it.

Sometimes, the original work may be inaccessible to you, for example, if only one copy exists and is unobtainable. In this case, the usual rule applies: you must be scrupulously honest. You would have to say (if you only had access to Jones's work) something like:

> Jones (1998) described the earlier work of Smith (1992) and Jenson (1993) in which they . . . His conclusions were that . . .

If Jones quoted Jenson, then you may want to repeat the quote, even though you have not read Jenson. They are not your words, and not Jones's words, and you are not sure they are Jensen's words, as you haven't read Jensen! So you must be very precise in what you say. The following would be acceptable:

> Jones (1998) quotes the work of Jenson (1993) stating that '. . .'

In carrying out your research, you will have had to spend some time tracking down the original source of an idea. You should always remember that others will have the same concern when reading your work.

 Reflection Point

Go to the home page of Wikipedia, the online encyclopaedia: http://en.wikipedia .org/wiki/Main_Page.

What kind of information source is Wikipedia? How authoritative are the authors? Take time to critically evaluate an article from Wikipedia.

When would it be appropriate to quote from Wikipedia?

In answer to the last point, it is usually only appropriate if the research is studying Wikipedia itself! This is because, as Wikipedia (2009) itself notes, 'citation of Wikipedia in research papers may not be considered acceptable, because Wikipedia is not considered a creditable source'.

Self reference

Referring to your own work is something that you need to think about. If your current work depends on work that you have previously reported in a published document, then you should refer to it, just as you would refer to any other published work. It is important that you only refer to such work if it is relevant and authoritative; authors who over-reference their own work soon lose the respect of their colleagues.

As we have note previously, cutting and pasting from your earlier work is not acceptable; this is sometimes called self-plagiarism. Although self-plagiarism must be avoided, it is likely that the same author might use similar phrases to describe similar concepts. You should be careful not just to 'rework' earlier texts. There is no justification for work that is not original.

Practicalities of referencing

Referencing is a key skill required for academic writing. We have already discussed standard rules to decide when to apply referencing, but there are also standards telling us how to display the reference. The style adopted may be specific to a general field of research, an institution or indeed a preference of the publisher. By maintaining a consistency of style, it is very easy for someone experienced in reading academic papers to identify where to find the follow up information they require. In some instances, you might want also to include a bibliography. Box 9.4 outlines the difference between a bibliography and a reference list.

There are two distinct aspects of a reference:

- in-text citation – where a quote or an idea has been used;
- the reference itself – this usually occurs at the end of the text in a list or within a footnote, providing full details of the source of information so it can be traced by others.

How these two aspects are displayed is dependent on the referencing system employed. Two styles in popular use are:

- Author/Date, for example Harvard; American Psychological Association (APA, 2010a) (this is the style used throughout this book);
- Numerical/Citation sequence, for example Vancouver.

Box 9.4   Bibliographies and Reference Lists

Bibliography: A list of background reading which may have influenced you generally, or been a source of information. It is not a reference or reference list, and is normally optional in academic writing.

Reference List: A list of all the material reproduced or referred to in an essay, which appears at the end of the essay. This is an essential element of academic writing.

In this chapter, we illustrate using the APA and Vancouver styles, but please note there are variations in layout. For example, APA uses a comma between the author surname and date in in-text citations (e.g. Agostini & Singh, 2008), while some other author/date versions do not (e.g. Agostini and Singh 2008). Variations are acceptable, provided that you are consistent in their use.

Author/date system

In-text citation

An 'in-text' citation is required at the point where an idea or quotation has been used in the writing. Each time an author is referred to, the surname and year of publication appear in the text close to that reference, for example:

> . . .as Agostini and Singh (2009) argue, postoperative physiotherapy regimes are effective following thoracic surgery.

The reference to Agostini and Singh in this instance is used as part of the sentence, therefore only the year the reference refers to is in brackets. Sometimes it is more convenient, and reads more fluently, to give the author's surname and date at the end of a sentence, especially when it does not form a natural part of the sentence, for example:

> . . . incentive spirometry can be effective for lung re-expansion after major thoracic surgery (Agostini & Singh, 2009).

Note also that in APA style, the word 'and' is used to connect authors' names outside brackets, but the symbol '&' is used within brackets.

 Action Point

Try these two different formats for referring to authors within the text.

Select a piece of text, assimilate the information, and construct two sentences referring to the information, one where you use the author's name within the sentence, with the year of publication in brackets, and the other where you are not using the author's surname as part of the sentence, and therefore the author's surname and year of publication both go in the bracket.

Reference list

The reference list appears at the end of your work. Its standards and conventions are designed so it is easy for others to trace the work to which you have referred. The list is constructed in alphabetical order by surname or organization. No matter how many times a reference source has been cited, it appears in the alphabetical list only once.

Example

In the text:
As Pritchard (2008) suggests. . .
In the reference list:
Pritchard, A. (2008). *Studying and learning at university.* London: Sage.

Where there are two authors, both names should be given each time they are cited in the text. For between three and six authors, all names should be included in the text the first time the sources are mentioned; thereafter, it is sufficient to give the first, followed by *et al.* (meaning 'and others'). However, all these authors must be included in the reference list at the end of the paper. Where there are more than six authors, use the first, plus *et al.* in the text; include the first six in the reference list plus *et al.* for others.

Example

In the text:
Pears and Shields (2003) argued that. . .
Rugg *et al.* (2008) argue that. . .
In the reference list:
Pears, R., & Shields, G. (2003). *Cite them right: The essential guide to referencing and plagiarism.* Newcastle-upon-Tyne: Northumbria University Press.
Rugg, G., Gerrard, S., & Hooper, S. (2008). *The stress-free guide to studying at university.* London: Sage.

If an author has published more than one item in the same year, and you refer to them both, these are distinguished by lower case letters: For example Pritchard (2008a, b).

Where no author is stated, the responsible organization or committee is stated, for example Department of Health (2007). Abbreviations are acceptable if explained in full the first time within the text, as in Department of Health (DH), 2007.

Reference list elements and examples

Note that APA style uses a hanging indent for each reference after the first line. Other versions of Author/Date system may not, but ensure you are consistent.

Book

Author's surname and initials. (Year of publication). *Title of the book in lower case italics.* City of publication: Publisher.

Example

Pritchard, A. (2008). *Studying and learning at university.* London: Sage.

If a book has more than one edition, make clear in the reference list which edition you have used, unless it is the first.

Example

Cottrell, S. (2008). *The study skills handbook* (3rd ed.). Basingstoke: Palgrave Macmillan.

Chapter within an edited book

Author's surname and initials (Year of publication). Title of the chapter appearing in book. In Initial and Surname of Book editor(s) (Ed[s].), *Title of the book in italics* (page numbers of chapter). City of publication: Publisher.

Example

Murphy, E., & Dingwall, R. (2001). Qualitative methods in health technology assessment. In A. Stevens, K. Abrams, J. Brazier, R. Fitzpatrick & R. Lilford (Eds.), *The advanced handbook of methods in evidence based healthcare* (pp. 166–178). London: Sage.

Journal article

Author's surname and initials. (Year of publication). Title of article. *Name of journal in italics, Volume number in italics* (issue number if available), page numbers.

Example

Lloyd, M. (2007). Developing academic writing skills: the PROCESS framework. *Nursing Standard, 21*(40), 50–56.

Electronic and internet sources

The key principles, when using and referencing electronic material, are to direct readers as closely as possible to the information cited, providing Uniform Resource Locator (URL) (web) addresses that work, or Digital Object Identifiers (see below) where available.

As the APA (2010a) indicates, you should include the same elements, in the same order, as for a printed reference, but add in as much information about the electronic source as needed for others to locate the sources themselves. For the latest guidance, consult the latest edition of the APA Publication Manual (2010a) or Concise Guide (2010b).

Retrieval dates

You should give the date you retrieved the material, if that material is likely to change. No retrieval date is necessary for content that is not likely to change, such as a journal article or book (APA, 2010a).

Digital Object Identifiers (DOIs) (http://www.doi.org/)

To resolve the problem of web site references frequently changing and moving, some publishers now assign documents a Digital Object Identifier (DOI®). The DOI system is used to label documents in the digital environment, so that if information about a digital document changes over time, including where to find it, its DOI name will not change. To find the source of a DOI, either type the number into a search engine such as Google, or go to http://dx.doi.org/ and type or paste the number into the box provided. You will then be taken to a web page associated with that document. When a DOI is available, include this instead of the URL in the reference.

Example

Where there is a DOI:
Edgley, A., Timmons, S., & Crosbie, B. (2008). Desperately seeking sociology: Nursing student perceptions of sociology on nursing courses. *Nurse Education Today, 29(1), 16–23*. doi: 10.1016/j.nedt.2008.06.001
Where there is no DOI:
Matzo, M., & Hijjazi, K. (2008). There's no place like home: Oklahomans' preferences for site of death. *Palliative care: Research and Treatment*, 1, Retrieved from http://www.la-press.com/journal.php?journal_id=86&issue_id=87
NB In these examples, the final version of the article is being referenced, so there is no need to include the retrieval date.

Material on a web site

Give the author or organization, date of publication (if available), document title or description, retrieval date and an accurate URL. Where no date is given, use (n.d.) after the author or organisation's name. In the example below, the retrieval date is given, as this is not necessarily a permanent location.

Example

British Nutrition Foundation (2008). *Healthy eating on a budget.* Retrieved June 12th 2009 from http://www.nutrition.org.uk/home.asp?siteId=43&sectionId=1348 &parentSection=304&which=4

 Action Point

1. Rewrite the passage below so that it is correctly referenced according to APA style.
Surprisingly, in such an established area as smoking research, there is disagreement. For example, investigators like Dr R Williams in his book 'The Effects of the Experimenter in Research' published in 2005 found positive effects in 85% of cases, while another investigator writing in a recent journal article found positive effects (Smith '03) in only 62% of cases. Even if the studies of the two most successful investigators are ignored the differences remain significant. (Jones, Walker and Evans 2007). Jones, Walker & Evans (2007) who recently wrote a chapter in a book by Frank Mitchell, have also noted that there is a need for further studies in this area.
A suggested answer is as follows:
Surprisingly, in such an established area as smoking research, there is disagreement. For example, Williams (2005) found positive effects in 85% of cases, while Smith (2003) found positive effects in only 62% of cases. Even if the studies of the two most successful

investigators are ignored, the differences remain significant (Jones, Walker, & Evans, 2007). Jones *et al.* have also noted that there is a need for further studies in this area.

2. Construct a hypothetical reference list for the sources cited.

Hypothetical reference list

Jones, B., Walker, K., & Evans, H. (2007). Research into smoking: The need for evidence. In F. Mitchell (Ed.), Smoking: *A beginner's guide to the evidence* (pp. 51–84). Oxford: Interesting Books.

Smith, A. (2003). A study to show the effects of the investigator in smoking research. *Journal of Smoking Research, 11*(3), 25–39.

Williams, R. (2005). *The effects of the experimenter in research*. London: Wicked Publishers Ltd.

Numerical/citation system

This is used in many medical texts and journals, but please note it is not the style adopted in this textbook, where we have used the APA (2010a) version of the author/date system throughout.

In-text citation

As with the Author/Date system, an 'in-text' citation is required at the point where an idea or quotation has been used. Each time a source is referred to, a number is added, usually as a superscript[1] or in brackets (1), which refers to the numerical position of the full reference in the reference list. Dates are not given in the text, and it is not always necessary to include the author's name.

Example

In text
Preparing a paper for submission involves synthesis of three key elements[1]
In reference list
1. Epstein D, Kenway J, Boden R. Writing for publication. London: Sage; 2005.

Reference list

The reference list appears at the end of your work. As with the Author/Date system, its standards and conventions are designed to enable others to trace the work to which you have referred. The list is constructed in numerical order. This means that if you refer to the same source more than once, it will appear in the reference list more than once, with a different number for each citation

Example

In the text:
As has been suggested[1] ...
In the reference list:
1. Pritchard A. Studying and learning at university. London: Sage; 2008.

The in-text citation will appear the same, no matter how many authors are involved. As with the Name/Date system, all the authors must be included in the reference list, except where there are more than six, when only the first six plus *et al.* need to be listed. If an author has published more than one item in the same year, and you refer to them both, these will be indicated by unique superscript numbers.

Reference list elements and examples

Hanging indents and italics are not used.

Book

Author's surname and initials. Title of the book. Edition if not the first. Place of Publication: Publisher; Year of Publication.

Example

1. Cottrell S. The study skills handbook. 3rd ed. Basingstoke: Palgrave Macmillan; 2008.

Chapter within an edited book

Author's surname and initials (Year of publication). Title of the chapter. In Surname and Initial of Book Editor(s) (Ed.), Title of book. Place of publication: Publisher; year of publication. page numbers of chapter.

Example

1. Murphy E, Dingwall R. Qualitative methods in health technology assessment. In: Stevens A, Abrams K, Brazier J, Fitzpatrick R, Lilford R, editors. The advanced handbook of methods in evidence based healthcare. London: Sage; 2001. p. 166–178.

Journal article

Note that Journal titles are shortened to their standard abbreviation, as per the most recent edition of Index Medicus (ftp://nlmpubs.nlm.nih.gov/online/journals/ljiweb.pdf); for example British Medical Journal becomes Br Med J.

Author's surname and initials. Title of article. Abbreviated journal title, Year of publication; Volume number (issue number if available): page numbers.

Example (Assuming this Article was the sixth Source to be Referred to in the Text)

6. Rickarda C, McGrailb M, Jones R, O'Meara P, Robinson A, Burley M *et al.* Supporting academic publication: Evaluation of a writing course combined with writers' support group. Nurs Educ Today 2009; 29 (5): 516–521.

Electronic and internet sources

The key principles are the same as for the Author/Date system. Specific examples are as follows:

E-book

Author's surname and initials. Title of book [medium, e.g. Online]. Edition. Place of publication: Publisher; Year of publication. [Date cited].Available from: URL.

Example

Harvey J. *et al.* Handbook of Practice Management [online] London: Royal Society of Medicine Press; 2000. [Cited 12 June 2009]. Available from: http://www.rsmpress.co.uk/bkhpm.htm.

Material on web site

Author or source, Title of web document or web page. [Medium] [date of citation]. Year. Available from: web site address.

Example

British Nutrition Foundation. Healthy eating on a budget [online]. [cited 2009 June 12]. 2008.. Available from: http://www.nutrition.org.uk/home.asp?siteId=43&sectionId =1348&parentSection=304&which=4.

Choosing your referencing style

These two major styles are only guides to good practice. Many organizations and publishers operate using variations of the styles demonstrated. It is, therefore, always important to check university regulations, style manuals, or journal author guidelines as appropriate, to check which system to use and for local nuances with punctuation.

From these examples it is easy to observe that Vancouver is more compact than APA, and may thus be preferred if there are many citations (such as in Medicine, where it is generally adopted). APA is easier to 'read' (you don't have to keep turning to the reference list, to check 'reference [5]'). When you do your own research, take time to look at how journal articles and textbooks are referenced. Which style do you find easier to use?

We hope that, now you have read this chapter, you will have considered the many different ways in which you might write for different audiences, and that you are aware of the significance of plagiarism and how to avoid it. In the next chapter, we consider further how you might reflect on and review your own work and its limitations, and how you might share what you are writing with others.

References

American Psychological Association (APA) (2010a) *Publication Manual*, 6th edn, APA, Washington.
American Psychological Association (APA) (2010b) *Concise Rules of APA Style*, 6th edn, APA, Washington.
Cottrell, S. (2008) *The Study Skills Handbook*, 3rd edn, Palgrave Macmillan, Basingstoke.
Doll, R. and Hill, A.B. (1950) Smoking and carcinoma of the lung: Preliminary report. *British Medical Journal*, 2 (4682), 739–734.
Fowler, H.W. (1998) *Fowler's Modern English Usage*, 3rd revised edn, Oxford University Press, Oxford.
Garfield, E. (2005) The agony and the ecstasy - The history and meaning of the Journal Impact Factor. Retrieved from http://www.garfield.library.upenn.edu/papers/jifchicago2005.pdf.

Hart, G. (2000) Readability indexes – a debate. Retrieved from http://www.geoff-hart.com/resources/ 2000/readability.htm.

Neville, C. (2007) *The Complete Guide to Referencing and Avoiding Plagiarism*, Oxford University Press, Oxford.

Ritter, R.M. (ed.) (2003) *The Oxford Style Manual*, Oxford University Press, Oxford.

Truss, L. (2003) *Eats, Shoots and Leaves: The Zero Tolerance Approach to Punctuation*, Profile Books, London.

Wikipaedia (2009) Academic Use. Retrieved from http://en.wikipedia.org/wiki/Wikipedia:Academic_use.

Turnitin (2009) Retrieved from: http://turnitin.com/static_jisc/ac_uk_products.html#originality_checking.

Further reading and resources

Anderson, I. (2009) Avoiding plagiarism in academic writing. *Nursing Standard*, **23** (18), 35–37.

Blamires, H. (2003) *Compose Yourself and Write Good English*, Penguin, Harmondsworth.

Copus, J. (2009) *Brilliant Writing Tips for Students*, Palgrave Macmillan, Basingstoke.

Cottrell, S. (2008) *The Study Skills Handbook*, 3rd edn, Palgrave Macmillan, Basingstoke.

Epstein, D., Kenway, J. and Boden, R. (2005) *Writing for Publication*, Sage, London.

Equator Network (2009) The resource centre for good reporting of health research studies. Retrieved from http://www.equator-network.org/.

Gimenez, J. (2007) *Writing for Nursing and Midwifery Students*, Palgrave Macmillan, Basingstoke.

Godwin, J. (2009) *Planning Your Essay*, Palgrave Macmillan, Basingstoke.

Levin, P. (2004) *Write Great Essays! Reading and Essay Writing for Undergraduates and Taught Postgraduates*, Open University Press, Maidenhead.

Lloyd, M. (2007) Developing academic writing skills: the PROCESS framework. *Nursing Standard*, **21** (40), 50–56.

Maier, P., Price, G. and Cowen, M. (2009) *Study Skills for Nurses and Health Care Students*, Pearson Education, London.

Murray, R. (2002) *How to Write a Thesis*, Open University Press, Buckingham.

Murray, R. (2004) *How to Write for Academic Journals*, Open University Press, Buckingham.

Pears, R. and Shields, G. (2003) *Cite them Right: The Essential Guide to Referencing and Plagiarism*, Northumbria University Press, Newcastle-upon-Tyne.

Pritchard, A. (2008) *Studying and Learning at University*, Sage, London.

Rose, J. (2001) *The Mature Student's Guide to Writing,* Palgrave Macmillan, Basingstoke.

Rugg, G., Gerrard, S. and Hooper, S. (2008) *The Stress-Free Guide to Studying at University*, Sage, London.

Soles, D. (2005) *The Academic Essay: How to Plan, Draft, Write and Revise*, Studymates, Abergele.

Williams, K. and Carroll, J. (2009) *Referencing and Understanding Plagiarism*, Palgrave Macmillan, Basingstoke.

10   Sharing Research Knowledge

Paula Roberts, Colin Macduff, Tim Smale and Helena Priest

Introduction

This chapter focuses on research implementation and dissemination strategies. Firstly, it discusses the need to consider the limitations of your work as well as its strengths, and ways to summarize and conclude written reports. It then considers ways to implement evidence based practice and empirical research results in practical contexts, from a book review to a journal article. Finally, it provides suggestions for writing abstracts, presenting research at conferences, and liaising with publishers and the academic press, in order to disseminate the results of good quality empirical studies.

Preparing to disseminate your work: Considering limitations

Even with thorough planning and attention to detail, no research study is perfect, and whether you have undertaken a large multi-site or small-scale study, it is important to acknowledge the study's limitations before you plan to disseminate it. Valid and reliable small-scale studies have a very important part to play in the contribution of knowledge and understanding in your field. However, not all studies are generalizable to other settings and this should be made explicit. Small-scale studies are limited by relatively small sample sizes and sometimes by elite bias (where participants are selected by purposive sampling or by using key informants). Although the selection of well informed and articulate respondents can generate rich data, samples may be unrepresentative due to potential subjectivity during the process of selection (Black, 1999). Similarly, with snowball sampling, often used in qualitative interviews, the representativeness of respondents cannot be established within the wider population. Consequently, the findings cannot be generalized *per se*.

Additionally, whilst you may have had a good sample size from your population, a study will have limited generalizability if you have only used one study site or organization. This must be acknowledged by stating, for example, that 'whilst useful insights have been gained, findings from this study cannot be generalized to other organizations'.

If you have conducted your own empirical study, you should make the limitations of the study explicit in your research report, presentations or any publications arising from the study.

The limitations will depend upon several factors relating to the design of the study, its resources, scope, depth and timeframe. It is important to be honest in detailing a study's limitations. You do this through your own assessment and critique of your study. Areas you may need to consider include:

- Literature search and review: Was your literature review sufficiently comprehensive to conclude that your research was necessary? How was your literature review delineated? Did you limit your review to UK/American literature? If so, why? What was the scope of your enquiry? What search engines did you use? Are you confident that your search strategy generated sufficient literature?
- Theoretical orientation of the study: Has your appraisal of the literature given you a sufficiently robust theoretical foundation upon which to structure your exploratory study, or from which to develop valid theoretical constructs?
- Did you ensure that you had the appropriate ethical/R & D approval for your study?
- Have you ensured anonymity for participants and organizations involved in your study?
- Was your study designed to generate sufficient data to obtain reliable results? For example, if you undertook focus group interviews, did you continue conducting focus groups until saturation occurred in the data; that is until the same ideas were being generated and there was repetition in the type of data being proffered? If you were developing measurement scales, were your theoretical item constructs based on a sufficiently large sample of respondents? Did you pilot your instruments? Were your measurement scales tested on sufficiently large samples to claim reliability? What measures have you taken to minimize bias in the sample? (For example, did you exclude pilot participants from your main study?) If you conducted a survey, what measures did you take to improve response rates and reduce non-response bias? (For example, did you use methods whereby results from later respondents (after reminders) are compared to those of early respondents?) Was your sampling strategy and frame sufficiently robust for the subsequent methodology and to generate valid and reliable results?
- Were your methods of data analysis rigorous? Did you undertake respondent validation and inter-coder reliability checks?
- Have you considered your own impact upon the data collection and analysis? Were you an integral part of the research team? Might your own interpretation of findings have had a bearing on the validity of results? Being a researcher within your own professional field has advantages and disadvantages, in that whilst you will have professional insight in your chosen field, and thereby will be able to authenticate responses and findings intuitively, your familiarity within your working context may obscure issues and ambiguities that others from outside the field may be prompted to question;
- Are your findings valid and reliable? Can you have confidence in presenting your data? Can you defend your research design and results? Can your results be generalized beyond your study? If so, what is the scope of generalizabilty?

While it is important to discuss the study's limitations, you should also discuss what can be gained from your study (however small, and whatever its limitations). In other words, you should try not to be too negative, otherwise readers may not appreciate the value of your work. Include a summary of the useful insights that have been gained whilst undertaking the study, which may be helpful for others in similar settings.

For example, you could report 'whilst this was a small-scale study undertaken in one healthcare setting and, therefore, results cannot be generalized to other settings, nonetheless some useful insights can be gained from the study, which may be helpful in other contexts' (and then discuss them). You should then summarize your study, detailing what the study can, and cannot, claim to offer.

In the same way, if you are reading and reporting on a research paper, you must consider the strengths and limitations of the study as you go through it. A good paper will have a section on limitations towards the end of the paper.

Summarizing your work and making recommendations

It is very important to summarize the findings of your study and to make explicit its main recommendations. Your readers will want this information in a succinct form, so that they can readily see where they could use the findings in the development of their own practice or organization. They will want to know not only that they can rely on the findings of the study, but also that your recommendations are based on sound interpretation of the results. In some forms of report, an executive summary is presented first; this summarizes the key aims, objectives, questions, methods, findings, implications and recommendations. In other forms of paper, an abstract precedes the paper itself; it is normally a paragraph of 200–300 words summarizing these same areas. Some journals require that the abstract is presented in a structured format using key subheadings, such as 'method', 'conclusion', 'recommendations', or 'application to practice'; journal author guidelines available from the journal's web site will indicate the required format for the abstract. Some journals also require a list of key words that will be indexed by the publication and will then facilitate literature searching (Chapter 4).

In summarizing your research, you need to bear in mind the audience; are you summarizing the findings for a research report, a poster, a seminar or conference paper, a published paper or your research thesis? It is useful at this point to refer back to the aims of your study, in order to frame the recommendations.

Disseminating evidence in your workplace

If you have undertaken a literature review as part of your studies, or are in the process of conducting an empirical study, you could offer to disseminate your ideas and findings to your local colleagues. You are now in an ideal position to influence good practice, and see the results of changes in practice. There are several ways in which you could do this: offer to host a lunchtime seminar for your clinical colleagues; incorporate your findings into clinical teaching; offer to give a presentation at the local research seminar series at your local university; or produce a summary paper for your clinical area's resource file.

Seminars

A good place to start sharing your work and ideas with others is by presenting at a local seminar or journal club relevant to your professional speciality. This does not need to be about research you've undertaken; it can be presenting developments in your clinical field, evidence based practice, or a topic you have investigated for a project. Many healthcare and educational providers host regular seminar programmes or journal clubs. To find out where these are being held, check web sites or contact the seminar organizer at your local NHS Trust or the relevant faculty/school at your local university. Write to the organizer with a 500 word abstract detailing your work, and offer to do a 15 minute presentation with 15 minutes for questions. Many seminar or journal club organizers will welcome such an offer.

Once you have booked a slot on the seminar series or journal club, then prepare your presentation. A good presentation should be clear, succinct and visually attractive, with accompanying handouts of the presentation.

Use a proprietary presentation package, such as *Microsoft Office PowerPoint*, and prepare the slides. It's important to familiarize yourself with the presentation package at this stage. It will guide you in how to create a new presentation, apply a range of attractive templates, graphics and annotations to your slides, and help you time your presentation. By using the 'notes' function, you can prepare more detailed notes on each slide to guide your talk, or to distribute as handouts. Once you are happy with your presentation, save it on a data stick to take with you to the seminar venue, and arrange with the organizer to e-mail your slides and notes files in advance of the presentation for pre-loading onto their equipment.

 Action Point

Write a 500 word abstract on a topic of interest, such as an update in evidence based practice in your field or a topic you have investigated for a project.

Forward it to your local seminar organizer for consideration for the next seminar series.

Conference presentations

Having gained some experience in giving papers at local seminar programmes, it is time to start disseminating more widely. There are many regional, national and international conferences to target. The professional journals and their web sites list forthcoming conferences. Each discipline/speciality usually has a special interest section with its own conference area. Additionally, there are many generic and interprofessional practice, education and research conferences to target. Conferences usually call for abstracts well in advance of the conference dates, so look out for calls for abstracts on web sites and in professional journals and flyers. Note the special requirements of the particular conference in relation to the sort of paper are you aiming to submit.

 Action Point

Go to one of the web sites below, as relevant to your field, and browse its forthcoming conferences section. Have a look at the section 'Call for Abstracts', and the requirements. Conferences usually have a range of ways to contribute; for example, you can choose to submit a poster presentation or a paper for a concurrent session or symposium:

Healthcare Conferences: http://www.healthcare-events.co.uk/
Royal College of Nursing: www.rcn.org.uk

Nurse Education: http://www.netnep-conference.elsevier.com/

Royal College of Midwives: http://www.rcm.org.uk/college/resources/events/

Medical and health-related conferences: http://www.gmc-uk.org/links.asp#doctors

Medical Education conferences: Association for the Study of Medical Education: www.asme.org.uk

British Psychological Society: http://www.bps.org.uk/

Chartered Society of Physiotherapy: www.csp.org.uk

Association of Operating Department Practitioners: http://www.aodp.org/

National Prescribing Centre: www.npc.co.uk/events

Royal Pharmaceutical Society of Great Britain: http://www.rpsgb.org/worldofpharmacy/events/

British Dental Association: http://www.bda.org/education/

Doctoral colloquiums

If you are a doctoral student (undertaking Doctorate in Philosophy (PhD) or Professional Doctorate), an extremely useful way of gaining academic and professional feedback on your work is to submit an abstract to present a paper at a doctoral colloquium. These are often attached to conferences and offer doctoral students the opportunity to present their work in a safe and supportive environment in which feedback is encouraged from the audience of peers and academic/professional colleagues. Doctoral colloquiums can often help with viva voce examination preparation and in developing the skills of defending your work with wider audiences.

Working papers

Presentations on working papers focus on work in progress; for example, presentations on pilot studies or the first section of a longer research study that you might present more fully once subsequent stages of the research have been conducted.

Concurrent papers

This means that several similar but individual papers are clustered for presentation within a theme, and several theme tracks are being hosted concurrently. Delegates at large conferences then select the presentations they wish to attend. You can usually expect up to 30 delegates at your presentation (occasionally many more if it's a popular topic).

Symposia

These are several individual themed papers, developed together around a particular topic. The sessions are usually pre-linked by group members coordinating their development and scheduling the various papers within the topic area. The abstracts and group of papers are then submitted together as a symposium presentation of three to five related papers.

Poster presentations

You may choose to submit your work as a poster presentation, or sometimes when you submit an abstract to present a paper, you are offered a poster presentation instead. This is often because the review committee feels your work would be best disseminated visually at the conference. Poster presentations offer the opportunity to develop your artistic and writing skills, and are a very useful way to disseminate your work, as you can discuss your work with delegates in a relaxed and informal way. Some conferences offer the opportunity to have a short presentation of posters, for example three minutes and one conference slide prior to the hosting of posters. You will be expected to register at the conference and to be available with your poster to discuss your work and answer questions.

Producing a poster

If you are offered a poster presentation, before you start to produce it check the required size, that is, will the board it is to be displayed on be portrait (vertical appearance) or landscape (horizontal appearance), so you can produce the poster accordingly. It is also a good idea to check if you are required to include information such as your institution's logo. When you have obtained the information about the size of your poster, you will need to check with your reprographics unit or local printer that they will be able to produce this size, and what margins you need to set around the border of your poster (these must then be set in the page properties of the program you are using).

Although there are many programs you can use to create a poster, the two most commonly used are *Microsoft Office Publisher* and *Microsoft Office PowerPoint*. These two applications allow you to create free floating text boxes and insert pictures with ease. Posters can also be created effectively using *Microsoft Word*. We will focus on producing posters with *MS Publisher*, available to use in many university libraries or purchase from *Microsoft* http://office.microsoft.com/en-gb/publisher/default.aspx. Packages are sometimes available for free download from *Microsoft* for a limited period.

When you are ready to start putting your poster together, you need to create a new document (File, New...). It is good practice to set the page properties (via the File, Page Setup menu) equal to the size required in the final poster. This is so that when you come to print the final poster you will reduce the risk of having pixelated images and diagrams. Pixelation is where an image is increased in size to the point where the individual pixels are visible and the image is therefore distorted.

Putting a poster together might sound like a difficult task and that it requires skill in graphical design, but it really does not. With *MS Publisher*, creating a poster is simple and fast. To produce a simple, but effective poster, you might only need to use two tools:

'Insert, Text Box' and 'Insert, Picture, From File...'

A Text Box is a free floating area where you can produce the textual content of your poster. This box can be resized/shaped and moved around on the page (by clicking on it with your computer mouse and dragging the box) until you are happy with its location. All text boxes are independent of each other and can be formatted differently, although the use of too many different formats is not recommended, as it will not give a uniform look to your poster. You can add as many text boxes as you need. Similar features are available on *MS Word*.

Inserted pictures (images) can be treated in a similar way to Text Boxes in that they can be resized and moved around the page. A point of caution is that when you resize a photo you should ensure sure that you do not stretch the image in only one direction. This will distort the image and could affect the resolution (clarity). This can be prevented by right clicking on the image with your mouse, then selecting 'Format Picture...' In the new menu, you need to select the Size heading and select the 'Lock aspect ratio' option. This will prevent the image becoming distorted. *Microsoft Publisher* has some useful inbuilt functions to help you edit your images, but if you have an image editing program (such as *Adobe Photoshop*) you may produce better results.

If you do not have an image editing program, all the tools required to edit your image can be found in *MS Publisher* on the 'Picture' toolbar. A similar toolbar is available in *MS Word* by selecting 'view/toolbars/picture'.

 Action Point

Locate the Picture Toolbar on your computer and list the options available.

You should have found the following symbols available for use:

- Insert New Picture;
- Insert Picture From Scanner or Camera;
- Colour (Allows you to change you picture to black and white, greyscale, etc.);
- More Contrast;
- Less Contrast;
- More Brightness;
- Less Brightness;
- Crop (Allows you to remove parts of your image);
- Line/Border style (Allows you to place a border around your image);
- Compress Pictures (Allows you to reduce the quality of the image to that of your printer and to remove the cropped areas of your image from the memory. This will reduce the size of your file but could reduce the quality of your poster when you come to print it);
- Text Wrapping (Allows you to define how text will react to the image being placed over it. This is not commonly used in Publisher as text and images are usually in separate boxes);
- Format Picture (Opens the Picture Properties menu);
- Set Transparent Colour (Allows you to select a colour in your image that you would like to be transparent. This is usually the white areas at the edge of your image);
- Reset Picture (Allows you to reset your picture to its original format, unless you have compressed the image).

To prevent your images from being pixelated, you will need to obtain the highest resolution images you can (you can test this by opening the image in an image editor and looking at its properties or by seeing how far you can zoom in before you can see the pixels).

Once you have inserted your images into your poster file, you can test how your image might look when printed. To do this, you need to change the view of your poster to represent its true size. For this go to 'View, Zoom, 100%'. This will make your poster appear on your screen the same size as it will be when printed. In this view, have a look at your images and text. If they are not clear, you will need to obtain better quality images, or consider making the images smaller.

Posters will usually have a white background or be printed onto coloured paper, but if you would like a coloured background or to use an image as your background, you can do this by going to 'Format, Background. . .' This will open a menu allowing you to alter your poster background to your liking. If you wish to make more advanced changes, you can click on 'More backgrounds. . .' In this menu, you will have greater control over your poster background. This menu will also allow you to change the transparency of your background image, thus giving the effect of a watermark and a more subtle image.

Once you have finished putting together your poster, or would just like to see how it will look, you can print out parts of your poster on any size paper you like and then put them together to represent your full size poster. This allows you to have a final check on how your poster will look, and to check the quality of the images you have used. To do this, you will need to select 'File, Print. . .' Here you need to select the 'tiled' option from the 'print options' area and alter any of the other options you wish to use (the default settings should be adequate in most cases). It is always best to preview what you are printing before you send it to the printer and to do this all you need to do is click 'Print Preview'. If you are happy, you can then click 'Print'. Your poster will then be printed onto multiple pages that you can stick together.

So, you have finished your poster and now need to send it for printing. You need to check with the printers which format they would like, and their preferred method of receiving your file (some can receive via e-mail and some will need it on a CD or memory stick). If you are required to save your poster as a pdf (portable document format) file, you will need to have a pdf creator. A readily available one is *Adobe Acrobat*, but you will find some very good free pdf creators online, such as *PrimoPDF*. Every pdf creator is different and you should read the help documentation before using it. You need to make sure that the pdf retains the quality of the original poster. In the options of most pdf creators you will need to specify the size of the pdf page (make this the same as your poster) and the compression percentage (try not to compress your poster as this will reduce the quality of your images).

If you plan to keep your poster or display it for a long period, you might wish to consider getting it laminated to protect it from damage.

 Action Point

Practise creating a poster using *MS Publisher* package now.

This can be about anything of interest, for example your favourite holiday spots, or your family tree. It is your design skills and formatting that are important at this stage. Once you have done this, try printing your poster to see how it looks.

Oral presentation tips

Use a proprietary presentation package such as *Microsoft Office PowerPoint* and prepare the slides to accompany your presentation. Wherever you are presenting (seminar, conference), start by introducing yourself and give a bit of information about your position, the organization you work for or are representing, and then signpost your session. Signposting is very important as it lets your audience know what is in your session and the approximate time it will take.

Signposting starts with the first slide, in which you introduce yourself, followed by the second slide, which should have bullet points giving an overview of the full presentation to follow. Each bullet point on the second slide is followed through sequentially in the presentation with a slide or two for each bullet point, to develop the information and act as an *aide memoire*. For example:

- An overview of the study;
- Aims and objectives;
- Research methods;
- Ethical considerations;
- Data collection and analysis;
- Discussion;
- Summary and findings.

Distribute your pre-prepared notes as handouts at this point, to give your audience the opportunity to make notes on them. As you progress your presentation, make eye contact with your audience, using your slides as prompts. Don't be tempted to read from pre-written notes or cards. Instead, have a good grasp of your subject area, then your talk will flow naturally. With research data, unless you have the written permission of your participants, and the organization you undertook the study in, you must make details anonymous; do not divulge the organizations in which the data were collected or identify your participants (see Chapter 6 on conducting ethical research). At the end of your presentation, thank your audience and invite questions. It is useful to distribute an evaluation questionnaire; this gives invaluable feedback on your presentation style and the content of your presentation, which you may adapt for future conference presentations.

Listing your presentations on your CV

Having given your presentation, it is important to include it on your Curriculum Vitae (CV). Some conference proceedings are published in hard copy form, others on a CD-ROM or on the Internet. Some have an ISBN number, which means they are published conference proceedings in the public domain. With subsequent presentations, list them in date order with the most recent at the top of the list. Have sections entitled: Seminar Presentations/Conference papers given/Poster presentations, and list your presentations as:

Surname, initial. (Year, date). *Title of presentation*. Paper (or poster) presented at Title of event, Venue, see examples in Box 10.1).

 Action Point

If you don't already have a Curriculum Vitae (CV), create one now (for help with this go to a search engine on the Internet and type in 'Writing a CV'). There are many sites offering invaluable advice and CV templates.

List your seminar/conference/poster presentations on your CV, most recent first.

Box 10.1   **Examples of Entries on CV**

Seminar Presentations

Smith, J. (2008, September 9th). *Implementing evidence-based practice in cardiac rehabilitation: a local case study*. Seminar paper presented at the Cardiac Care Journal Club, (Name of) NHS Trust.

Conference Papers

Priest, H., Roberts, P.M., Dent, H., Blincoe, H., & Armstrong, C. (2007, July). *Interprofessional education within mental health care contexts*. Paper presented at the Royal College of Nursing International 1st Joint Education Forum, Brighton, UK.

Poster Presentations

Roberts, P.M., Priest, H., Dent, H., Blincoe, H., & Armstrong, C. (2007, July). *Shared learning in mental health care education*. Poster session presented at the Association for the Study of Medical Education (ASME) Scientific Meeting, Keele University, UK.

Disseminating your work through publications

Book reviews

A book review is a summary of a book written by another author or authors. The summary usually gives an overview of the book's contents, intended readership, strengths and weaknesses (including value for money!), what is innovative and what is not covered. Writing a book review in a field relevant to your work is often a good way to start writing for publication.

   Action Point

Go to your local library; browse the professional/academic journals in your field. Make a list of all those that publish book reviews. Read the book reviews and note the style of the reviews. How do these differ with different reviewers? What makes a good book review?

   Action Point

Contact the editor of a professional/academic journal that publishes book reviews. Offer to become a book or journal reviewer, giving details of your professional field. When you have book reviews accepted and published, list them on your Curriculum Vitae.

Professional journals

Professional journals are targeted at readers in a specific field or professional discipline. They are often published frequently, for example weekly, and contain a wide range of news and information, including short articles, peer reviewed articles, job advertisements and conference information.

The advantages of publishing in a professional journal are that the review and publication time is relatively short, as the journal has a more frequent publication schedule. Professional journals usually have a much larger circulation than academic journals, thus your work will be readily available to your professional group. Some professional journals offer you a fee for publication of your article. The downside is, if you need your work to count towards university research assessment exercises, not all professional journals have an Impact Factor (Chapter 9). The impact factor is a measure of the esteem of a journal within its field, calculated annually by a statistic: the total number of citations received by that journal in that year to articles published over the previous two years, divided by the total number of citable items published by the journal in that two year period. Journal Citation Reports (JCR, http://thomsonreuters.com/content/press_room/sci/448197) indicate this impact factor, or see journal home pages.

If you are new to academic writing, you could try writing a short article about current trends within your field, or an innovation in your workplace, and submit it for consideration in a professional journal. Check the guidelines for publication within the journal you intend to target. Such journals often welcome practise based articles by students. Do not submit your work for consideration to more than one journal at the same time. You should not identify any person or organization without the appropriate approvals being granted. It is useful to make summary boxes with key points/action indicators for the readership. The article should clearly signpost what the readership can expect to gain from reading it, and there should be clear bullet points of the main messages in summary boxes. It is also important to acknowledge the limitations of the review/research, and specify ways in which the findings can be implemented in practice, with examples. Articles in professional journals focus on implementation and improving practice, so ensure your article offers the readership something they can use to improve their practice, either at individual and/or organizational level.

Short articles are generally not peer reviewed, that is forwarded to other similar colleagues within your professional field for their opinions. If the editor feels your article is topical and of interest to the readership, there is a good chance it will get published. Having short articles published gives you the confidence to tackle bigger papers.

More substantive articles, such as literature reviews, are usually forwarded in the first instance to the editor, who then decides if they should go forward for peer review. Articles which are innovative, relevant and of interest to the readership are usually forwarded to peer reviewers. Generally, two peers are selected from a range of relevant reviewers who undertake reviews for the journal. The peer review process is usually 'double-blind', that is you don't know who the reviewer is and the reviewer doesn't get to know who you are, as your paper will be made anonymous prior to being sent for peer review, and the return comments from the reviewer will be similarly made anonymous. You may be asked to make minor amendments, which are often very easy to do, or sometimes you are asked to undertake a major rewrite of the article, which may entail restructuring, or adding more up-to-date information.

The first time you submit an article for publication is very exciting, and if it gets accepted that's fantastic, but very often you are asked to make amendments. Don't despair or get disheartened. This is absolutely normal, although the first time you get a reply from the editor asking you to revise your article it can be very disappointing. Keep going! You will receive the detailed comments of the reviewers to help you with this. The editor will give you a deadline and it is important that you adhere to this, as articles need to be scheduled for publication. A good tip is to make a cover sheet indicating exactly how you have addressed the reviewers' comments, to enable the editor to see if revisions have been satisfactorily addressed, or if the article needs to go for further review (sometimes with new reviewers). Occasionally, reviewers conclude that the paper is not acceptable, either because of content, clarity or relevance. It could be that your paper is more acceptable to another journal with a different focus. Take on board the comments of the reviewers, amend your paper and try elsewhere. However, be cognizant of the timeliness of information and the relevance to the professional context of the time. If articles are very context specific they may have a limited timeline or shelf-life, or you may need to add more up-to-date literature if you submit to another journal after having waited for a decision from one publisher.

 Action Point

Go to your local university health library and browse the journal section. Identify which journals are professional journals and which are academic journals within your field. Ask your health librarian for help. Make a list of the relevant professional and academic journals within your field.

 Action Point

Choose a professional journal that is relevant to your area of practice. Look up the guidelines for publication (sometimes these are within the journal or you will find them on the journal's web site).

Write a short article (300–500 words) about a practice innovation within your field, taking note of the ethical considerations outlined in Chapter 6. Submit it for consideration in your chosen professional journal.

 Action Point

Undertake a systematic literature review of a topic of interest (Chapter 5). Prepare a paper for publication in a professional journal of your choice. Check the guidelines for publication and ensure you meet the journal's criteria in terms of style and word length. Submit your paper for consideration.

Academic journals

Academic journals are published less frequently than professional journals, for example quarterly or bi-monthly, and tend to publish a collection of peer reviewed articles on research topics within a particular field. For example, literature reviews, published research findings and other papers which are either innovative or groundbreaking. The submission process is much longer. It can take up to eighteen months from submission to publication. It is good, therefore, to gain some experience of writing for professional journals prior to writing for academic journals, as you need to experience some early success to build your confidence.

Writing in an academic journal

Sometimes papers in academic journals are single authored; this might be the case if you were publishing your PhD literature review or findings, although you may wish to include your supervisor(s) as co-author(s). However, more often, papers are co-authored by all members of the research team who have worked together on a research study. Collaborative research teams may work across research sites, in several organizations, across a wide geographical area, or several countries. The Internet has enabled researchers to be based in diverse locations yet still to collaborate on studies and papers for publication.

Writing with others

It is good practice to try writing with colleagues, as they can bring new perspectives, ideas and constructive criticism to your work. The key to success is to find colleagues who are like-minded in terms of enthusiasm, commitment and available time. It can be a real pleasure to work together on articles for publication and this affords the opportunity for networking, with the additional benefit of sharing the effort needed for completion. Always agree on who will do what at the outset and prepare an overall plan. To comment on your colleagues' work as you go along, use the Comment function on *Microsoft Word* – highlight an area of text, go on the top menu, select Insert, Comment, then write your comment. A comment box appears as a balloon at the side of your work, which you can then save for your colleague to see. You can also edit these comments and remove them by right clicking your mouse on the comment balloon.

   The Internet enables you to e-mail files and work on shared drafts very easily, but you should always try to get together to discuss your work as you go along, as such meetings can generate a shared understanding of your article, and additional good ideas. Always save and date your file, so that you know which version you are working on, for example, File name: Asthma Review 12.06.09.; then when you or a your colleague works on it subsequently, they will then save the work as Asthma Review 20.06.09., and so on.

 Action Point

Collaborate with a colleague (or two) to write a joint article for a journal. Review what went well, and what would you change next time.

Writing research reports

If you are undertaking an empirical research study, it will be a requirement of your sponsoring organization, Research Ethics Committee (REC) and Research and Development board of local NHS Trusts (if the research involves the NHS) that you submit interim reports and a final report.

Research reports often form the foundation of peer reviewed academic articles, but are often much more detailed. It is important to frame the research report for the audience in question. If the report is for an REC committee, the ethical considerations undertaken will need to be detailed. Some organizations will provide a template for your report. Make a note of when research reports are due, so that you meet the deadlines required.

Writing a dissertation

Writing a dissertation is a task that requires careful planning. The key to success is time management. You should plan the overall structure of the dissertation and break down its components into manageable time slots. If it is a Masters or PhD thesis, you should allow time following completion of writing for formatting, proof reading and copy-editing (Chapter 5). You should have collated your reference list as you worked (rather than trying to find references at a later stage). Reference manager programs (such as RefWorks [http://www.refworks.com/] and Endnote [http://www.endnoteweb.com/]) are available to help you format, store and retrieve references and insert them into your writing. A useful guide to help you prepare your dissertation is the American Psychological Association (2010) Publication Manual, which offers invaluable advice on grammatical style, presentation, referencing, headings, and so on. See also the resources section for a list of materials that can help you to structure and survive your dissertation!

Writing a book

Writing a book can seem a very daunting task, but can be extremely enjoyable, as it gives you the opportunity to be more creative and expansive than is possible when writing journal articles. If you are considering writing a book, browse the different styles available in your local health library. You should also get a good feel of the type of book published by different publishing houses. Some publishers specialize in academic textbooks, others specialize in monographs. When you have a good idea of the type of book and publishing house you would like to work with, download the book proposal guidelines from the publishers' web site. Make early contact with the commissioning editor to discuss your ideas. They are often a source of very good advice that can save you a lot of time. There are several types of book you could consider writing.

Monographs

Monographs are single-authored books. Usually, they follow on from doctoral study, whereby you adapt your study for a book. There are relatively few subject monographs compared with authored books and edited works.

Edited works

An edited work (such as this book!) may be a textbook with different chapter authors or a collection of published papers brought together and edited by one or more editors. The editors have overall responsibility for ensuring the clarity and coherence of subject matter and grammatical style between chapter authors, and may indeed write or contribute to chapters themselves. Whilst it may appear a good way to expedite a book, the editor's role can be very challenging, for example in recruiting chapter authors, keeping everyone to task and editing their work. However, a good edited book can offer a breadth and depth of material which would not otherwise be possible if written by single or conjoint authors.

Online publishing

Online publishing is becoming a popular means of getting material disseminated. The advantages are that your work is in the public domain quickly, as your article, once accepted, can be published within an on-line journal very rapidly. Your article is potentially available to a very wide international audience, and on-line archives enable your article to be retrieved from the Internet in the future.

 Action Point

Ask your health librarian (and see Chapter 4) to help you locate some online journals. Log on to the Internet and read some online journals relevant to your speciality. For example, see:

British Medical Journal Online: http://journals.bmj.com/;
Evidence-based Medicine Online: http://ebm.bmj.com/;
Evidence-based Nursing Online: http://ebn.bmj.com/.

Online publishing: Dissertations or theses

Online publishing is also an increasingly attractive way of getting larger scale academic work to a wide audience. University libraries and other institutions in the United Kingdom have developed Institutional Repository(IRs) that allow peer reviewed, academic outputs including Masters' and PhD theses, conference proceedings and reports to be available in electronic format on the World Wide Web. One of the main advantages of the IR is that web search engines are much more likely to pick up and list your output than if you simply display your dissertation on your own personal web page.

Presenting your work in electronic format via an IR also gives you opportunities to be creative about the type of content you can include. For instance, a video clip of an interview or a physiological process can often say more than pages of description. This means it is best to think about how you will present your thesis or dissertation as early as possible in your academic studies. No matter when you are thinking of publishing online, the advice of library staff can be invaluable. They can help you consider your target audience, matters of permission and copyright, and how best to present and publicize your work. Within the United Kingdom, the Intute web site (http://irs.ukoln.ac.uk/) allows you to search for the IR of most relevance to you. An international search is also possible via The Directory of Open Access Repositories (http://www.opendoar.org/index.html). To access a wide selection of international work in many different disciplines, use the Networked Digital Library of Theses and Dissertations (http://www.ndltd.org/).

Action Point

Log on to the Internet to look at examples of online dissertations and theses. For a nursing example, follow the pathway from the link below:

Macduff, C. (2007). *An analysis of the development of family health nursing in Scotland through policy and practice 1998-2006.* (Doctoral Dissertation, The Robert Gordon University, Aberdeen, 2007). Retrieved from http://www.rgu.ac.uk/nursing/research/page.cfm?pge=27219

Conclusion

This chapter has given an overview of how to critique, summarize and disseminate your work in a variety of forums and through various media. It is hoped that by developing your dissemination skills in a progressive way as suggested, you will have developed your confidence and abilities and feel able to write good quality abstracts that get you offers to present your work, present papers and posters at conferences, and liaise with publishers to disseminate your work in journals and the academic press. Most importantly, it is hoped that you disseminate the results of your work for the benefit of others within your own professional field, not only at conferences, but also in your own workplace, to help others implement and review evidence based practice. Arguably, not to do so is unethical, given that you have engaged the time and cooperation of people who will be expecting that others will benefit from their participation in your work.

 Action Point

Suggest *three* potential challenges in disseminating or implementing the findings or recommendations of research into practice.

References

American Psychological Association (APA) (2010) *Publication manual of the American Psychological Association*, 6th edn, APA, New York.
Black, T.R. (1999) *Doing quantitative research in the social sciences*, Sage, London.

Further reading

Presentation skills

Bienvenu, S. (2000) *The Presentation Skills Workshop: Helping People Create and Deliver Great Presentations*, American Management Association, New York.
Briggs, D.J. (2009) A practical guide to designing a poster for presentation. *Nursing Standard*, **23** (34), 35–39.
Chivers, B. and Shoolbred, M. (2007) *A Student's Guide to Presentations. Making your Presentation Count*, Sage, London.

Hamlin, S. (2006) *How to Talk so People Listen: Connecting in Today's Workplace*, HarperCollins, London.
Happell, B. (2009) Presenting with precision: Preparing and delivering a polished conference presentation. *Nurse Researcher*, **16** (3), 45–56.
Kaul, A. (2005) *The Effective Presentation: Talk your Way to Success*, Sage, London.
McCarthy, P. and Hatcher, C. (2002) *Presentation Skills: The Essential Guide for Students*, Sage, London.
Maier, P., Price, G. and Cowen, M. (2009) *Study Skills for Nurses and Health Care Students*, Pearson Education, London.
Rotondo, J. and Rotondo, M. (2001) *Presentation Skills for Managers*, McGraw-Hill Professional, New York.
Shephard, K. (2005) *Presenting at Conferences, Seminars and Meetings*, Sage, London.

Writing for publication

American Psychological Association (APA) (2010) *Concise Rules of APA Style*, American Psychological Association, New York.
Craswell, G. (2004) *Writing for Academic Success: A Postgraduate Guide*, Sage, London.
Epstein, D., Kenway, J. and Boden, R. (2007) *Writing for Publication*, Sage, London.
Hall, G.M. (1998) *How to Write a Paper*, BMJ Publishing, London.
Jackson, H. (2005) *Good Grammar for Students*, Sage, London.
Kitchin, R. and Fuller, D. (2005) *The Academic's Guide to Publishing*, Sage, London.
Lester, J.D. and Lester, J.D. Jr (1999) *The Essential Guide to Writing Research Papers*, Longman, New York.
Levin, P. (2004) *Write Great Essays*, Open University Press, Buckingham.
Murray, R. (2004) *How to Write for Academic Journals*, Open University Press, Buckingham.
Peat, J., Baur, L. and Keena, V. (2002) *Scientific Writing*, BMJ Publishing, London.
Peck, J. and Coyle, M. (2005) *The Student's Guide to Writing*, 2nd edn, Palgrave, Basingstoke.
Peck, J. and Coyle, M (2005) *Write it Right. A Handbook for Students*, Palgrave, Basingstoke.
Thody, A. (2006) *Writing and Presenting Research*, Sage, London.
Wallace, M. and Wray, A. (2006) *Critical Reading and Writing for Postgraduates*, Sage, London.
Wolcott, H.F. (2009) *Writing up Qualitative Research*, 3rd edn, Sage, London.

Writing dissertations

Bryant, M.T. (2004) *The Portable Dissertation Advisor*, Sage, London.
Churchill, H. and Sanders, T. (2007) *Getting your PhD. A Practical Insider's Guide*, Sage, London.
Hart, C. (2004) *Doing your Masters Dissertation*, Sage, London.
Oliver, P. (2003) *Writing Your Thesis*, Sage, London.
Roberts, C.M. (2004) *The Dissertation Journey: A Practical and Comprehensive Guide to Planning, Writing, and Defending Your Dissertation*, Sage, London.
Murray, R. (2002) *How to Write a Thesis*, Open University Press, Buckingham.
Roberts, P.M. (2000) Practical issues in 'writing up' a research thesis. *Nurse Researcher*, **7** (4), 14–23.
Rudestam, K.E. and Newton, R.R. (2007) *Surviving Your Dissertation. A Comprehensive Guide to Content and Process*, 3rd edn, Sage, Thousand Oaks, CA.
Walliman, N. (2004) *Your Undergraduate Dissertation: The Essential Guide for Success*, Sage, London.
Wellington, J., Bathmaker, A., Hunt, C. *et al.* (2005) *Succeeding with Your Doctorate*, Sage, London.

Publishing on the Internet

O'Dochartaigh N. (2002) *The Internet Research Handbook. A Practical Guide for Students and Researchers in the Social Sciences*, Sage, London.
Macduff, C. (2008) Think out loud: Publishing your dissertation or thesis on line. *Nursing Standard*, **22** (21) 62–63.
Stein, S. (1999) *Learning, Teaching and Researching on the Internet. A Practical Guide for Social Scientists*, Pearson Educational Ltd, Essex.

Useful web sites

- Creative Commons (a not-for-profit corporation dedicated to making it easier for people to share and build upon the work of others, consistent with the rules of copyright): http://creativecommons.org/about;
- Equator (Information for authors of research reports) http://www.equator-network.org/resource-centre/authors-of-research-reports/authors-of-research-reports/;
- Intute: Repository search: http://irs.ukoln.ac.uk/;
- The Directory of Open Access Repositories: http://www.opendoar.org/index.html;
- Networked Digital Library of Theses and Dissertations: http://www.ndltd.org/.

Part 2

Research in action

11 Combining Research Methods: Case Studies and Action Research

Rebecca Jester

Introduction

In Chapters 7 and 8, we focused on the unique features of quantitative and qualitative research. In this chapter, we aim to demonstrate how research methods can be integrated and combined to address specific research questions. The chapter will provide an overview of two specific research designs: action research and case studies, together with examples from research projects conducted by the author. This chapter does not aim to provide an in-depth philosophical debate related to case study and action research approaches, but rather a practical discussion of the merits, limitations and application of these two approaches. We begin by discussing the concepts of 'mixed methods' and 'triangulation', first introduced in Chapter 2.

Mixed methods approaches

Traditionally, within health and social research, individuals have aligned themselves with either the quantitative or qualitative paradigm. However, in reality, many real world research projects benefit from mixing or combining methods. Mixed methods research can be accomplished either by using specific approaches to research, such as action research or case study, as discussed within this chapter, or by adopting a phased approach within a study. This might involve the first stage being exploratory within the qualitative paradigm, and the results from this being used to form specific hypotheses for testing within an experimental design, such as a randomized controlled trial. Equally, a quantitative approach (say, a questionnaire) might be used to gather data from a wide range of people, with the results being used to develop a qualitative interview schedule for use with a small sample of respondents.

Triangulation

Very often a research study is undertaken with multiple datasets, mixed methodology or with different researchers, such as at different sites. Triangulation is a very useful technique that enables you to enhance and verify concepts. As Ramprogus (2005, p. 4) suggests, 'triangulation. . .tries to reconcile the differences of two or more data sources, methodological approaches, designs, theoretical perspectives, investigators and data analysis to compensate for the weaknesses of any single strategy towards achieving completeness or confirmation of findings'. However, triangulation must be exercised with caution; it is no substitute for robust and well-established methods of establishing validity. Rather it is used to confirm or affirm, and therefore verify findings.

Combining methods in practice

The author's research interests focus on applied clinical studies related to the care and treatment of trauma and orthopaedic patients. Applied clinical research often develops from the identification of clinical problems and the need to develop robust evidence to support practice, policies and protocols. Often, clinical research questions necessitate the use of multiple methods, which may include both quantitative and qualitative approaches. Furthermore, if research findings are to be used to underpin practice, and managers and health care professionals are to be convinced to change practice based on research evidence, it is important for them to be active partners in the research process instead of being passive recipients of research findings and decisions. Healthcare practitioners and managers are bombarded with policy directives, efficiency targets and new policy on a daily basis and often feel that the pace of change is overwhelming. From observation, many practitioners and managers are reluctant to engage in the process of implementation of research findings because they do not understand the research process or data analysis, or how to interpret and implement the findings. We must strive, therefore, to support healthcare professionals to be at least competent and confident appraisers of research relevant to their practice. Action research and case studies are two practical approaches that put the patient/client and/or healthcare staff at the centre of the research process, and indeed necessitate their active participation. Being involved should help to demystify research and improve understanding and translation into clinical practice.

However, mixed methods approaches are not without their challenges. Collins, Onwuegbuzie and Qun (2007) identify four challenges to mixed methods research: representation, legitimization or validity, integration and politics. The challenge of integration of qualitative and quantitative approaches is the most complex to tackle, and Collins *et al.* (p. 269) pose the question: 'Is it appropriate to triangulate, expand, compare or consolidate quantitative data originating from a large, random sample with qualitative data from a small, purposive sample?'

As researchers, we need to weigh the benefits of mixing approaches within a single study against the challenges and complexities that it involves. Most importantly, the approaches taken must be justified as the most effective method of answering the research question/s, and we must not permit our individual biases toward particular paradigms to influence those decisions. We now illustrate two ways in which methods can be integrated within a single research design: action research and case studies.

Action research

Action research has been used within the social sciences since the 1940s. Kurt Lewin (1890–1947) is generally thought to be the originator of the term 'action research' as a method of researching a social system, while at the same time attempting to change the system being studied. Many students and healthcare practitioners are familiar with Kurt Lewin's work related to change management theories and, specifically, force field analysis (Value Based Management, 2009). This begins to highlight the symbiotic relationship between generating new knowledge through the research process and using this knowledge to change practice or systems.

Action research is a form of enquiry that describes, interprets and explains a social situation while at the same time implementing an intervention aimed at change, improvement and involvement. It is problem-focused, context-specific and future-orientated, and founded on partnership between all researcher(s) and participants (Waterman, Tillen and Dickson, 2001).

 Action Point

From the description above, identify key words and concepts that indicate action research may be a useful approach in contemporary healthcare research. Think about the words you have selected, and why.

Characteristics of action research

The words you have selected may relate to the key characteristics of action research presented below, which are adapted from Waterman and Hope (2008):

- collaboration and participation;
- developmental;
- change and improvement;
- practical and context specific;
- cyclical;
- involves reflection and reflexivity.

Within the context of contemporary healthcare research, most funding bodies (such as Research for Patient Benefit; National Institute for Health Research (NIHR), 2006) strongly encourage or indeed insist upon research designs and approaches that include the active partic- ipation of patients/service users/carers and practitioners. There is an increasing realization that many research studies do not influence clinical practice or policy, and there is a need to increase emphasis on implementation of good quality research. The cyclical nature of action research also lends itself to healthcare, as there is a constant need to evolve our evidence based practice and policy. There are several models of action research, including the early action research cycle developed by Kemmis and McTaggart (1982) which includes: identification of the problem; in- vestigation of problem concepts and study of the related literature; designing the plan of action to solve the problem; putting the plan into action and monitoring changes to practice; reflection, changes and modifications to the solution. This model is illustrated within the case study of applied action research, later in this chapter. Subsequent models include that of Hart and Bond (1995), which includes: the stages of identifying a problem; using research methods to assess the problem; planning and implementing change; and evaluating the outcome of change.

Types of action research

Hart and Bond (1995) identify four types of action research:

- experimental;
- organizational;
- professionalising;
- empowering.

A number of authors, including Grbich (1999), purport that these four types of action research run along a continuum, whereby at the experimental end the researcher leads in all aspects of research design and process and usually conducts the study at the behest of senior managers within an organization who perceive the need to 'fix a problem'. The organizational approach remains researcher-centric, but does include greater negotiation and consultation with those working at grass roots, that is, practitioners. Professionalising approaches begin to embrace approaches to the design and process of the research, where often the need to change practice through research is identified by the practitioners and/or service users/carers themselves, with the researcher acting as a guide and facilitator. The empowering approach views the participants as co-researchers who contribute equally to decisions about what the problem is and which approaches of design and process are needed. Ultimately, the empowering approach aims to lead to emancipation of grass roots practitioners, service users and carers, enabling them to break free from top-down approaches to improve services and instigate change to policy and practice.

The empowering/emancipatory approach aims to foster a culture of collective enquiry, reflection and problem solving. These are important benefits, as once the action research project has ended, change and continual improvement need to be sustained by practitioners, managers and service users/carers.

Case Example 11.1:   Pre-operative Fasting

The author, whilst engaged as a lecturer practitioner within a specialist orthopaedic hospital, was approached by a number of ward based nurses who were concerned about pre-operative fasting policy and practice within the organization. The custom was to withhold all fluids and food for patients from midnight prior to surgery the following day, irrespective of what time the patient was scheduled to have their surgery. A critical incident where a patient's surgery was cancelled due to severe headache bought on by dehydration prompted the nurses to raise their concerns. The issue of concern was raised with the senior consultant anaesthetist and the author, although a novice to the technique, believed action research was the best approach to be taken.

Kemmis and McTaggart's (1982) model of action research was chosen to guide the process.

Identification of the problem

Patients were being starved for excessively long periods prior to surgery. There were also frequent changes made to theatre lists by surgeons, and often these changes were not communicated in a timely manner to ward staff and patients. Nurses perceived that post-operative nausea and vomiting were in part due to the excessive fasting practices.

Investigation of problem concepts and study of the related literature

The literature review revealed that it was safe for healthy adult patients to drink clear fluids up to two hours prior to surgery and consume food or milk up to six hours before. The researcher then conducted a survey of fasting times, with a convenience sample of 110 elective adult orthopaedic patients over a period of one month. This survey revealed that the mean fasting time was 11.94 hours and far exceeded the recommendations from the literature review. The literature review had also highlighted reasons why patients are starved for excessive periods pre-operatively, including:

- lack of knowledge by nurses about the physiology of gastric emptying in healthy adults;
- practice based on custom rather than on evidence based research;
- changing of theatre lists leading to uncertainty about what time patients would be anaesthetized.

Designing the plan of action to solve the problem

In collaboration with the senior anaesthetist, three interlinked actions were agreed. Firstly, anaesthetists were asked to start prescribing the time patients could consume both food and fluids. Secondly, the author implemented an educational package for ward based nurses to improve their knowledge of evidence based fasting practice (Jester and Williams, 1999). Thirdly, pre-admission letters to patients informed them of the new fasting practices and they were encouraged to drink clear fluids up to two hours prior to their surgery, for example, at 6.30 a.m. for those on the morning list and 11 a.m. for those on the afternoon list.

Putting the plan into action and monitoring changes to practice

Following a three month period during which nurses were asked to report problems with the implementation of the new fasting practices, a follow up survey was conducted on 106 adult elective orthopaedic patients within the same clinical areas as before. The follow up survey revealed that the mean fasting time had reduced by 5.40 hours from the initial survey, but this still meant that patients were, on average, not taking clear fluids for around six hours prior to their surgery. The survey also demonstrated that 60 of the 106 patients were prescribed a last drink by an anaesthetist, while 46 were not. Of the 60 patients who had a prescription for the last time of clear fluids, nursing staff did not give the drink at the prescribed time to six patients for the following reasons:

- three patients were asleep and were not woken up for a drink;
- one patient refused the drink offered;
- one patient had their position on the list moved up;
- no reason was given for one patient.

(Jester and Williams, 1999)

Reflection, changes and modifications to the solution

This stage was used to explore why only 60 of the 106 patients had been seen by an anaesthetist and had the last time for clear fluids prescribed. This highlighted that for patients admitted on the day of surgery, the anaesthetist often did not arrive at the hospital in time to see patients before he/she needed to be in theatre. Discussions with nursing staff also highlighted the fact that frequent changes to theatre lists made nurses fearful of encouraging patients to drink clear fluids up to two hours prior to surgery. This was because surgeons would be unhappy if they called for patients who could not go to theatre because they had been given a drink. The reasons for frequent changes to the list were investigated and this revealed that it was often because of surgeons' preferences, or occasionally because the correct instruments were not available in theatre.

In this case illustration, it can be seen that action research was truly cyclical because more work was needed to improve communication between theatre staff and ward based staff. Furthermore, improving efficiency around availability of equipment was required, as was the need for the empowerment of nurses to advocate for their patients' rights.

 Action Point

Reflecting on Case Example 11.1, what approach to action research was adopted? (Take into consideration there may be an amalgam of approaches.)

The approach taken in the worked example was predominantly professionalising, as the clinicians identified the problem, namely excessive pre-operative fasting periods for elective orthopaedic patients. However, it can also be viewed as adopting elements of the organizational approach, as the research methods were determined by the researcher, rather than in consultation with the clinicians.

 Action Point

If you were replicating the study, what would you do differently, and why?

To answer this question, you need to consider possible limitations of the study and how these might be addressed. Limitations appeared to include the following:

- A further element of data collection was required at the stage of 'problem concepts investigated and related literature studied', as the author did not explore the unique issues affecting fasting practices within the organization. That is, there was an over-reliance on the literature;
- Not all staff groups were represented in the action research process; specifically, there were no surgeons in the project team and, because they were highly influential within the organization, their support was needed to minimize changes to theatre lists and to avoid conflict when nurses adopted the new fasting policy;
- There was no patient involvement; it would have enriched both the data collected and the implementation of improved policy to elicit patients' views and preferences related to preoperative fasting practice.

Limitations of action research

There are a number of criticisms of action research, which include the emphasis on action and outcomes and the need to instigate change, rather than to generate theory or a new body of knowledge. Also, the researcher may have a conflict of interest if the action research is at the behest of senior managers (e.g. at the experimental/organizational end of the continuum). However, action research is one of the few approaches that offers the potential for clinicians, users and carers to be engaged in all aspects of research design and process, which greatly increases the chance that the findings of the research will be implemented and sustained within the practice setting.

Case studies

Robson (2002, p. 178) defines a case study as 'a strategy for doing research which involves an empirical investigation of a particular contemporary phenomenon within its real life context using multiple sources of evidence'. Case study methodology involves the in-depth recounting and analysis of experience. It can be used to study phenomena in health and social care at an individual level, such as one client or patient, or part of or a whole organization, such as the trauma and orthopaedic unit or an acute hospital. The researcher can adopt either a retrospective (looking back) or prospective (looking forward) approach to the case study. Yin (2003) proposes that case studies are most useful when the researcher wants to ask *how* and *why* questions. Case study is not an approach usually used to test a hypothesis or determine cause and effect; it is mostly concerned with the subjective richness of individual or organizational experiences of a phenomenon (Zucker, 2001). Thus, qualitative approaches to data collection and analysis are often used. However, case study approaches can also adopt quantitative approaches; for example, single-subject experiments involve the individual or unit of research being exposed to an intervention/treatment and data being collected both before and after implementation of the treatment. Furthermore, case studies can be used for exploratory, descriptive or explanatory purposes; the specific approach taken will depend on the nature of the research question(s) and the degree of control the researcher has over the phenomena being studied. Case studies are strong in reality and allow the researcher to study the phenomenon within its social, political and economic context.

 Action Point

Suggest some data collection methods that would be suitable for both prospective and retrospective approaches to a case study of an individual or part of or a whole healthcare organization.

Some of these are summarized in Table 11.1.

Characteristics of case studies

Whether the case study involves an individual or part or all of an organization, there are certain characteristics that must be identifiable, which include:

- clearly articulated research questions;
- propositions;
- unit(s) of analysis;

- a determination of how the data are linked to the propositions;
- criteria to interpret the findings.

(Yin, 2003)

Table 11.1   Approaches to data collection in case study methodology.

Prospective	Retrospective
Participant and non-participant observation of direct patient care, team meetings, case conferences, and so on.	Examination of case notes, care plans.
Interviews with patients, relatives or staff.	Minutes of meetings.
Examination of a patient, reviewing clinical investigation results such as blood tests or urinalysis.	Analysis of critical incident reports.
Taking photographs, video or tape recordings.	Reviewing photographs, floor plans, x-rays, and so on.

To understand these characteristics, let us relate them to a worked example (Case Example 11.2).

Case Example 11.2:   Delays in Internal Fixation of Hip Fractures

A study by Williams and Jester (2005) identified that despite Department of Health guidelines stating older patients with hip fractures should undergo internal fixation surgery within 24 hours of admission to hospital, many patients faced prolonged delays that adversely impacted on their morbidity and mortality. The author drew up a research proposal for a case study as a follow up to the original study, to provide an enrichment of the reasons for this phenomenon.

Articulating the research question

This was defined as 'why do patients continue to face delays to undergo internal fixation of their hip fracture?'

Propositions

Based on review of the literature, previous research in the area and experience of working with older patients with hip fracture, the proposition was that delays to surgery are caused by lack of dedicated theatre time for this patient group and that they were viewed by staff as less urgent than younger trauma patients.

The unit of analysis

To capture a rich in-depth view of the phenomenon, a single case study of a patient admitted for internal fixation of their hip fracture was adopted. The data collection methods included: participant observation with the researcher working as a member of the nursing team; interviews with nurses, anaesthetists and orthopaedic surgeons; analysis of medical and nursing notes and care plans; and analysis of clinical investigations such as blood results and chest and hip X-rays.

A determination of how the data are linked to the propositions

Data related to how long the patient waited for surgery, the number of times their theatre slot was postponed, and why, were collected and correlated with data related to how trauma theatre lists are determined and by whom, resources available in terms of theatre slots, and availability of orthopaedic surgeons and anaesthetists. A focus group with nurses, surgeons and anaesthetists determined their views and attitudes as to why the delays were occurring. The participant observation element allowed the researcher to elicit the real attitudes of staff to this phenomenon.

Criteria to interpret the findings

Rigour of interpretation and analysis is essential when dealing with both quantitative and qualitative data. Criteria adopted included triangulation of the data between the perceptions of staff and the realities of the patient journey and using iterative approaches to analysis with reference back to literature and organizational policy. Data related to physiological status of the patient, such as urea and electrolyte results, were treated as within-subject repeated-measures data. Data analysis also included comparing the case to prior predictions outlined at the propositions stage.

 Action Point

What are the potential weaknesses in the approaches to data collection and analysis used in this case study?

Suggested limitations to the approach taken include the following:

- The focus group with staff may not elicit their true attitudes, as within a group there will be the strong possibility of social desirability bias with participants saying what they think is both socially/professionally acceptable and conforming to hospital/Department of Health policy;
- Using a single case of one patient will limit the generalization of the findings, and rigour would be improved by studying several cases, including an extreme case, a normal case and a deviant case.

Conclusion

Reflecting on the two illustrations within this chapter, we find that both benefited from a mixed methods approach. Firstly, the action research project to improve pre-operative fasting involved a quantitative element with the collecting of numerical data (length of fasting) and compared that statistically before and after the implementation of the new fasting guideline. In addition, a qualitative approach was used with the focus group to elicit staff perceptions of why evidence based fasting practice was not in place at the commencement of the study. The second example of the case study included both a within subjects comparison of blood results across time with the single 'case', a focus group with staff to elicit their attitudes to delays in surgery for older hip fracture patients, and further qualitative data collection and analysis through the process of participant observation and generation of field notes.

 Reflection Point

Thinking about your own area of practice, what clinical or organizational problems might lend themselves to study using a mixed methods approach?
What data sources might you use?
Why would this be approach be preferable to either a single quantitative or qualitative approach?

References

Collins, M., Onwuegbuzie, A. and Qun, G. (2007) A mixed methods investigation of mixed methods sampling designs in social and health science research. *Journal of Mixed Methods Research*, **1** (3), 267–294.
Grbich, C. (1999) *Qualitative Research in Health*, Allen & Unwin Ltd, St Leonards, Australia.
Hart, E. and Bond, M. (1995) *Action Research for Health and Social Care: A Guide to Practice*, Open University Press, Maidenhead.
Jester, R. and Williams, S. (1999) Pre-operative fasting: putting research into practice. *Nursing Standard*, **13** (39), 33–35.
Kemmis, S. and McTaggart, R. (1982) *The Action Research Planner*, 2nd edn, Deakin University Press, Melbourne.
NIHR (NHS National Institute for Health Research) (2006) *The Research for Patient Benefit Programme*. Retrieved from http://www.nihr-ccf.org.uk/site/programmes/rfpb/default.cfm.
Ramprogus, V. (2005) Triangulation. *Nurse Researcher*, **12** (4), 4–6.
Robson, C. (2002) *Real World Research: A Resource for Social Scientists and Practitioner-Researchers*, 2nd edn, Blackwell Publishing, Oxford.
Value Base Management (2009) *Force field analysis*. Retrieved from http://www.valuebasedmanagement.net/methods_lewin_force_field_analysis.html.
Waterman, H., Tillen, D. and Dickson, R. (2001) Action research: a systematic review and assessment for guidance. *Health Technology Assessment*, **5** (23), 1–166.
Waterman, H. and Hope, K. (2008) Action research, in *Nursing Research: Designs and Methods* (eds R. Watson, H. McKenna, S. Cowman and J. Keady,) Churchill Livingstone, Edinburgh.
Williams, A. and Jester, R. (2005) Delayed surgical fixation of fractured hips in older people: impact on mortality. *Journal of Advanced Nursing*, **52** (1), 63–69.
Yin, R,(2003) *Case Study Research: Design and Methods*, 3rd edn, Sage, London.
Zucker, D. (2001) Using case study methodology in nursing research. *The Qualitative Report*, **6** (2). Retrieved from: http:www.nova.edu/ssss/QR/QR6-2/zucker.html.

Further reading

Dellinger, A. and Leech, N. (2007) Toward a unified validation framework in mixed methods research. *Journal of Mixed Methods Research*, **1** (4), 309–332.

Fenech Adami, M. and Kiger, A. (2005) The use of triangulation for completeness purposes. *Nurse Researcher*, **12** (4), 19–29.

Greenwood, D.J. and Levin, M. (2007) *Introduction to Action Research. Social Research for Social Change*, Sage, Thousand Oaks, CA.

Magnusson, C., Finnerty, G. and Pope, R. (2005) Methodological triangulation in midwifery education research. *Nurse Researcher*, **12** (4) 30–39.

Williamson, G. R. (2005) Illustrating triangulation in mixed-methods nursing research. *Nurse Researcher*, **12** (4), 7–18.

Teddie, C. and Tashakkori, A. (2009) *Foundations of Mixed Methods Research. Integrating Quantitative and Qualitative Approaches in the Social and Behavioural Sciences*, Sage, Thousand Oaks, CA.

12 Involving Vulnerable People in Research

Helen Combes and Ranil Tan

Introduction

I like discussions, and when I am asked questions, I try to answer them ... In the serious play of questions and answers ... they depend only on the dialogue situation

(Foucault, 1984).

In accordance with the words of Foucault, in this chapter we are hoping to open up a dialogue about research, which we hope will include the voices of vulnerable people. Our aim is to encourage and enable people working within health and social care professions to find ways of working in partnership with vulnerable people, to enable them to ask questions they may have about their health and the health of their communities, and to find answers to those questions. A range of examples from research with people with learning difficulties and mental health problems will enable us to consider whether and how we can truly develop research methodologies which include, encourage and respond to the questions of vulnerable people.

We have used the term 'learning difficulties' in this chapter in line with the People First organization's statement: *'At People First (Self Advocacy) we believe that people labelled as having a learning disability are disabled by society. We choose to use the term 'learning difficulty' instead of 'learning disability' to get across the idea that our learning support needs change over time.'* (www.peoplefirstltd.com), and because this is the term preferred by the people who took part in some of the research described.

Firstly, we define vulnerability and describe the historical context in which research, especially within the National Health Service (NHS) and other contexts, has been conducted and developed. Secondly, case examples (Case examples 12.1–12.3) will be presented and summarized and readers will be asked to consider a range of clinical and ethical dilemmas that have emerged through the research projects being conducted.

Who is vulnerable?

There are points during all of our lives when we feel vulnerable or at risk of being hurt through the actions of others. For the purpose of this chapter, however, we will define vulnerability as a systematic and prolonged process of devaluation, which has occurred for some groups throughout Western History. Historically, certain groups of people have been disenfranchised or placed on the margins of communities; such groups include people suffering from mental health problems and learning disability, travelling communities, homeless people, asylum seekers and refugees, amongst many others (Involve, 2004). Of course, this vulnerability is influenced by context and there will be situations in which these people are more susceptible to wounding (and others where they are not). One principle stressed in this chapter is that through our research we have the potential to do further harm to people, or render them more vulnerable. One such example is the war crimes, argued at the time to be of scientific interest, committed during World War II in concentration camps. People being held in the camps were subject to huge atrocities leading to them being disfigured or killed to advance the ideology of Hitler's third Reich; this is an extreme example of elitist research. After the war, these atrocities were investigated and this led to the advancement of The Nuremberg Code of Medical Ethics (1949), which forms the basis of contemporary ethical codes around conducting research with human participants.

History of research with vulnerable groups

Since the UK National Health Service was launched in 1948, the political context in which research is carried out within that service has changed; early research tended to focus on the specific interests of particular medical consultants and academic experts working within a healthcare and research context. In 1952, the Medical Research Council undertook the first randomized controlled trials (Chapter 7), looking at the effectiveness of the drug Streptomycin in pulmonary tuberculosis, and since this time much research conducted within a medical context has used and relied upon randomized controlled trials as the gold-standard (Stolberg, Norman and Trop, 2004). This preference presumes that all questions that come under the auspices of health and medicine are best subjected to an experimental or positivist method.

During the 1980s, under the Thatcher Government, the NHS adopted a business model, becoming more target focused; the NHS was required to demonstrate cost effectiveness, and audit and evaluation become essential elements of providing care and therapy to people in the NHS. 'New Labour', under the leadership of Tony Blair, continued to have this interest, but highlighted the role of the customer in the research agenda (and in the future of service provision and evaluation). The subjective view of the NHS 'customer' is increasingly being sought, not only in evaluating clinical outcomes, but also about the kinds of questions that it should be asking.

In contrast to Health Service research, various charitable trusts have established different ways of conducting research with vulnerable groups. The Joseph Rowntree Foundation (www.jrf.org.uk), for example, was established in 1904. Its aim, at that time, was to look at the relationship between inequalities in health and poverty; the work of the Foundation continues, as a charitable trust, focusing upon the impact of poverty on quality of life. The research it funds is broad and includes work around community inclusion, children in poverty and older people.

Within the NHS, research should no longer be in the interests of the powerful, but should increasingly be participatory and reflect the needs of the individuals and communities funding that service (the tax payers). This political agenda has important repercussions and implications for services that work with disempowered and vulnerable people in under-resourced communities. It raises a number of ethical and methodological issues about how to include vulnerable people in conducting participatory research that gives those people and their community power and control over the research process.

Service user involvement and participatory research

In this context of participation and inclusion, it is apparent that service users must be at the forefront of the research process, before services are developed and become established, and that the views of those people must, in turn, influence the governance and indeed the Government's agenda. When conducting research, we need to work very closely with people who, through their contact with society and services, have become devalued and are at risk of becoming further devalued. In addition to this, as health and social care workers (or skilled helpers) we have a duty of care to ensure that through our work (and indeed through the dissemination and sharing of that work) we inflict no further harm or further marginalize individuals or groups of individuals. To do this as researchers and clinicians we have to be open to new models and ways of conducting research. Such research needs to be conducted in close partnership with the people and communities we serve and creative in its use of research methodologies, which have the potential to become vehicles for service development in themselves (Oliver, 2002).

Ethical issues

Any research which is looking at the lives of vulnerable people or includes vulnerable people needs to be subjected to ethical scrutiny (Chapter 6). Sometimes these processes can seem to hinder progress, but their principle is to protect the public and it is therefore important to ensure that all research questions and methods are subject to ethical scrutiny.

If you are working in either social care or healthcare settings then your research proposal should be scrutinized by an appropriate ethical committee. Most materials for submission to these committees are available online (Chapter 6) and the Patient Advice and Liaison Service (PALS) can help researchers develop their consent forms and information sheets in a user-friendly style. It is important to ensure that the people you are working with have the capacity to give their informed consent to participate in the research. When there are questions about their capacity to give consent, it is important to ensure that they have an identified person who will help them to understand the research, the method and feedback mechanisms, and to help them to identify questions they may have of the researcher. For researchers interested in working with people with learning difficulties, for example, the Department of Health (2001) has developed a range of resources.

An ethical reviewer will want to be sure that the researcher has given participants adequate information, that the researcher has gained the consent of the participants, and that they are free to withdraw from the study should they choose. The committee will also want to ensure that the research is using the correct methodology to answer the question; they may also be interested in how the information will be disseminated and shared with others. The committee requires regular updates on the progress of the research and it is important that someone takes on the role of Chief Investigator and agrees to provide these updates to the committee on a regular basis.

Case Example 12.1:   Using Q Methodology to Help People Identify Valued Activities in Their Lives

This research project aimed to get people with learning difficulties involved in both the research process and in setting service goals and objectives around the things they would like to be able to do (Combes, Buchan and Hardy, 2004).

As an assistant psychologist, the first author had worked in a setting which was introducing individual planning into its service. She was invited to a meeting where the person who was being reviewed had limited verbal skills. She wondered about how to find ways to get this person's views on how they would like to develop, how could services find ways to get to know the valued life direction that the person themselves wanted to live? In this example, the person had found it hard to stay in the meeting and came in and out of the meeting at will. The researcher wondered how the person could be included in the meeting to ensure they had been involved in planning for their future home, friends and leisure activities. In addition to this question, she had also wondered about the extent to which families and staff supporting the person were truly representing the views of the person, rather than their own, in the meeting.

A literature review showed that there was a paucity of established methods to ensure that the views of people with limited verbal skills could be included in planning. Such inclusion was (and continues to be) a challenge to services. Recommendations had been made about how to use pictures in meetings, but no paper had shown how pictures could be ascribed a value by the person; values tended to be assumed through behavioural indicators. If someone refused an activity, for example, then it was assumed that it was an activity they did not value or want to do. The researcher felt that there may be many other reasons that a person might not participate in an activity other than because they did not value it. For example, someone might refuse to swim, but it might be because they do not think they have the skills to swim, do not feel safe or do not like the swimming pool.

Q methodology, devised by William Stephenson (1902–1989), involves people sorting or ranking variables presented as statements written on cards. It had been used by Carl Rogers (1954) to identify goals for person-centred therapy, and on reading the literature it seemed that this method could be adapted to use pictures, which could then be sorted by people without reading ability or with limited verbal skills. It seemed that Q methodology could enable us to identify, in partnership with the service users and their families, a range of valued activities and to represent these activities through photographs. It should then be possible to ask each person and his or her circle of support to rank the extent to which they valued these activities.

A proposal was made to the local research ethics committee, using Q methodology as the principal tool to investigate whether people with moderate to severe learning difficulties could identify and rank a range of valued activities and whether the staff caring for them and their family members would be able to represent their views accurately.

When the first author began to work in a service where they were committed to rolling out person-centred planning (PCP), she asked if she could help to devise a way to involve the person in identifying their valued activities. The PCP team invited her to a meeting where they found out about the research project; they then identified potential participants. Once participants had been identified, the researcher obtained their consent to participate. This consent was obtained by telling local home managers about the research and giving them a research information sheet, written in simpler language, supplemented with pictures. They contacted potential service users and the researcher then met the service user and their key worker. The service user either signed or stated the advantages and disadvantages of taking part in the research. They were then given a 'cooling-off period' and left a consent form on which they could place a mark. The key worker re-contacted the researcher once consent had been obtained.

The researcher then arranged a focus group meeting which included the person with learning difficulties and their circle of support. The two service users chose the venue for the meeting and lunch was provided for everyone. The members of the focus group were asked to identify, firstly, the things that they believe people are valued for in Western Society and then the things that they valued in people. Once these values were identified, the focus group considered what kinds of activities might represent these values. Once a list of activities had been developed, the focus group began to identify photographs or pictures that might represent these activities. The service users brought along photographs of activities they enjoyed and these were used to stimulate discussion about values. The researcher found pictures to represent these activities and sent them out to the focus group, which replaced photographs where they felt the meaning was ambiguous. Thirty-six pictures were identified. Once this task was done, each picture was put on card.

Each member of the focus group then completed a card sort. Firstly, they sorted the cards into 'values' and 'does not value'. They were then asked to state which activity they thought the focus person valued most. This was given the highest ranking. This was completed for all picture 'statements'; each card was given a ranking. All members of the focus group completed a sort, including the focus person. It took the focus person longer, but everyone was able to rank all of the activities from highly valued to least valued. To ensure reliability, the card sorts were completed in the same setting three weeks later. For one person, there was a correlation between sort at time one and two of 0.454 (a low correlation); for all participants, however, the sorts were highly correlated. The ranking of valued activities was then shared in advance of the next planning meeting and goals were identified which ensured that people were being given the opportunity to participate in those activities which they enjoyed.

Getting started

At the start of the research enterprise, it is important first to establish allegiances with local groups and communities with whom you share a common value base and interest, and with whom you feel you can have an open and honest dialogue about the strengths and potential pitfalls of the research. This can occur through your routine clinical practice, when contacting people within systems and organizations with ideas and questions that they would like to explore with others. These questions could range from issues about service provision to inequalities in health, employment and wealth. From these initial enquiries, a focus or research group could be established to which interested parties should be invited to attend. The time and venue should be set to enable service users to participate and, sometimes, additional resources will be required to ensure that this can happen.

Reflection Points

Did this research truly include people with learning difficulties?
What could the researcher have done to ensure that the participants were giving their informed consent to the study?
What other things could the researcher have done to ensure their voice was heard?
What methodologies might you adopt to ensure that people with moderate to severe learning difficulties and limited verbal skills are involved in planning their lives?

This study showed that people with learning difficulties could ascribe value to photographs of activities, but that at least for one of them this statement of value may not be reliably assumed. It also showed that carers and families completed sorts that were highly correlated to the person's own sort. This might demonstrate that the findings (views of others) were reliable, but what are the risks in assuming that because the views of the family were highly correlated in the first instance (but not on the second sort) that they understood the needs and values of the person whose life they were planning?

Of course, this study is now quite old and people continue to develop innovative ways to ensure that the views of people with disabilities are involved in planning their lives (for example, using 'Talking Mats', a low technology communication framework involving sets of symbols; http://www.talkingmats.com/). Indeed, while this research endeavoured to include the views of vulnerable people (and to be participatory), it does not appear to have had their questions at the heart of the research enterprise. Researchers have a duty to develop and build upon innovative methodologies to ensure that the voices and perspectives of vulnerable people are heard.

Participatory research with vulnerable people

Traditionally, exponents of participatory research have viewed qualitative methodologies as providing the best context for enabling and including the perspectives of vulnerable people, and there are many examples of qualitative methods being used to help us to understand the experiences of vulnerable people who wish to access or receive health and social care services. Participatory research methods should bring the voice of the community to the fore. The second author completed a qualitative research project which endeavoured to find out what people who had accessed an early intervention service for people with psychosis felt they were recovering from. It was hoped that the findings from this might help Early Intervention in Psychosis services to identify how best to help people during the recovery process.

Qualitative methodologies are seen as appropriate for exploring people's experiences and the meanings ascribed to them (Banister *et al.*, 1994; Chapter 8). The second author became interested in using this approach to research when working with people experiencing psychosis. In particular, he was interested in the area of recovery from a first episode of psychosis, and the way in which service users described and understood the recovery process. As part of his research he examined what people with first episode psychosis were recovering from and the implications of this for clinical practice, systems and the wider environment.

Case Example 12.2: Recovery and Early Psychosis: A Grounded Theory Study

The concept of recovery within mental health services has been appropriated by professionals and may not truly represent the language and experiences of service users (Turner-Crowson and Wallcraft, 2002). Therefore, the second author used a qualitative methodology to explore what young people within an early intervention service thought they were recovering from. Grounded Theory (Chapter 8) was used because it leads to the emergence of a theory from the data rather than relying on predetermined analytic constructs, categories or variables. Furthermore, it is concerned with the social context from which meaning is derived, which was particularly relevant when considering the concept of recovery.

Semi-structured interviews were conducted with eight participants. Grounded Theory was applied to the design and analysis; sampling and coding ceased when saturation of the data was reached. A theoretical model was developed using Strauss and Corbin's (1990) framework. A core category of 'Distress' was elicited which was evident in all participants' accounts of their recovery. Overall, six categories were identified and it was proposed that individuals were recovering from the distress of past experiences, uncertainty, a challenged identity, being in a psychiatric system, the reactions of others and social disadvantage. There was a clear finding that recovery from early psychosis is complex and does not simply involve recovery from a single experience. Encouraging people to share their stories (particularly those that are in vulnerable positions) is one way of empowering someone through their recovery journey (May, 2004).

Giving a voice to people's experience

Initially, there were ethical questions about whether people should be asking participants about the distress they had experienced, particularly as many service users would have talked about their experiences to numerous professionals during the course of their contact with services. As with most qualitative methods, the use of interviews meant that it would be difficult to predict what participants would say and how they may react when talking about their experiences. An article by Becker-Blease and Freyd (2006) was particularly poignant, discussing the ethics of talking about abuse (one of many sensitive areas that came up during interviews with participants). Becker-Blease and Freyd particularly note the 'wall of silence' that can surround abuse, where family, friends, professionals and wider society can ignore the issues of abuse because of the feared impact it may have on an individual as well as themselves. However, what too often happens is that stories of trauma and abuse become dismissed, leaving individuals feeling misunderstood, ignored and isolated. The research aimed to give participants the opportunity to talk openly and comfortably about their recovery without feeling silenced.

One of the difficulties of carrying out this research was that as participants reflected upon their experiences it was difficult to explore those experiences in depth. This presented the researcher with a dilemma around knowing whether it was ethical to probe people around these distressing events or whether it was important to continue to explore the research question. The researcher was guided by what participants decided to talk about rather than taking a very directive approach. Clearly this may have meant participants did not report all their experiences (e.g. talking about distressing events may have been minimized), which, it could be argued, weakens the researcher's findings. Re-interviewing participants in order to determine whether there were additional areas that needed to be explored further may have been a helpful way to ensure participant's experiences were being fully represented within the results.

Language

Using a qualitative methodology requires us to pay attention to the language that participants use. In these interviews, it was important to note how participants described their recovery. When asked the question 'what do you feel you are recovering from?' only one participant used the word 'psychosis'. None of the participants used the word 'schizophrenia' and only one participant used the word 'symptoms'. What was much more apparent in their stories were the rich descriptions participants gave about what they felt their recovery had involved. The omission demonstrates that understanding recovery purely in terms of a decrease or absence of symptoms can prevent us from really engaging with the important issues that vulnerable people face. If the absence of symptoms is our only measure, then there is an apparent misfit between the way professionals and service users understand recovery. Noticing how service users use language, the way in which they describe their experiences as well as what they choose not to say, are extremely valuable ways to learn more about the way a person understands their life and the difficulties they have encountered. Relying on a particular professional understanding of psychosis may mean we are using language that is both unhelpful and inconsistent with the way service users have conceptualized their experience.

Interpretation within qualitative research

If there are biases in the way that a researcher interprets participants' accounts, there is a possibility that the interpretation will be inaccurate. Two ways in which this can be minimized is through using theoretical sampling (Chapter 8) or by summarizing the emergent themes and asking participants to comment on and validate the findings.

It was also important to reflect on the process of carrying out the research from the position of a Trainee Clinical Psychologist. This involved appreciating the differences between being a therapist and a researcher. As a therapist, rapport, engagement, containment and learning about an individual's experience may take several sessions. As a researcher, exploring someone's experience was limited to one interview. At times, this meant asking about sensitive areas which in the therapeutic milieu may not have been addressed until later sessions. Clearly, the purposes of a therapist and researcher are different; however, the effect a researcher may have on how a participant understands their experience is important. Acknowledging, for example, a link between experiences (through the research process) may have challenged the person's current understanding of their experience. Remaining inquisitive and being mindful of the language used within interviews can help the researcher to remain empathic. Regular research supervision can provide a context in which these apparent disparate aims can be explored and accommodated.

 Reflection Points

How could participants have been included earlier in the research process?
How do we ensure we are not wounding people further through the research process?
What techniques ensure that we are truly 'grounding' our analysis in participants' accounts of their experiences?
How could service users be involved in further developing the proposed model?

Focus groups and service user empowerment

Many organizations are beginning to establish research focus groups (Chapter 8) to help vulnerable groups of people identify the kinds of questions they are interested in researchers and service systems investigating. The Joseph Rowntree Foundation and the Norah Fry Research Centre (http://www.bristol.ac.uk/norahfry/) emphasize both empowerment and participation of vulnerable people in research. They sponsor research that includes the voice of the communities they serve at all levels. Local healthcare trusts are beginning to apply similar rules to research produced in their areas (Oliver *et al.*, 2004).

Focus groups provide us with an ideal opportunity to identify the questions that vulnerable people might have about their services. In this next section we will outline a research project which endeavoured to do just this, and which also tried to help people with a learning difficulty to develop the skills to be able to undertake important elements of the research process themselves.

Case Example 12.3:   The Burton Street Research Group

The Burton Street Project is a community project that provides a range of activities to people living in its vicinity. As part of this, it provides opportunities for people with learning difficulties to participate in local community activities and work schemes. The first author ran some groups in this community project as part of her clinical work. When one of these groups had finished, members of the group seemed to have a lot of questions about services and how they were provided, as well as about the lives of other people with learning difficulties, their different work opportunities, friendships and values. We began to think of ways to explore these questions and decided to form a research group, which would meet in the evenings at Burton Street. A time and day that was convenient for the majority of people was identified and Burton Street agreed to our using their premises for the research group. We received a nominal amount of funding for the research, which meant that equipment could be purchased, attendance fees paid and expenses incurred on behalf of the research group reimbursed.

Four professionals were involved at this stage, three clinical psychologists and a researcher from the local university. Nine people from Burton Street attended the first meeting. We decided to start by helping people to learn research methods (and get some experience of doing some research) and identified a curriculum to do this. It started with practising core research skills: looking/observing, listening and asking questions. We then had a session on ethical issues in research and one on making sense of numbers. Finally, the group practiced their interviewing and questioning skills and we spent a further session identifying themes from a range of textual resources – newspaper clippings and magazine articles. During the final session we reflected on what had been taught and asked people what questions they had begun to ask since the course had developed. Each person had a research question they wanted to develop. All of this demonstrated to us that everyone had skills in specific areas and that all of these skills could be developed and strengthened within a research programme. The provision of funding was contingent on a paper being written by the group. This was published in 2007 (Abell *et al.*, 2007).

Reflection Points

What potential problems might there be around the anonymity of group members?
What issues might emerge around carrying out the research?

Conclusion

All of the studies outlines in this chapter, as part of their endeavour, have tried to include the voices of vulnerable people at the heart of the research. Some studies have asked people what they feel they are recovering from, rather than what others may believe they are recovering from. Two of the studies have had focus groups as part of their methodology. One used photographs to facilitate hearing or seeing the subjective views of a vulnerable group. They are each limited in the extent to which they have really enabled people to participate in their plans or have enabled the voices of vulnerable people to be heard (McClimens, 2004). None of them have used novel methodologies such as Photovoice (2008), which enables everyone to see things through the eyes or the lens of vulnerable groups. All of these studies have been completed from within a health and social care setting. They have required the researchers to get to know their community and to hear about what their community wishes to learn. Of course, who ultimately profits from this research is debateable (Clements, Rapley and Cummins, 1999), and as yet the authors have not seen the lives of those people who they have worked with significantly altered to make a long-standing difference to how they are valued. The authors hope that they have brought those voices to the foreground for a while, but remain sceptical about whether it is their lives and reputations which have been advanced through the research process or whether it has really enriched the lives of the people they have worked with.

References

Abell, S., Ashmore, J., Beart, S. *et al.* (2007) Including everyone in research. The Burton Street Research Group. *British Journal of Learning Disabilities*, **35** (2), 121–124.

Banister, P., Burman, E., Parker, I. *et al.* (1994) *Qualitative Methods in Psychology: a Research Guide*, Open University Press, Buckingham.

Becker-Blease, K.A. and Freyd, J.J. (2006) Participants telling the truth about their lives: The ethics of asking and not asking about abuse. *American Psychologist*, **6** (3), 218–226.

Clements, J., Rapley, M. and Cummins, R.A. (1999) On, to, for, with – vulnerable people and the practices of the research community. *Behavioral and Cognitive Psychotherapy*, **27**, 103–115.

Combes, H.A., Buchan, L. and Hardy, G. (2004) Using Q-methodology to involve people with learning disabilities in person-centred planning. *Journal of Applied Research in Intellectual Disabilities*, **17** (3), 149–159.

Department of Health (2001) Seeking Consent: Working with People with Learning Disabilities, Department of Health, London.

Foucault, M. (1984) Polemics, Politics and Problematizations: Interview with Paul Rabinow. Retrieved from http://www.foucault.info/foucault/interview.html.

Involve (2004) Involving marginalised and vulnerable people in research: A consultation document. Retrieved from http://www.invo.org.uk/pdfs/Involving%20Marginalised%20and%20VullGroups%20in%20 Researchver2.pdf.

May, R. (2004) Making sense of psychotic experience and working towards recovery, in *Psychological Interventions in Early Psychosis: A Treatment Handbook* (eds J.F.M. Gleeson and P.D. McGorry), John Wiley & Sons, Ltd, Chichester, pp. 245–260.

McClimens, A. (2004) What difference does it make who is speaking? Audience, ownership and authority in learning disability research. *Journal of Learning Disabilities*, **6** (1), 71–88.

Oliver, M. (2002) *Using emancipatory methodologies in disability research*. 1st Annual Disability Research Seminar, National Disability Authority, Dublin. Retrieved from http://www.nda.ie/cntmgmtnew.nsf/0/87418679FAE58B0E80256F02004753E9?OpenDocument.

Oliver, S., Clarke-Jones, L., Rees. R. *et al.* (2004) Involving consumers in research and development agenda setting for the NHS: developing an evidence-based approach. *Health Technology Assessment 2004*, **8** (15), 1–148.

Photovoice (2008) Retrieved from http://www.photovoice.org/.

Rogers, C.R. (1954) *Psychotherapy and Personality Change*, University of Chicago Press, Chicago, IL.

Stolberg, H.O., Norman, G. and Trop, I. (2004) Randomized controlled trials. *American Journal of Roentgenology*, **183** (6), 1539–1544.

Strauss, A.L. and Corbin, J. (1990) *Basics of Qualitative Research: Grounded Theory Procedures and Techniques*, Sage, Newbury Park, CA.

Turner-Crowson, J. and Wallcraft, J. (2002) The recovery vision for mental health services and research: A British perspective. *Psychiatric Rehabilitation Journal*, **25** (3), 245–254.

The Nuremberg Code (1947) cited in *Doctors of Infamy: the Story of the Nazi Medical Crimes* (eds A. Mitscherlich and F. Mielke) (1949), Schuman, New York, pp. xxiii–xxv.

Further reading

Munro, E.R., Holmes, L. and Ward, H. (2005). Researching vulnerable groups: Ethical issues and the effective conduct of research in Local Authorities. *British Journal of Social Work*, **35**, 1023–1038.

Tee, S.R. and Lathlean, J.A. (2004) The ethics of conducting a co-operative enquiry with vulnerable people. *Journal of Advanced Nursing*, **47** (5), 536–543.

Turner, M. and Beresford, P. (2005) *User controlled research. Its meaning and potential. Shaping our lives and the centre for citizen participation*. Brunel University/Involve. Retrieved from http://www.invo.org.uk/pdfs/UserCon_Rptfinal%20web081205.pdf.

Usher, K. and Holmes, C. (1997). Ethical aspects of phenomenological research with mentally ill people. *Nursing Ethics*, **4** (1), 49–56.

Resources

(Patient Advice and Liaison Service) (PALS), http://www.pals.nhs.uk/
Participatory approaches to research on poverty:
http://www.jrf.org.uk/knowledge/findings/socialpolicy/334.asp.
http://www.ushmm.org/wlc/article.php?lang=en&ModuleId=10005168.
For more information about Q methodology see http://www.qmethodology.net/ and http://www.qmethod.org/about.php.

13 Involving Older People and Carers in a Research Project: The 'Virtual' Steering Group

Sue Ashby and Sian Maslin-Prothero

Introduction

Case Example 13.1 describes the involvement of five service users representing older people as equal members of a research project steering group. A brief summary of the underpinning policy and the specific significance of service user involvement in research are outlined, followed by details of the research area and the service user involvement in the project. Unexpected events

---

Case Example 13.1:   Policy Underpinning Service User Involvement in Research

Within England, the launch of The NHS Plan (DH, 2000) demonstrated a commitment by the Government to make service users and carers the focus of services. Whilst previous policy suggested that improvements could be achieved by service user evaluation (DH 1997, 1998a, b, 1999) the NHS Plan asserted: 'All NHS Trusts, Primary Care Groups and Primary Care Trusts will have to ask patients and carers for their views on the services they have received (DH, 2000, Section 10.23). Person-centred care became an important concept in health and social care policy with the publication of the Department of Health (DH) White Paper 'Our Health, Our Care, Our Say' (DH, 2006a), calling for increased public engagement in the planning and delivery of health and social care services. The document directed organizations to ensure that local people are involved and that services respond to their requirements. Service user involvement is gaining acceptance internationally as being central to healthcare research, policy and practice (Royal College of Nursing, 2007), and DH funded research must involve service users at all levels. This includes initial planning, commissioning, researching and dissemination of findings (NHS Executive, 1998; Consumers in NHS Research Support Unit, 2000; NHS Executive Trent, 2001). To be successful, user involvement must be genuine and address the issues most central to users' concerns (Maslin-Prothero, 2003). Research ethics committees require evidence of meaningful user involvement, and will seek justification if users are not being involved. Indeed, many research applications have to be accompanied by a lay summary of the research in clear and straightforward language that can be read easily and understood by non-professionals. The challenge to researchers is to ensure that elements of 'tokenism' are not introduced into studies and that service users are fully supported and given the opportunity to participate as fully as possible within the complex range of activities involved in conducting quality research.

encountered during the project are reviewed, together with the benefits and opportunities that arose, concluding with a discussion of how an established relationship with service users can facilitate continued involvement to improve health and social care services. As there is no commonly agreed language to describe people who use health and social care and related services, the term 'service user' is used in this chapter to signify patient, customer, client and carer of people who use these services.

Participatory action research

With this underpinning policy in mind, a project was designed to evaluate and develop inter-professional working between health and social care staff in statutory and voluntary sectors, at a local and national level, in relation to older people receiving intermediate care. Participatory Action Research (PAR) is an egalitarian approach that discards the differentiation between researcher and participant, viewing all as co-participants and co-researchers. The aim is to remove the power differential that traditionally exists between researcher and participant, and to empower people who historically would have been the passive subjects of research to direct the research process. Its emphasis is on the contribution of all and the belief that at all carry equal value. The PAR approach ensures that everyone has a voice and the right to be heard; and decisions are made by consensus. An important aspect of PAR is to educate and develop members of the community who are acting as co-researchers, providing them with the tools to participate, sustain and implement initiatives (Koch, Selim and Kralik, 2002). PAR challenges the traditional concept of research and views people as thinking, feeling individuals with rights and responsibilities.

In practice, PAR is a cyclical process that employs periods of exploration, action and review. Each individual is seen as an expert in their own area. For example, researchers may know about methodology, funding opportunities and grant applications, whilst members of the community will have insider knowledge crucial in many areas of the research, such as experience of accessing and using services.

The intermediate care research project

This research aimed to evaluate and develop, through appropriate training, interprofessional working amongst health and social care professionals in primary and secondary care settings in the United Kingdom. Its focus was on intermediate care services for older people. The Department of Health (DH, 2001) defines intermediate care as the layer of care that sits between primary care and specialist services, to help prevent unnecessary hospital admission, support early discharge and reduce or delay the need for long-term residential care. Intermediate care involves multidisciplinary working across the interface between primary and secondary care, the independent sector and voluntary agencies, aiming to provide a timely and seamless continuum of care centred around the person's individual needs; the care is mainly provided for people over the age of 65 (DH, 2001).

The United Kingdom (UK) Government advises that intermediate care is a crucial element in improving services for older people (DH, 2006b) However, it has been acknowledged that service users/carers have to date had little involvement in the development of intermediate care services (Barrett *et al.*, 2002; National Health Service (NHS) North West Regional Task Force for Older People, 2002). It is recognized that the diversity of care provided by this type of service, together with the diverse and often complex needs of the older person, presents challenges to the involvement of this group of service users; it is also acknowledged that different people may want different levels of involvement (Roberts, 2002). It is, therefore, important to develop means of ascertaining the views and preferences of individual older people and their carers effectively in the provision of intermediate care (Social Care Institute for Excellence [SCIE], 2005), and the training that professionals providing that care receive.

Using a combination of participatory action research (PAR) and action learning enabled a reflective process of progressive problem solving, led by stakeholders and individuals working in teams or as part of a community of practice. The key stakeholders in this project were clients and their carers, and statutory, voluntary, and independent health and social care staff working in intermediate care. The approach was based on collaboration and partnership with practitioners, academics and service users (Koch and Kralik, 2006). The key stages of the project are outlined in Table 13.1.

The principles guiding this study were voluntary recruitment, collaborative decision making and looking, thinking and acting (Day, Higgins and Koch, 2009). Looking came from the systematic literature review and scoping exercise. Thinking came from interpretations of key issues and findings in steering group meetings (see below). Action entailed developing an

Table 13.1 Intermediate care project timetable.

Timeframe	Activity
Year 1, January–June	• Approach and appoint local and national Steering Group members (including users and carers); • Apply for Multicentre Research Ethics Committee approval; • Begin to collect contact details of key stakeholders re intermediate care teams operating locally; • Start systematic literature review; • Develop questionnaire to scope Intermediate Care provision; • Arrange Steering group meetings for duration of project; • Develop web site.
Year 1, July–December	• Apply for Research Governance approval; • Get MREC and Association of Directors of Social Services (ADSS) approval; • Collect contact details of key stakeholders re intermediate care teams operating across the UK; • Complete systematic literature review; • Pilot study – collect information from intermediate care teams in locality; test questionnaire.
Year 2, January–March	• Collect information from intermediate care teams across the UK; • Select sites for case studies (to represent the four UK countries and both rural and urban communities, and both affluent and deprived areas); • Administer questionnaire to 10 selected sites; • Develop, deliver and evaluate short interprofessional educational intervention (based on findings) to10 UK sites; • Re-administer questionnaire following intervention.
Year 2, March–April	• Analyse data from evaluation of educational intervention and questionnaires; • Interviews and focus groups with stakeholders; • Analyse data from scoping exercise; • Develop outline for and commence writing final report.
Year 2, May–June	• Complete report, submit to funders and disseminate to stakeholders.

interprofessional educational intervention, and implementing this across 10 sites in the United Kingdom. However, other outcomes may be less tangible, such as increased self advocacy for the service users (Kramer, 2007).

Service user involvement in the steering group

The research team sought meaningful engagement at the earliest opportunity, believing that as the development and direction of the study would be focused on issues of importance to service users, they would provide an invaluable perspective. A Steering Group was established to manage and inform the research study; it comprised academics, practitioners, older people, carers and representatives from the voluntary sector, all with an equal remit to manage and inform the study.

Effective communication was needed to facilitate full and effective engagement, respectful of individuals' commitments, time and geographical location. To support this, electronic communication was adopted, resulting in a 'virtual' steering group (Ashby, Maslin-Prothero and Rout, 2007). This consisted of six-weekly meetings conducted initially via e-mail and later via a password-protected web site developed for the study, accessible to all members of the steering group, where 'virtual' steering group meetings could take place. The virtual steering group strategy was:

- Exchange of information will be via e-mail and web site.
- Information and meeting agendas will be posted to all steering group members at six-weekly intervals.
- There will be a fourteen day period for people to respond.

This process was augmented by face-to-face meetings with service user members, prior to scheduled virtual meetings, to ensure full understanding of the points to be raised for discussion and opportunities for agenda items to be raised. For example, technical language relating to information technology and healthcare could be clarified, and areas of significance to the service users highlighted and raised; this was very much a multidimensional exchange of knowledge and experience. These pre-meetings also built confidence, developed trust and understanding and provided a comfortable and accessible environment to facilitate training. Training was developed in tandem with the research, and was dictated by the individual requirements of steering group members. Service users explored the background to intermediate care, intermediate care provision, research governance, ethics and consent, whilst all members benefited from support surrounding computer software and the shared experiences of being in receipt of or caring for people in receipt of intermediate care.

This staged action learning approach enabled service users to examine documentation at their own pace. This was supported with hard copies of information and opportunities for discussion prior to feeding back their comments to the steering group (Ashby, Maslin-Prothero and Rout, 2007). Language can be powerful, and the principles of PAR are to make the work and any written material accessible to as many people as possible. A glossary was developed pertinent to the needs of the group. Comments were received regarding participant questionnaires, consent forms and patient, carer and staff information leaflets, which were developed, agreed and incorporated by the steering group prior to submission of documentation for ethical approval.

Service user involvement was not only invaluable in directing and informing the research study, but also provided several development opportunities for the service users. From very early involvement, it was recognized that this group of older people had little knowledge and understanding of intermediate care services, yet brought many examples of lived experiences of health and social care needs, expectations and actual service provision. As they developed understanding of intermediate care services, many questions were raised around choice, availability and accessibility of resources, communication with professionals and attitudes towards older people in society today. A digital video recording (DVD) of the service users' experiences, in which they referred to themselves as being 'invisible', was made for circulation to student health and social care professionals, which gave out a powerful message of the vulnerability of older people.

As their confidence grew, the service users were keen to share experiences and their involvement with the research study. An opportunity arose for a service user, facilitator and researcher to present a 'poster talk' at the INVOLVE Conference 2006 in Hertfordshire, UK, based upon experiences of being involved with this research project. INVOLVE focuses on actively involving service users in all stages of research, from initial applications for funding through to analysis of research findings (Involve, 2007). This resulted in networking with fellow service users and sharing experiences; two other service users presenting at the conference came to visit the service user representatives of the steering group.

Ethical issues

Prior to commencement of data collection, appropriate ethical, research governance and access permissions were sought and obtained. Informed consent was obtained prior to any research activity. There were no apparent risks to individuals as a result of participating in this research, but support mechanisms were in place and available to all participants, if required.

Issues surrounding service user involvement

The research study took place over an eighteen month period. During this time, one of the service user representatives experienced deterioration in their personal health, and was no longer able to contribute to the steering group. This affected the dynamics of the group, as all had contributed and worked as a team. It made the focus of the study even more pertinent to them as they reflected upon the reality of their own health and social care needs. Shortly following this, another member experienced a distressing situation involving their spouse; this was exacerbated by further upsetting circumstances and the death of their spouse. The situation surrounding this event was extremely sensitive and uncomfortably pertinent to areas of the research. Although upset and concerned for their colleague, the group found that through their shared experiences and relationships, support was gained from one another. The group supported this member and a 'debriefing' session took place to reflect on their experience; it was agreed to produce, at an appropriate time, a narrative of this experience that could be used to educate professionals about the significance of effective communication and involvement when planning and providing care to meet the complex needs of older people and their carers.

Opportunities and developments

The motivation and enthusiasm of this group of service users to influence the development and delivery of older people's services has continued beyond their initial agreement to be involved in the research study. As the study drew to a close, with completion of data collection and analysis of findings, members remained actively involved in sharing their experiences and in supporting the research team in disseminating their experiences and the findings of the research study at an International Nursing Research Conference in 2008 (www.rcn.org.uk/research2008).

A further development was the contribution of the service users to a Service User Strategy produced by the local university's School of Nursing & Midwifery. The four remaining service users joined a task group to develop and present this strategy, which was met with keen interest from School staff. The strategy aims to develop a framework through which the School can ensure a visible commitment to involving users and carers in education, clinical practice and research.

Reflections

This reflection is based on the experience of one of the researchers (the first author) who facilitated and chaired the service user group throughout the life of the project. Warelow (1997) advises that reflection begins in a search for questions rather than a search for answers; questions were certainly generated from the perspective of the service users, which from very early on in the project influenced research documentation. The project would have been deprived of that development if their unique experiences and perspectives had not been captured and applied.

The research team ensured that all members of the steering group had equal status for the duration of the project, and reinforced this through Terms of Reference and inclusion in related publications. Service user involvement was simultaneously at a strategic level (contribution to research protocol), operational level (influence on research documentation, such as wording of patient consent forms) and individual user and carer level (powerful messages from lived experiences). The service users had not been involved in the initial funding application; however, the bid acknowledged the limited service user involvement in the development of intermediate care provision and the significance of drawing on their unique experiences as service users.

Ensuring service users are recognized and valued for their time has its difficulties; to achieve equal status, they should be paid for their time and any costs incurred. These costs should be explicit in bids for research funding. Difficulties can arise, however, when payments conflict with the service users' statutory financial benefits. Organizations such as INVOLVE, National Institute for Health and Clinical Excellence (NICE), and the Royal College of Nursing offer guidance on good practice in reimbursing service users. This good practice was followed by provision of travel expenses, hospitality and compensation for any carer costs incurred.

Conclusion

The commitment, energy and enthusiasm of the service users has been an invaluable contribution to the research study, and their contribution has continued as the group has shared experiences and developed skills empowering them to undertake other research. Using a staged approach to respond to their specific needs saw them grow in confidence, and gain trust and respect from all members of the steering group. Partnerships with education, health and social care providers, and the voluntary care sector have all been established, as has a continuing interest in being involved in improving services for older people.

Acknowledgements

The research project referred to in Case Example 13.1 was funded by the Burdett Trust for Nursing. Thanks are extended to: Amelia Rout, Researcher; Jane Snape from the Beth Johnson Foundation; and service users Margaret Brandreth, Mary Peake, Ben Mountford, Joan Walker and Margaret Williams.

References

Ashby, S.M., Maslin-Prothero, S.E. and Rout, A.C. (2007) Involving service users and their carers as equal partners in a project using electronic communication. *Annals of the New York Academy of Sciences*, **1114**, 362–368.

Barrett, J., Goh, H., Todd, C. *et al.* (2002) A description of an intermediate care service using routinely collected data. *Journal of Nursing Management*, **10** (4), 221–227.

Consumers in NHS Research Support Unit (2000) *New National consumer advisory group for cancer research.* Consumers in NHS Research Support Unit News, 2, Autumn.

Day, J., Higgins, I. and Koch, T. (2009) The process of practice redesign in delirium care for hospitalised older people: A participatory action research study. *International Journal of Nursing Studies*, **46** (10), 13–22.

Department of Health (DH) (1992) Social Care for Adults with Learning Disabilities (Mental Handicap). LAC (92)15, HMSO, London.

Department of Health (DH) (1997) *The New NHS. Modern, Dependable*, The Stationery Office, London.

Department of Health (DH) (1998a) *A First Class Service*, The Stationery Office, London.

Department of Health (DH) (1998b) *Our Healthier Nation. A Contract for Health*, The Stationery Office, London.

Department of Health (DH) (1999) Patient and Public Involvement in the New NHS, Department of Health, London.

Department of Health (DH) (2000) *The NHS Plan. A Plan for Investment. A Plan for Reform*, The Stationery Office, London.

Department of Health (DH) (2001) *National Service Framework for Older People*, The Stationery Office, London.

Department of Health (DH) (2006a) Our Health, Our Care, Our Say: a New Direction for Community Services, Department of Health, London.

Department of Health (DH) (2006b) *A New Ambition for Old Age: Next Steps in Implementing the National Service Framework for Older People*, Department of Health, London.

Involve (2007) *Promoting public involvement in NHS, public health and social care research*. Retrieved from http://www.invo.org.uk.

Koch, T., Selim, P. and Kralik, D. (2002) Enhancing lives through the development of a community-based participatory action research program. *Journal of Clinical Nursing*, **11**, 109–117.

Koch, T. and Kralik, D. (2006) *Participatory Action Research in Healthcare*, Blackwell Publishing, Oxford.

Kramer, J.M. (2007) Using a participatory action approach to identify habits and routines to support self-advocacy. *Occupation, Participation and Health*, **27** (4) (Fall Supplement).

Maslin-Prothero, S. (2003) Developing user involvement in research. *Journal of Clinical Nursing*, **12**, 412–421.

National Health Service Executive, Institute of Health Services Management & National Health Service Con-federation (1998) In the Public Interest: Developing a Strategy for Public Participation in the NHS, NHS Executive Quality and Consumers Branch, Leeds.

National Health Service (NHS) North West Regional Task Force for Older People (2002) Intermediate Care: First Impressions; Key Messages from Older People. Report of a Meeting for Older Members of the Local Members of Local Implementation Teams (LITS) Conducted in Liverpool, National Health Service Executive North West, Manchester.

National Health Service Executive Trent (2001) Consumer Involvement in NHS Research and Development, National Health Service Executive, Trent, Sheffield.

Roberts, K. (2002) Exploring participation: older people on discharge from hospital. *Journal of Advanced Nursing*, **40** (4), 413–420.

Royal College of Nursing (2007) User Involvement in Research by Nurses, Royal College of Nursing, London.

Social Care Institute for Excellence (SCIE) (2005) Involving individual older patients and their carers in the discharge process from acute to community care: implications for intermediate care. Briefing paper 12. Social Care Institute for Excellence. Retrieved from http://www.scie.org.uk/publications/briefings/briefing12/index.asp.

Warelow, P. (1997) A nursing journey through discursive praxis. *Journal of Advanced Nursing*, **26** (5), 1020–1027.

Resources

Involve: www.invo.org.uk.

InvoNET: www.invo.org.uk/invoNET.asp.

The NHS Centre for Involvement: www.nhscentreforinvolvement.nhs.uk.

National Institute for Clinical Excellence (NICE) Patient and Public Involvement Policy: http://www.nice.org.uk/getinvolved/patientandpublicinvolvement/patientandpublicinvolvementpolicy/patient_and_public_involvement_policy.jsp.

14 Involving People with Intellectual Disabilities in Research: Participation and Emancipation

Mike Gibbs and Sue Read

Introduction

This chapter aims to demonstrate how people who use health and social care services can become actively involved in the research process, with illustrations drawn from the authors' experiences of conducting research involving people with intellectual disabilities. The discussion goes beyond simply involving service users as 'research participants'; rather, the focus is on how they can be involved in the process of designing and conducting the research itself.

It is acknowledged that service users are not a homogenous group, and consideration needs to be given to the processes and purpose of involvement in each individual case (Sergeant and Steele, 1998). To facilitate active and full engagement in research, the nature of the research itself, the level of proposed involvement and the background of service users need to be considered, to ensure appropriate support and training (dependent upon the level of their involvement). Ethical considerations such as access, diversity, consent and confidentiality apply equally to service users, even when they are not considered participants of research. The National Research Ethics Service (NRES, Chapter 6) can advise on requirements specific to individual research studies, as can the Cochrane Collaboration Consumer Network and, especially, Involve, a National Health Service (NHS) organization that promotes public involvement in NHS, public health and social care research (INVOLVE, 2007).

Terminology

Firstly, as discussed in Chapter 13, there is no commonly agreed language to describe people who use health and social care and related services. The term 'service user' is used in this chapter to signify patient, customer, client and carer of people who use these services.

Secondly, as discussed in Chapter 12, the terminology used to talk about people with disabilities is varied and conflicting. In the United Kingdom, the Department of Health (1992) adopted the term 'learning disability' to identify those people with an IQ (measure of intelligence) below 70. Other organizations, such as *People First* (www.peoplefirstltd.com), prefer the term 'learning difficulty' (see Chapter 12 for definition). In the USA, 'learning disability' means a disorder of the basic processes involved in understanding or using language, such as dyslexia, or in doing mathematical calculations. As the term 'intellectual disability' has been adopted by the World Health Organization (WHO), it is this term that is used in this chapter, whilst recognizing that it is at odds with the terminology selected for use in Chapter 12.

In the United Kingdom, intellectual disability is understood to mean impaired intelligence and social functioning, which started before adulthood, and which has a lasting effect on development (DH, 2001). In essence, this means people have a reduced ability to assimilate new or complex information or to learn new skills, and have difficulties in coping independently. Read and Morris describe people with an intellectual disability as individuals who 'find it harder to learn, understand and communicate ... [which is] caused by the way the brain develops ... that is life-long and usually has a significant impact on a person's life' (Read and Morris, 2009, p. 12).

Intellectual disability can develop because of genetic defects, metabolic disorders or infections; it can occur because of difficulties during childbirth resulting in lack of oxygen to the brain; or it can be the result of an injury to the brain in childhood. Recently, the World Health Organization has stated that this population 'are frequently the most vulnerable group and, on many occasions, are exposed to human rights violations and deprived of minimum services and dignity' (WHO, 2007).

Research and people with intellectual disabilities

Research relating to people with intellectual disability has, in the past, been conducted *about* them, not *with* them or *by* them (Kiernan, 1999). Since the 1990s, however, the UK Government has striven to include service users generally in research and evaluation, but much more needs to be done to include people with intellectual disabilities and to actively overcome barriers to their participation. These barriers and challenges include negative attitudes of professionals, imbalances in power relationships and lack of resources (Gilbert, 2004). There are now real efforts to overcome such challenges. Research funding bodies are setting conditions that people with intellectual disabilities are included in research and evaluation, and governments are insisting on participation in policy implementation. Increasing participation has now created tensions for the 'traditional' researcher; involving people with intellectual disabilities in research may actually challenge current research methods and accepted processes, and these will all require change and adaptation.

The intellectual disability research context has been greatly influenced by normalization theory (Nirje, 1980, 1985; Wolfensberger, 1972) and the social model of disability (Oliver, 1990, 1996), which have led indirectly to the inclusion of people with intellectual disabilities in research and evaluation. The concept of normalization has its roots in human rights; it is based on humanistic values, insisting that people with intellectual disabilities should have a voice in activities that affect their lives. To this end, they need to have access to relevant skills and knowledge. The principles of normalization are based on the interrelationship between deviance and social exclusion. 'Difference' is considered deviant, which can lead to stigma. Normalization aims to reduce deviance and thus reduce stigma. Normalization principles tend to focus on service delivery and enhancement in order to improve the lifestyle of individuals and thus reduce stigma, rather than on attempting to change social attitudes. Walmsley (2001) gives a coherent account of the relationship between normalization principles and inclusive research. Interestingly, normalization theory was developed by non-intellectually-disabled academics; at no time were people with intellectual disabilities asked for their opinion.

In contrast, the social model of disability (developed predominantly by people with disabilities) is a political theory linked to exclusion from employment, poverty and social control, which aims to change structures in relationships between non-disabled people and disabled people. The social model, when applied to research, suggests that people with disabilities are part of the research process, aiming at social change and the emancipation of the people involved (Gilbert, 2004).

In research, the ideal scenario would be that people with disabilities would be the principal researchers in research that concerns them; they would have skills in formulating questions, gaining ethical approval, collecting and analysing data, creating a discussion from the findings and disseminating such findings through publications, conferences and networking. The concept of involvement has come a long way from research being 'done on' or 'done to' people with intellectual disabilities. However, whilst some people with intellectual disabilities have been involved in all parts of the research continuum, it has often been as passive collaborators as opposed to true, equal partners. This may be asking a lot of people with reduced intellectual capacity but, despite this, the research community is progressing this agenda and there are now a number of published reports that demonstrate that people with intellectual disabilities can be equal partners in the research process. Participatory research, in this context, means that people with intellectual disabilities are involved as more than just research subjects or respondents. Emancipatory research goes further and is about the systematic demystification of the structures and processes that create disability and the establishment of a workable 'dialogue' between the research community and people with disabilities, in order to facilitate their empowerment (Barnes, 1992, p. 122).

Participatory research

Northway (2008, p. 25) describes the key features of participatory action research as:

- a focus on countering oppression;
- promoting participants at all stages of the research process;
- the production of useful knowledge to promote change;
- a different role for the researcher.

Involving marginalized groups in the research process can often be perceived as difficult, because it has been done so infrequently (Read and Corcoran, 2009). Research is a tool that, if used appropriately, can send explicit messages to those who participate, including people with an intellectual disability. Inviting and involving people in research suggests that those participants have a contribution to make and that participants' contributions will be useful and meaningful. Simply providing the time and creating the space suggests that the work is worth doing (Read and Corcoran, 2009). Such messages also affirm how much we, as researchers, value the time, experiences and contributions that participants (including people with an intellectual disability) have to offer (Read and Corcoran, 2009). Case example 14.1 and 14.2 demonstrate how participation might be achieved, albeit in different ways.

There is a range of published material available that helps us to understand the benefits of participatory research for the service user and the service provider. When considering involving people with an intellectual disability in research, it is important to consider several factors, as shown in Figure 14.1.

Accessing appropriate participants is important, and sometimes this will involve approaching gatekeepers of services for their advice and support. The researcher needs to decide in what capacity each individual will contribute to the research, and what each participant can potentially offer. This has to be done with an openness and honesty that promotes transparency of involvement and treats and respects individuals with full adult status. Organizing the contact in

---

Case Example 14.1:   Involving People with Intellectual Disabilities in Research Development

On gaining a post doctoral fellowship, one of the authors took the opportunity to complete phase one of a three-phase research project, which aimed to develop a quantitative tool to identify the need for bereavement support for people with intellectual disability. The research team included one of the authors, a psychologist and an information technologist. Phase one of this work involved working with a small group of adults with an intellectual disability within a local advocacy service, in order to identify suitable kinds and formats of images and to confirm the set of images to be taken forward to the second (pilot) phase.

Involving people with intellectual disability at this early stage was seen as crucial to the development of appropriate materials, due to both the nature of the intellectual disability itself and the sensitivities of researching bereavement. In order to empower group members within the research process, all participants were perceived as co-researchers. That is, they would be supported to drive the research and would be fairly rewarded (i.e. paid) for all of their input. In the locality, advocacy groups had been involved in numerous initiatives with one of the researchers, exploring loss, death and dying, and were familiar with collaborative working and research as 'finding out work' (Read and Corcoran, 2009). A series of meetings between the three researchers, a working group of four people with intellectual disabilities and two advocates was convened. An advocate, that is, a person paid to help and give voice to people with intellectual disabilities, facilitated access to these working groups and ensured that the participants were well prepared for the meetings and supported throughout the process.

The objective of the working group was to explore and discuss sample visual images depicting aspects of loss, grief and death, in order to identify suitable kinds (e.g. generic vs personal, abstract vs concrete) and formats (photographs, pictures, cartoons, etc.). These images were included in initial versions of the tool to be taken forward to phase two of this work. Four days were allocated to this process, over a four month period; it was anticipated that several meetings would be needed to reach a consensus amongst the people with an intellectual disability. The agreed-upon images would be tested in the final advocacy group session.

---

whatever capacity is crucial to effective outcomes and, in the authors' experiences, some people with an intellectual disability have very busy schedules. Research attendance and participation may be compromised due to the location of meetings, access, transport and cost. Participants in Case example 14.1 volunteered from a local advocacy service and the meetings were held in the advocacy service rooms to alleviate confusion and promote accessibility.

Gates and Waight (2007) address some of these issues, in their reflections on using focus groups with people with intellectual disabilities. Whilst Fraser and Fraser (2001) demonstrated how focus groups can be used as an effective means to help people with intellectual disabilities to promote their own social inclusion, they acknowledged that special arrangements may be required for groups to be successful. Additionally, Aldridge (2007) has recognized that researchers need to draw together the principles and processes of research and the invaluable part played in the research process by people with intellectual disabilities.

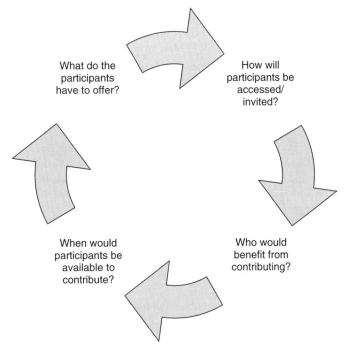

What do the
participants
have to offer?

How will
participants be
accessed/
invited?

When would
participants be
available to
contribute?

Who would
benefit from
contributing?

Figure 14.1   Factors to consider when involving people with an intellectual disability in research.

Emancipatory research

There is limited literature available on emancipatory research involving people with intellectual disabilities. However, Ham *et al.* (2004) give a clear account of how people with intellectual disabilities can become active, valued researchers. This case study describes the experiences of a number of people with intellectual disabilities, working as co-researchers, who experienced the ethical committee approval process (Chapter 6), and details their account of recognizing that they were actually researchers who were about to embark on a research project, thus becoming truly included in the research process.

The research team consisted of six people working as co-researchers, three of whom had intellectual disabilities. One of their aims was to learn more about the research process and develop their skills as researchers, in order to be involved in future research projects. The other team members were professionals experienced in the research process. It had become apparent to the research team that there was little published material that asked people with intellectual disabilities themselves about their health and what they wanted from health services. The research team met over several months to plan how they were going to develop a study relating to this.

The overall aim of the study was 'to ask other people with intellectual disabilities what they thought about health and what helps them to be healthy'. The team decided to adopt a focus group approach to data collection. This approach had been taken in a separate study on similar issues and the team felt it most appropriate. As the study was to involve data collection from people with intellectual disabilities, the experienced researchers within the team identified the need to gain ethical approval. The team began to construct the discussions and complete the

---

Case Example 14.2:   Supporting a Person with an Intellectual Disability to Develop his Own Research

Carl West[*] is a young man with intellectual disabilities, who is a paid worker in a local advocacy service. Part of the work Carl did was to facilitate groups, work with various health professionals to understand what it is like to have an intellectual disability and help other individuals to speak out and express their feelings, needs and wants.

Carl was recently taken ill and was taken to hospital for emergency treatment. His experience at the hospital was not very good and he refused some tests that could have been important to him and his long-term health and well-being. On reflection, he wished he had been patient and had tolerated the tests, but they weren't explained to him very well at the time and he was confused, uncomfortable and a little frightened. When sharing his story with other people around him, he found that their experiences of hospital were all very different, and he decided to 'find out' about other people's experiences and record their answers. Carl was helped to write his aim and helped to invite people to participate in his 'finding out' work. He conducted his own research and eventually interviewed 12 people who had various intellectual disabilities and who agreed to talk with him, so that he could record their experiences on paper.

Carl's work was not supported by public funding; it was simply an interest that he developed from personal experiences (as is true of much research). However, because the advocacy support workers helping him actively listened to what he said, really heard what he wanted to do, saw the value in what he wanted to find out, and were able to capture his enthusiasm and curiosity, Carl was able to conduct his study.

[*] Carl requested that his full name be used here.

---

ethical application forms. As this was felt to be a complex process, they developed a simpler form initially to help all the research team become involved in the ethical approval process. The use of clear language, symbols and photos helped with the construction of the ethical approval documentation. Prior to the local Research Ethics Committee meeting, the research team practiced how they were going to present their proposal to the committee. After gaining ethical approval, the co-researchers felt a great sense of achievement, to the extent of one of them saying 'I'm a researcher!' (Ham *et al.*, 2004).

Case example 14.2 also shows how inclusive research can go beyond participation to facilitate true emancipation in the research process.

Challenges to inclusion

Whether it be research involvement including consultation, collaboration or service user control (Consumers in NHS Research Group, 2001), there remain a number of challenges that any research team involving people who have intellectual disabilities must overcome. These include communication skills, training and support, practical skills and time.

Communication skills

More than 50% of people with intellectual disabilities are reported to have some form of communication impairment (Kerr, Richards and Glover, 1996). Therefore, reciprocal communication may be challenging and research teams need to be inventive in developing communication tools for effective involvement. The case examples show clearly how, sometimes, aspects of the research process need to be adjusted to facilitate appropriate skills and knowledge of service users. A further example of this is described by Aldridge (2007), who used photographs as communication aids in her research.

Training and support

To participate effectively in all aspects of the research continuum, people with intellectual disability need constructive and informative opportunities to understand about the research process and all that it entails. Perry and Felce (2004) reported a pilot study that trained a gentleman to interview his peers on their quality of life; the study demonstrated that people with intellectual disability can benefit from training and be competent data collectors. Training can be of great benefit to the service user researcher. It can help to put research processes into context and give them the necessary skills to 'research'. Within intellectual disability, it must be recognized that each person will be working at differing degrees of ability and all researchers must be cognizant of this. Richardson (2002) stated that to facilitate participation in data analysis it is necessary to create conditions in which participants feel comfortable about speaking and controlling meetings themselves.

Practical support

All aspects of costs and financial overheads for research need to be considered seriously and built into any funding application. Such costs might include travel and overnight expenses or costs to pay a carer to sit with another family member, so that the person can attend a meeting or other research activity. However, most, if not all, people with intellectual disabilities receive financial support from the government, and payments and other types of reimbursement must be negotiated with those involved, for danger of adversely affecting the person's overall income.

Time

People with intellectual disabilities may have significantly impaired ability to understand new and complex information. This does not mean that with the correct support and guidance they cannot become researchers themselves, they may simply require more time and resources to assist them in using their new skills. Having a research mentor might help individuals to orientate themselves into this role more easily.

Conclusion

As we have seen in Part One of this book, research is grounded in theory. There are rules and governance guidelines to follow, regardless of which research methods are used to elucidate and discover new knowledge. The process of research is, to some extent, pre-determined from identifying methods, analysis, the process of presentation and the original thought on how to approach the subject matter; research has its respected, accepted and refined approaches across the academic world. However, this chapter demonstrates that perhaps the research processes need to adapt and change in order to accommodate the involvement of service users.

Northway (2003) suggests that as the roles and skills of people with intellectual disability within the research process increase, then the research moves from a participatory mode, where they are equal partners in research, to emancipatory research, where it is the person with intellectual disability controlling the research process, as evidenced in Carl's story. Some writers argue that the two modes are interchangeable; others that they are at opposite ends of a continuum. Walmsley (2001) uses the all-encompassing phrase of 'inclusive research' to encompass both participation and emancipation. Whatever perspective we adopt, people with intellectual disabilities can take an active role in the research process and have much to contribute if they are given the opportunities to do so.

Acknowledgements

We would like to thank the following people for their contributions to this chapter: Dr Richard Stephens, University of Keele, co-researcher in Case example 14.1; Mr Carl West for permission to include his name and story; and Professor Ruth Northway for permission to cite the 'I'm a researcher' paper.

References

Aldridge, J. (2007) Picture this: the use of participatory photographic research methods with people with intellectual disabilities. *Disability and Society*, **22** (1), 1–17.

Barnes, C. (1992) Qualitative research: Valuable or irrelevant? *Disability and Society*, **7** (2), 115–125.

Consumers in NHS Research (2001) Getting Involved in Research: a Guide for Consumers, Consumers in NHS Research, Eastleigh.

Department of Health (DH) (1992) *Social Care for Adults with Learning Disabilities (Mental Handicap). LAC (92)15*, HMSO, London.

Department of Health (DH) (2001) Valuing People. A New Strategy for Learning Disability for the 21st Century, DH, London.

Fraser, M. and Fraser, A. (2001) Are people with intellectual disabilities able to contribute to focus groups on health promotion? *Methodological Issues in Nursing Research*, **33** (2), 225–233.

Gates, B. and Waight, M. (2007) Reflections on conducting focus groups with people with intellectual disabilities: Theoretical and practical issues. *Journal of Research in Nursing*, **12** (2), 111–126.

Gilbert, T. (2004) Involving people with learning disabilities in research: issues and possibilities. *Health and Social Care in the Community*, **12** (4), 298–308.

Ham, M., Jones, N., Mansell, I. *et al.* (2004) I'm a researcher!' Working together to gain ethical approval for a participatory research study. *Journal of Intellectual Disabilities*, **8** (4) 397–407.

Involve (2007) Promoting public involvement in NHS, public health and social care research. Retrieved from http://www.invo.org.uk.

Kerr, M.P., Richards, D. and Glover, G. (1996) Primary care for people with a learning disability – a Group Practice survey. *Journal of Applied Research in Intellectual Disability*, **9** (4), 347–352.

Kiernan, C. (1999) Participation in research by people with intellectual disability: Origins and Issues. *British Journal of Intellectual Disabilities*, **27**, 43–47.

Nirje, B. (1980) The normalization principle, in *Normalization, Social Integration, and Community Services* (eds R. Flynn and K. Nitsch), University Park Press, Baltimore, pp. 31–49.

Nirje, B. (1985) The basis and logic of the normalization principle. *Australian & New Zealand Journal of Developmental Disabilities*, **11** (2), 65–68.

Northway, R. (2003) Participatory research, in *Contemporary Intellectual Disability Practice* (eds M. Jukes and M. Bollard), Quay Books, Salisbury.

Northway, R. (2008) Participative approaches to research, in *Nursing Research. Designs and Methods* (eds R. Watson, H. McKenna, S. Cowman and J. Keady), Churchill Livingstone, London.

Oliver, M. (1990) *The Politics of Disablement*, Macmillan, Basingstoke.

Oliver, M. (1996) *Understanding Disability: from Theory to Practice*, Macmillan, Basingstoke.

Perry, J. and Felce, D. (2004) Initial findings on the involvement of people with an intellectual disability in interviewing their peers about the quality of life. *Journal of Intellectual and Developmental Disability*, **29** (2), 164–171.

Read, S. and Corcoran, P. (2009) Research: A vehicle for listening and promoting meaningful consultation with people with an intellectual disability. *BPS Qualitative Methods in Psychology Newsletter*, **6**, 28–37.

Read, S. and Morris, H. (2009) Living and Dying with Dignity: The Best Practice Guide to End of Life Care for People with a Learning Disability, Mencap, London.

Richardson, M. (2002) Involving people in the analysis: Listening, reflecting, discounting nothing. *Journal of Learning Disabilities*, **6** (1) 47–60.

Sergeant, J. and Steele J. (1998) Consulting the Public: Guidelines and Good Practice, Policy Studies Institute, London.

Walmsley, J. (2001) Normalisation, emancipatory research and inclusive research in intellectual disability. *Disability and Society*, **16** (2) 187–205.

Wolfensberger, W. (1972) The Principle of Normalization in Human Services, National Institute on Mental Retardation, Toronto.

WHO (2007) Atlas: Global Resources for Persons with Intellectual Disabilities, World Health Organization, Geneva.

Resources

Cochrane Collaboration Consumer Network: www.cochraneconsumer.com.
Involve: www.invo.org.uk.
InvoNET: www.invo.org.uk/invoNET.asp.
The NHS Centre for Involvement: www.nhscentreforinvolvement.nhs.uk.

15 Researching with Children and Young People

Jacqueline Collin and Geraldine Lyte

Introduction

Childhood is the term used internationally to define the period of human growth and development from birth until the age of eighteen years (United Nations (UN), 1989). Within this range, the terms 'child' and 'children' are typically applied to the pre-teen years, while the term 'young person' represents the adolescent years and transition to adulthood (Hughes and Lyte, 2009). There are wide-ranging variations in physical, psychological and social growth and development amongst the childhood population. Child development theories have proposed broad commonalities, or expected norms, by identifying stages or benchmarks for development through which children and young people are expected to progress (Berk, 2009). The extent to which individuals progress, and whether the array of child development theories adequately represent this process for all children and young people, can, in turn, be influenced by factors such as family dynamics, culture, gender, ethnicity, health and epidemiology and socio-economics. Consequently, children and young people, even from the same family unit, can attain developmental milestones at different rates and can react differently to common influencing factors like those cited above (Berk, 2009; Davies, 2004).

For researchers who plan to work with children and/or young people as part or all of their research population, an appreciation of concepts and theories related to childhood and child development is fundamental to the planning and conduct of the research. Of special importance, however, are knowledge, understanding and application of professional concepts and theories to guide researchers in the involvement of children and young people and family/carers in research. Conceptual and theoretical developments in nursing, particularly the seminal work for children's nursing initiated in the United Kingdom by Anne Casey (Casey, 1988), have been influential in proposing child, young person and/or family-centredness as well as partnership, negotiation, and shared decision making as core elements for effective involvement in healthcare and research. This is echoed in the UK National Service Framework for Children, Young People and Maternity Services (Department of Health (DH), 2004a), which includes promotion of self-expression and freedom of choice and, in some circumstances, depending on age and developmental stage, autonomy in decision making and consent to treatment (Birbeck and Drummond, 2007).

In this chapter, we focus on a popular approach for involving children and young people in research: the qualitative interview (Chapter 8). This includes an overview of the process and key ethical considerations for involving children and young people in research. Finally, we present an example of a small-scale research project involving children aged six and seven years, which illustrates the process.

Overview of the qualitative interview process for use with children and young people

Coyne (1998) argues that methodology enabling children and young people to be acknowledged as the most important source of evidence on how they live and experience their lives should be pursued. In particular, research methods need to promote self-expression, self-determination and partnership in decision-making appropriate to age and/or developmental status (Birbeck and Drummond, 2007; UN, 1989).

A range of child-centred methods are employed in research with children and young people (Crivello, Camfield and Woodhead, 2009); these include the use of diaries, photography, draw-and-tell, mapping, time use charts, drama and role play, video clips and radio workshops. Methods are selected that are not only relevant to the setting and the context of the research, but also appropriate to the age, gender and ethnicity of those participating, and which interest them in the research process whilst addressing the research question (Mauthner, 1997).

Qualitative interviews are an especially useful method of exploring children's and young people's views and perspectives. Evidence is emerging to provide practical guidance on data collection using semi-structured interviews specifically with children and young people. Kortesluoma, Hentinen and Nikkonen (2003) suggest that all aspects of the interview process must be thought through clearly and included in the research design, such as:

- whether to interview individually or in a group situation;
- where the interview is to take place and how long it will take;
- how the content of the interview will be determined;
- how it will be structured;
- whether other methods need to be employed to facilitate the interview.

In addition, the researcher needs to be aware of the developmental needs of children and young people, their cognitive and physical abilities (Docherty and Sandelowski, 1999), their usual way of communicating, social and cultural aspects of their background, and the way in which they would normally interact with adults. The importance of addressing these issues relates directly to the power imbalance between child and researcher that presents particular challenges when undertaking qualitative interviews with children and young people.

Deciding whether to use individual or group interviews will also reflect the specific nature of the research question and the context in which the research is to take place. There are a number of benefits and limitations within both approaches. Key points informing selection of the most appropriate type of interview are outlined in Table 15.1.

A related issue is the location of the interview. Hill, Laybourn and Borland (1996) reflected on the context of interviews that had taken place in homes and at school. They concluded that individual interviews undertaken at school were the ones in which children and young people appeared the most relaxed and open, surmising that they were less anxious because they knew that parents could not overhear their responses. However, other researchers argue that privacy is not always desired and that researchers need to be responsive to the individual situation. Irwin and Johnson (2005) advocate the use of 'kinetic conversations', where younger children can play or walk whilst being interviewed.

The format of the interview will be determined by the degree of structure imposed. The more exploratory a study, the less structure will be evident, whereas semi-structured interviews

Table 15.1   Individual versus group interviews with children and young people (adapted from Coyne, 1998; Fontana and Frey, 1998; Docherty and Sandelowski, 1999; Cree *et al.*, 2002; Irwin and Johnson, 2005).

Individual interviews	Group interviews
Not suitable for children under the age of six	Children over the age of four
Responses are more thoughtful	Spontaneous responses
Privacy can lead to expression of deeper feelings	Potential to develop 'group think'
Quieter children have more opportunity to respond	Some individuals may verbally dominate
Some children may be more reticent to respond in a one to one situation with a stranger	Peer support particularly if younger children are interviewed in friendship groups

enable the researcher to focus on issues of specific relevance to the research question. There is a degree of openness within a semi-structured interview so that children are able to talk about issues important to them, encouraging a child-led dialogue that maintains the child's frame of reference. The interviewer can clarify meaning or probe further to enhance understanding. The success of a qualitative interview depends largely upon the researcher's positive interaction with them and their ability to gain confidence; 'the purpose is to get the children to talk about what they know' (Kortesluoma, Hentinen and Nikkonen, 2003, p. 440).

Ordering of questions will help to facilitate positive responses; it is useful to structure questions around everyday experiences to provide some familiarity (Backett and Alexander, 1991). Using open-ended questions starting with 'how', rather than 'what', encourages children and young people to talk around subject areas and minimize the risk of single word answers. However, Irwin and Johnson (2005) maintain that with younger children a series of direct questions, particularly at the beginning of an interview, is beneficial, providing opportunities for the child to speak and allowing the researcher to explore information proffered. Language should also be contextually and developmentally appropriate (Kortesluoma, Hentinen and Nikkonen, 2003).

To augment the interview process with younger children, visual methods can be employed as ice beakers or to promote a less threatening dialogue between the researcher and child. Such approaches, it is argued, help to facilitate discussion and enable children to be active participants in the research process (Pridmore and Bendelow, 1995). These are particularly useful with young children or those with limited verbal skills. A tool frequently used is the *draw and write* technique, popularized in research with children in the 1980s because it incorporates a familiar activity (Backett–Milburn and McKie, 1999). Key features of draw and write are shown in Table 15.2.

Ethical considerations when researching with children and young people

As with all healthcare research, ethical approval for research involving children and young people is fundamental in ensuring that procedures for obtaining consent, and ensuring competence to consent, participate, make decisions and/or be autonomous in the process, have been addressed. Other factors including anonymity, confidentiality and possible risks or potential harm

Table 15.2   Draw and write technique.

Benefits associated with this technique	Issues to be considered
It is fun and an enjoyable participatory activity for children of all ages. 'Natural appeal' (Bradding and Hortsman, 1999)	Some children do not like drawing
Children draw what is relevant and important to them	Children may draw what they feel competent to draw and omit some things because they don't feel they can draw it well enough (Backett–Milburn and McKie, 1999). If drawing in a group situation there may be conferring between children leading to a consensus about what to draw and limiting individual expression
Flexible activity, can be used on its own or as one of several research methods and can be applied in different settings; for example, part of an interview schedule, as an icebreaker, eliciting children's views about specific experience, used in school or home (Sartain, Clarke and Heyman 2000)	It should not be viewed as an easy option and needs good facilitation and be well structured
An opportunity using a familiar medium to express feelings, fears and thoughts about sensitive issues (Hill, Laybourn and Borland, 1996)	Should not be considered a non-invasive approach, support for children should be identified within the research design
Developmentally appropriate method	Children's ability to communicate is developmentally led but also heavily influenced by their social, cultural and economic backgrounds (McPherson and Thorne, 2000); drawing skills are developmental
Reveals children's understanding where verbal ability may be limited (Hortsman *et al.*, 2008)	To avoid misinterpretation pictures need interpretation by the drawer and should not be considered direct translations of the child's thinking (Backett–Milburn and McKie, 1999)
Shifts the focus from the adult researcher's question to the child's experiences and frame of reference	Power imbalance between the adult and child will need to be addressed throughout the research design; for example, environment, consent, conversational style of questioning (Hortsman *et al.*, 2008)
Child-centred and non-threatening approach (Bradding and Hortsman, 1999)	How methods are used by researchers will determine whether it is a child-centred and participatory method
Provides richer data than writing alone (Pridmore and Lansdown, 1997)	Helps children with limited literacy skills to participate in research

resulting from involvement in research need to be considered (Kodish, 2005). Consequently, all proposed research within the NHS or Social Care is submitted and approved by research ethics committees, in accordance with the Research Governance Framework for Health and Social Care (DH, 2005). Primary considerations are:

- informed consent;
- the child's level of competence to provide informed consent, participate and/or make decisions alone or in the presence of an appropriate adult;
- anonymity and confidentiality.

Informed consent is a critical factor in the ethical assessment of research proposals and this includes assessment of participant information, judging individuals' competence to consent, and ensuring that consent has been obtained on a voluntary basis (DH, 2005). The process of informed consent for children and young people determines their understanding of what they are being asked to do, and requires provision of an information sheet with a full explanation of all aspects of the research, written at a level appropriate for maximum understanding by the child or young person. This may be achieved in pictorial form, prose or a combination of pictures and prose. For younger children, in particular, this will also necessitate the development of information sheets for parents or significant others who may need to participate in the consent process on behalf of or in conjunction with a child for whom they have parental responsibility (DH, 2004b).

The issue of competence to provide informed consent can be complex where children and young people are concerned. Competence is generally determined based on a participant's understanding and voluntary agreement to take part in a study, but for children and young people this may need to be balanced against their parents' or carers' role in the decision-making process (Alderson, 2000). On the one hand, a parent/carer's right to decide what is in the best interests of their child should be considered by the researcher. On the other hand, if the principles of involvement of children and young people in matters directly concerning them, such as self-expression and partnership in decision making, are to be realised, then provision is needed in the consent process for this.

There are two key guiding principles for researchers. The first emerged as case law in 1985, when Victoria Gillick, the mother of a child under 16, made a legal bid that parental consent should be required in decision making concerning contraception for the under 16s. Mrs Gillick lost the case on the basis that children under the age of 16 may be deemed competent if they can demonstrate understanding, intelligence and discretion in acting in their own best interests (David, Edwards and Alldred, 2001). Since then, the term 'Gillick-competent' has been used when referring to assessment of competence of children and young people to make decisions in their own interests (David, Edwards and Alldred, 2001). The second guiding principle is provided by the United Nations Convention of the Rights of the Child in 1989 (UN, 1989), where it was declared that if a child is capable of forming their own views, then they have the right of expression of those views in matters that affect them directly (Article 12).

Gaining consent from children and young people for research is, therefore, still a relatively new phenomenon and competence to consent will be affected by a range of factors including age, social and cultural contexts and life experiences. Even where they are deemed competent, they may still be subject to a dual-consent process, whereby their parents/carers provide consent to access them (Morison, Moir and Kwansa, 2000). Access to children and young people is only possible with the agreement of adult gatekeepers who consider themselves as acting in the best interests of children. There is debate about the positive and negative functions of gatekeepers and the degree to which they are protective or acting as censors (Cree, Kay and Tisdall, 2002). Hood, Kelley and Mayall (1996) describe a 'hierarchy of gatekeeping', ranging from organizations to parents and leading eventually to children and young people. Education researchers may sometimes approach children and young people through education establishments such as secondary schools, where the school acts as gatekeeper and parental consent is not always sought (David, Edwards and Alldred, 2001).

Regardless of the means by which competence is assessed and consent gained, direct access can also be subject to other checks. In healthcare research, this involves the right of healthcare organizations to check a researcher's criminal record status with the Criminal Record Bureau

(CRB) as part of their conditions of access. This can include an 'enhanced disclosure', whereby checks are made related specifically to the protection of vulnerable people. Researchers who are also healthcare practitioners are likely to be familiar with this process, as CRB checks are now standard within recruitment processes. However, CRB clearance in one NHS area does not assume CRB clearance in others, and this is an important consideration for gaining access.

Finally, it is essential that consent to participate is voluntary, so that at any time during a research study, a child or young person can feel able to withdraw without explanation, and without fear of challenge and/or coercion by a parent/carer or researcher to continue (Birbeck and Drummond, 2007; Greene and Hogan, 2005; Punch, 2002). Other key considerations are to assure confidentiality in the treatment of information and anonymity in the research, particularly in dissemination and publication of findings. In qualitative research, where samples are typically small, the possibility of being able to identify a participant is greater than if they were one of several hundred people responding to fixed questions in a survey (Silverman, 2005). In qualitative interviews, a participant may inadvertently refer to something about themselves that could identify them to others. It is the responsibility of the researcher to ensure that, as far as possible, all identifying elements are removed, such as personal details and locations, taped conversations and reference to others by name. In addition, the use of verbatim quotations in reports and publications may mean that absolute confidentiality cannot be assured, and prospective participants need to be aware of this. One way researchers can attend to this is to return to participants with transcripts of what they have said, thus giving them the opportunity to withdraw their consent for particular parts of the transcript to be published (Chapter 8). Some children and young people may also be inhibited if speaking in front of parents/carers and so the presence or absence of a parent/carer needs to be negotiated with the two parties, especially when data is collected in the family home.

To illustrate some of the issues raised in this chapter, Case example 15.1 is an example of how recruitment, consent, choice of methods and data collection were managed within a small research project undertaken by the first authors.

Case Example 15.1:   Interviewing Children Using the Draw and Write Technique

The study explored the views of children about who contributes to keeping them healthy. Data collection took place at their school. The draw and write technique was used as an exploratory tool for data collection from all children, and as a focus for a follow-up group interview with four children.

Recruitment

A small purposive sample was used. Gatekeepers were parents, the Head Teacher and class teacher. The school was selected out of convenience. The researcher had a contact at the school and the time limit for the project was short. Access was negotiated with the Head Teacher and class teacher prior to parents and children being contacted. Twenty-seven children were invited to participate. The children were all in the same class and aged six and seven years old. Six children were absent on the day of data collection (two were sick and four were on holiday). One parent did not want their child to participate. Twenty children took part.

Consent

The researcher respects that children have a right to self-determination and, consequently, the right to decide whether to participate in the research. This has to be balanced with the legal obligation to secure parental consent. To address these issues, a letter was sent home with the children explaining the nature of the study and how information would be used. Parents were asked to complete and return an enclosed form should they *not* want their child to be invited to participate. Subsequently, the class teacher and researcher were available to answer parents' queries and concerns at a parents' evening at school. Contact details of the researcher were also provided. One parent asked for further details and one parent declined consent for their child to participate.

Following parental consent, and in recognition of the concept of free choice and self-determination, some researchers advocate the need for children's assent. Assent can be sought following consent to participation from parents. This assures children about time, expectations, benefits and an explanation of their right to withdraw from the study at anytime without explanation to the researcher, thus ensuring that consent is ongoing and not a one-off procedure (Lindeke, Hauck and Tanner, 2000). The researcher asked each child if they would like to take part in the research, providing explanations about the nature and purpose of the study, what would be expected of them, what would happen to the pictures they drew, and how information gathered by the researcher would be used. All children approached agreed to participate. They may have agreed because children of this age usually comply with adult requests. However, developmentally this is an age of industry, with children often demonstrating a willingness to join in activities.

Choice of methods

Two methods of data collection were selected, the 'draw and write technique' and the qualitative, semi-structured interview. This reflects the need for flexibility of methods during data collection. The use of introductory material can be used to orientate children to the research subject area and focus dialogue on the research topic during the interview. Hence, children interviewed in this study were asked to draw pictures that were subsequently used to guide the interview. The use of drawings helped the children relax, provided the opportunity to develop rapport, and focused their thinking around the subject area of the interview. Ownership of the drawings was clarified with the children; it was decided that the children would retain their original work on the day of data collection. The drawings would, therefore, be available to take home and share with parents. The researcher would make photocopies of the children's work.

The benefits and limitations of using this technique are presented in Table 15.2. A key point is that the simplicity of administering and collecting data should not underestimate the complexity of interpretation, because analysis of pictures needs careful consideration to avoid adult interpretation and misrepresentation. For example, in this study the researcher noted that a child had drawn a heart in response to the question 'who keeps you healthy?' (Figure 15.1a). It was initially thought they had included the heart as an organ. However, the child explained that it represented God's love. Another depiction of God with a heart also indicated God's love (Figure 15.1b).

Semi-structured interviews are a valuable source of information regarding children's thoughts and views (Ireland and Holloway, 1996). Coyne (1998), in emphasizing the alien environment of the interview situation to children, suggests they may feel more secure being

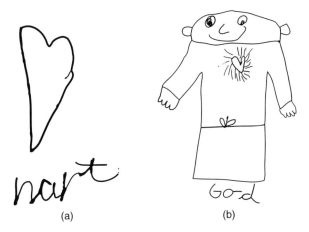

(a)   (b)

Figure 15.1a–b God's Love.

interviewed with children from their own age group. The children in this study were familiar with the environment in which they were interviewed and were also in the same age group and knew each other well. This peer support can reduce the power differential that inevitably exists between interviewer and interviewee, and between adult and child (Cree *et al.*, 2002)

Procedure for data collection

The researcher had spoken to the children individually, providing information about the study and invited them to participate. The venue for data collection was the classroom. One child was not included, after parents refused consent. Arrangements were made with the teacher prior to data collection for this child to be engaged in another activity. On the day of data collection the child approached the researcher and asked to draw pictures with the other children. The difficulty was adhering to the parent's decision without making the child feel excluded, while respecting the views of the child. The decision made following discussion with the class teacher was to allow the child to draw pictures of anything they wished. None of these would be included in the study; they would be retained by the pupil at all times. However, it could be argued that the inevitable cross fertilization of ideas between children as they draw pictures in close proximity to one another means that although the child's drawings did not appear in the study, it is possible that some of their ideas may have. The child's parents were informed of the decision. The established relationship the parents had with the teacher was clearly important in that they trusted the decision to have been fair. However, the researcher is aware that different parents in similar situations may have drawn different conclusions.

Immediately before the draw and write session, information about the study was again repeated to the whole class, stressing that there were no right or wrong answers. Children were encouraged and given the opportunity to ask questions. The children usually sat in predetermined groups, but during the study they were able to choose where to sit, and indeed organized themselves into four groups. All children had three sheets of paper on which to draw. They wrote their names and ages on the back of the paper so that the researcher could return the pictures to the children. The children were asked to draw whatever they liked in response to three requests. Each request was made individually before moving on to the next, that is each picture was collected before the next one was started. Children could write on their pictures if they wanted to. The requests were:

1. draw a picture of things that keep you healthy;
2. draw a picture of things that are not healthy;
3. draw a picture of people who keep you healthy.

The researcher went to each group and discussed with the children some of the images they were drawing. At the end of the drawing session, each group nominated one child to talk to the researcher about their third picture. The four nominated children were interviewed together. Prior to the interview the children had playtime. The researcher went with the children into the playground and was available to children. They took the opportunity to talk about their pictures and ask questions. They appeared comfortable with their visitor.

After playtime, the group interview was carried out with four children, two girls and two boys. The researcher was taken to a quadrant with classrooms on each side. There was a pond and a table with two benches. There was no negotiation with the school about the location for the interviews and the researcher felt compromised as she needed to focus the children on the interview and away from the interesting pond. It is important to have strategies to maintain the motivation of participants. Unexpected issues such as an aeroplane flying overhead also limited the quality of the recording. The researcher introduced herself and asked the children their names. Explanation of the structure and purpose of the forthcoming discussion was given. The recording equipment was placed centrally. For a short time before commencement of the interview the children were shown the audiotape and encouraged to hold it and see how it worked; they were shown how to turn it on and off so that they could discontinue recording if they wished to at any point during the interview.

The researcher focused on the third picture and asked the children to talk about the people they had drawn. The children interrupted one another as they became excited to contribute and it was difficult on occasions to encourage them to take turns without controlling the situation and reinforcing the adult–child power differential. The interview lasted 20 minutes. At the end of the interview the children asked if they could listen to themselves. They were amused and pleased by the sound of their voices. Notes were made by the researcher at the end of the interview with regard to events that had taken place.

Findings

It is not the purpose of this chapter to discuss fully the findings or implications of this research. However, findings from the third picture and the interview will be highlighted to illustrate some of the benefits and limitations of the draw and write technique when used to support a qualitative interview with children (Table 15.2).

Generally, busy pictures identifying a range of 'people' were organized by the researcher for convenience and presented in eight categories, including health professionals, family, school, activities, sports people, religious figures, organs and others. The group interview focused on this picture, providing valuable insight and maintaining focus on the childrens' experiences. Children of six and seven years old are strongly influenced by the here and now of their experiences, as well as by information gained from their families, hence their observations largely represented images they were familiar with. The importance of religious figures to the children relates to the context of the research that was conducted in a Faith School. Children

Table 15.3 Activities of adults that contribute to keeping children healthy.

Provision of healthy things	Mummy and Daddy, God, Jesus
Teaching	Gym person, Classroom assistant, PE Teacher, PE Students
Caring and helping	Class teacher, Classroom assistant, Jesus, PE Students, Mummy and Daddy, God (Holy Spirit)
Facilitator of activity	Gym person, Class teacher, PE Students, PE Teacher, Mummy and Daddy
Intervention	Dentist, Nurse, Health Visitor, Operation person, Classroom assistant

identified activities that adults carried out in keeping them healthy (Table 15.3). The functions identified are a starting point in gaining meaningful insight into children's perception of who keeps them healthy and what they perceive to be healthy. Three children out of twenty identified themselves as contributing to their own health. Health professionals were the most frequently represented people within the pictures. Family members were the next largest group.

The health professionals largely represent stereotypical images of nurses, doctors and dentists. Major changes in the nursing profession relating to dress, roles and service delivery are not recognized amongst the pictures of traditional uniforms, and 'needle and syringe' images still apparently dominate the minds of these children (Figures 15.2a–c).

The children interviewed linked being hurt with the role of the nurse, reflecting that their usual encounter with a nurse is either when they are ill or injured or for immunizations. 'They stick needles in you'; 'they help doctors do the operations and they're very important'. They did not distinguish between different types of nurses but stated a variety of places nurses work, including hospital, clinic, the dentists (Figure 15.2(c)) and school. The children's pictures illustrated similar people in similar ways but they also clearly reflect individuality that is unique to children's experiences, reflecting the cultural and social influences on their lives.

The interview supports this. Children were more articulate about individuals they were familiar with, for example the classroom assistant, who is an important person to the children whilst they are in school. All the children commented excitedly on some aspect of her role. Pastoral care for children in primary schools is an accepted part of the role of the teaching staff and this is reflected in both the pictures and interview. The children interviewed identified a range of functions carried out by the classroom assistant, including teaching, caring and helping and intervening directly if the children were hurt. However, only one child drew this person, reinforcing the limitations of the draw and write method if used in isolation. Within this study, the researcher has attempted to address this issue, selecting an approach that enables the voices of children to be heard directly, with the researcher acting as a mediator in the interpretation of data. However, it is generally agreed within the research community that the skill of the researcher in using qualitative methods will determine whether research methods are child-centred and participatory.

Conclusion

In this chapter, we have focused on some of the key considerations for researchers who wish to include children and young people in research, and particularly in qualitative interviewing. The exemplar of incorporating draw and write provides highlights of how these considerations applied to one group of children in their early school years. The children provided a wealth of

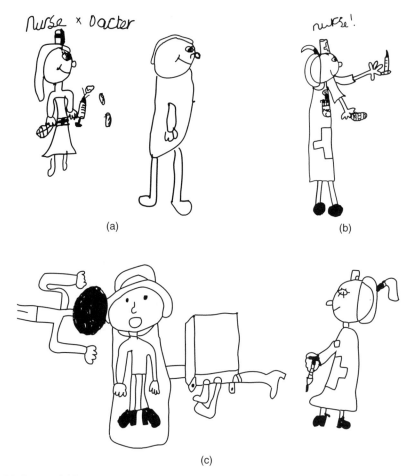

(a)   (b)

(c)

Figure 15.2a–c Children's perspectives of health professionals.

information through their pictures and dialogue, making a useful and insightful contribution to adult understanding of children's perceptions of what keeps them healthy, what they understand as not healthy, and who is significant in keeping them healthy. The draw and write technique, used in conjunction with semi structured interviews, was relevant to the age group and school context in which it was used, and children appeared happy to participate and proud of the pictures they produced. The children were also keen to show them to the researcher and this represents the importance of setting aside sufficient time within the data collection period to recognize and respect the children's contribution fully. Using the children's pictures to guide the interview was extremely useful in maintaining the focus of discussion and generating enthusiastic responses.

Methodological issues experienced during the study have developed our understanding of the complexities of the research process, including the need for creativity and flexibility in planning for the expected and in responding thoughtfully to the unexpected. Because children and young people of all ages increasingly act as participants in research, it is important for each study to consider developmental, ethical and methodological influences for their participant group, and remind themselves that even children and young people in the same age range may respond differently to this process.

Acknowledgements

We would like to acknowledge the children, their families and school staff for their contribution to the illustrated study. We would also like to acknowledge Linda Milnes, University of Manchester, for her input on ethical issues.

References

Alderson, P. (2000) *Young Children's Rights: Exploring Beliefs, Principles and Practice*, Jessica Kingsley Publishers, London.

Backett, K. and Alexander, H. (1991) Talking to young children about health: methods and findings. *Health Education Journal*, **50**, 134–137.

Backett-Milburn, K. and McKie, L. (1999) A critical appraisal of the Draw and Write technique. *Health Education Research: Theory and Practice*, **14**, 387–389.

Berk, L.E. (2009) *Child Development*, 8th edn, Allyn & Bacon/Longman, United States.

Birbeck, D.J. and Drummond, M.J.N. (2007) Research with young children: Contemplating methods and ethics. *Journal of Educational Enquiry*, **7** (2), 21–31.

Bradding, A. and Horstman, M. (1999) Using the write anddraw technique with children. *European Journal of Oncology Nursing*, **3** (3). 170–175.

Casey, A. (1988) A partnership with child and family. *Senior Nurse*, **8** (4), 8–9.

Coyne, I.T. (1998) Researching children: Some methodological and ethical considerations. *Journal of Clinical Nursing*, **7**, 409–416.

Cree, V.E., Kay, H. and Tisdall, K. (2002) Research with children: sharing the dilemmas. *Child and Family Social Work*, **7**, 47–56.

Crivello, G., Camfield, L. and Woodhead, M. (2009) How can children tell us about their wellbeing? Exploring the potential of participatory research approaches within 'Young Lives'. *Social Indicators Research*, **90** (1), 51–72.

David, M., Edwards, R. and Alldred, P. (2001) Children and school-based research: 'Informed consent' or 'educated consent'? *British Educational Research Journal*, **27** (3), 347–365.

Davies, D. (2004) *Child Development: A Practitioner's Guide*, 2nd edn, Guilford Press, New York.

Department of Health (DH) (2004a) The National Service Framework for Children, Young People and Maternity Services, HMSO, London.

Department of Health (DH) (2004b) The Children Act, HMSO, London.

Department of Health (DH) (2005) Research Governance Framework for Health and Social Care, HMSO, London.

Docherty, S. and Sandelowski, M. (1999) Focus on qualitative methods: Interviewing children. *Research in Nursing and Health*, **22**, 177–185.

Greene, S. and Hogan, D. (eds) (2005) *Researching Children's Experience: Approaches and Methods*, Sage, London.

Fontana, A. and Frey, J.H. (1998) Interviewing: The art of science, in *Collecting and Interpreting Qualitative Materials* (eds N.K. Denzin and Y.S. Lincoln.), Sage Publications, Thousand Oaks, pp. 47–73.

Hill, M., Laybourn, A. and Borland, M. (1996) Engaging with primary aged children about their emotions and well being: Methodological considerations. *Children and Society*, **10**, 129–144.

Hood, S., Kelley, P. and Mayall, B. (1996) Children as research subjects: a risky enterprise. *Children and Society*, **10**, 117–128.

Horstman, M., Aldiss, S., Richardson, A. and Gibson, F. (2008) Methodological issues when using the Draw and Write technique with children aged 6 to 12 years. *Qualitative Health Research*, **18**, 1001–1011.

Hughes, J. and Lyte, G. (eds) (2009) *Developing Nursing Practice with Children and Young People*, Wiley-Blackwell, Oxford.

Ireland, L. and Holloway, I. (1996) Qualitative health research with children. *Children and Society*, **10**, 155–164.

Irwin, L.G. and Johnson, J. (2005) Interviewing young children: Explicating our practices and dilemmas. *Qualitative Health Research*, **15**, 821–831.

Kodish, E. (2005) *Ethics and Research with Children: A Case-based Approach*, Oxford University Press, New York.

Kortesluoma, R.L., Hentinen, M. and Nikkonen, M. (2003) Conducting a qualitative child interview: Methodological considerations. *Journal of Advanced Nursing*, **42** (5), 434–441.

Lindeke, L.L., Hauck, M.R. and Tanner, M. (2000) Practical issues in obtaining child assent for research. *Journal of Pediatric Nursing*, **15** (1), 99–104.

Mauthner, M. (1997) Methodological aspects of collecting data from children: Lessons from three research projects. *Children and Society*, **11**, 16–28.

McPherson, G. and Thorne, S. (2000) Children's voices: Can we hear them? *Journal of Pediatric Nursing*, **15** (1), 22–29.

Morison, M., Moir, J. and Kwansa, T. (2000) Interviewing children for the purposes of research in primary care. *Primary Health Care Research and Development*, **1**, 113–130.

Pridmore, P. and Bendelow, G. (1995) Images of health: Exploring beliefs of children using the Draw-and-Write Technique. *Health Education Journal*, **54**, 473–488.

Pridmore, P. and Lansdown, R. (1997) Exploring children's perceptions of health: Does drawing really break down barriers? *Health Education Journal*, **56**, 219–223.

Punch, S. (2002) Research with children: The same or different from research with adults? *Childhood*, **9** (3), 321–341.

Sartain, S., Clarke, C. and Heyman, R. (2000) Hearing the voices of children with chronic illness. *Journal of Advanced Nursing*, **4**, 913–921.

Silverman, D. (2005) *Doing Qualitative Research*, 2nd edn, Sage, London.

United Nations (1989) Convention of the Rights of the Child, United Nations, Geneva.

Further reading

Twycross, A. (2009) An interprofessional approach to the ethics of undertaking research with children. *Nurse Researcher*, **16** (3), 7–20.

Resources

Criminal Records Bureau: www.crb.gov.uk.

16   Researching Organizations: Evaluating a 'Partnership for Older People Project'

Roger Beech, Brenda Roe, Michelle Russell, Bernard Beech and Deborah Gent

Introduction

This chapter considers the evaluation of one UK Council's 'Partnership for Older People Project' (POPP). To support the evaluation, a range of research methods, both quantitative and qualitative, was needed. The purpose of this chapter is to illustrate the role and value of a mixed methods design when evaluating organizational initiatives of the type introduced in this project.

After a discussion of the policy context and nature of the POPP, the subsequent section of the chapter outlines the aims of the evaluation, the methods used, why they were chosen and how they were implemented. Rather than providing comprehensive findings, selected results are presented to illustrate how the information generated by the different methods complimented and enhanced each other. The role of the information in supporting decision making in relation to the delivery and 'benefits' of the POPP is also illustrated.

Beyond this project, it is recognized that a mixed methods design is needed when developing and evaluating complex service interventions (Medical Research Council, 2008). The final section of the chapter offers further reflections on the role of mixed methods designs within studies of this type.

The partnership for older people project

England, in common with other western states, is facing an increase in the proportion of its population that is elderly (Department of Health, 2006). This demographic shift is likely to place increasing pressure on services delivering health and social care for older people.

The initial policy response by central government was to increase services for providing intermediate care (Department of Health, 2000; Chapter 13). Such services aim to reduce pressures on acute hospital services, either by providing an alternative to acute hospital admission or by facilitating the timely discharge of acute hospital patients (Beech *et al.*, 2004; Beech, 2005; Roe, 2005).

However, intermediate care services primarily target individuals who have suffered an 'acute' event. More recent policy documents have recognized that, alongside services for responding to 'illness', there is a need to increase the supply of 'services' for promoting the health, well-being and independence of older people. The aim of this expanded service remit is to prevent or delay older people needing more costly services, such as those delivered in acute hospitals (Department of Health, 2006, 2008). However, these policy documents also recognize that there is a need to increase the evidence base surrounding the nature and impact of such services.

The Council in which this project took place is one of 29 localities from across England which, following a process of competitive bidding, received funds to establish and pilot initiatives for promoting and maintaining the health and well-being of older people (PSSRU, 2008). The aims of the POPP were to:

- provide a range of needs-led services requested by older people;
- encourage investment in preventative approaches that promote older people's health, well-being and independence;
- offer more 'low level' care and community support with a view to preventing or delaying older people needing to access higher intensity and more costly forms of care.

(Beech *et al.*, 2008).

To identify the types of schemes that needed to be developed or expanded to address these aims, project leads from the Council held meetings with older people, their colleagues in social care departments and representatives from the health and independent sectors. The information presented in Table 16.1 provides a brief summary of the nature of the schemes that emerged

Table 16.1   An overview of the Council's POPP schemes.

Name of scheme	Purpose of scheme	Agency responsible for delivering scheme
Time Limited Contact	This scheme aimed to prevent changing times escalating into crisis situations for older people.	Pensioners Link
Free counselling for individuals and groups	This scheme aimed to prevent client 'symptoms' accelerating into serious mental health problems or stress related physical illness.	Pensioners Link
Rapid Intervention Project	This scheme provided a flexible respite service, at short notice, to enable carers to manage an urgent situation.	Crossroads Care Scheme
Holistic Home Assessment Team	In this scheme, Community Health Development workers visited people who had a health concern that did not require input from a specialist health professional.	Primary Care Trust
BME Carers and BME Mental Health	This scheme addressed mental health issues impacting upon older members of the ethnic minority community.	Primary Care Trust
Handy Person Project	A Handy Person undertook small household jobs for people, with home safety and security being major areas of priority.	Age Concern
Gardening Project	This scheme aimed to ensure that the gardens of people with a disability or over 50 were maintained when personal circumstances made it impossible for them to cope or get help with essential gardening.	Groundwork
Care and Repair Project	This existing scheme was expanded to allow it to meet a rising demand of enquiries from elderly and disabled home owners.	Arena Options Care and Repair
Stop and Lock Project	This scheme focused on upgrading the security of homes by fitting locks, bolts and window alarms.	Police
The Stepping Out Project	This scheme included free health talks, activity sessions and health walks.	Leisure and Culture Trust
Assistive Technology Project	This scheme supplied and installed a range of new technologies for promoting home safety and independence.	Adult Services Department

from these discussions. These schemes could be accessed by individuals who were aged 50 and over. Relative to a 'traditional' age boundary of age 65 and over, the Council's wider definition of an older person stemmed from a view that changes in lifestyles and improved access to services amongst the 'younger' old might prevent or delay 'health' problems in later life.

Table 16.1 also provides details of the agencies that were primarily responsible for the delivery of the schemes. As can be seen, a focus on health and well-being meant that a range of agencies needed to be included.

Evaluation aims

To generate learning about their initiatives, POPP sites were required to undertake local evaluation activity (the main focus of this chapter). The overall aim of the local evaluation was to generate information to guide the development of the schemes. This developmental rather than judgemental focus reflected the fact that many of the schemes that formed the POPP were newly introduced and would evolve during the lifetime of the evaluation. Hence, the role of the evaluation was to generate on-going learning about areas of 'success' and areas requiring modification.

Research governance and ethical approval

Studies of this type need research governance approval from the key organizations involved in the delivery of the project and ethics approval from a relevant committee. Research governance approval safeguards the interests of organizations (for example, are any inputs required by their employees adequately resourced) and ethical approval the interests of research participants (for example, are there adequate procedures for obtaining their informed consent to participate in the study). In this study, research governance approval was obtained both from the Council and from the local Primary Care Trust. Ethics approval was obtained from the NHS Research Ethics Committee that covered the Primary Care Trust.

Methods

The research strategy adopted was in keeping with guidance from the Medical Research Council (Medical Research Council, 2008). That guidance describes differing phases in the development and evaluation of complex interventions and the evolving role that research projects play within these phases. The differing phases are:

- developing the intervention;
- piloting the intervention and assessing its feasibility;
- formally evaluating the intervention;
- reporting the results of the evaluation.

Evaluation research within the initial phase helps stakeholders to clarify the nature and purpose of an intervention and in the second phase to establish the processes and procedures for its delivery. When these processes and procedures have been confirmed, evaluation of the impacts of an intervention can commence.

Research embraced each of these phases. Discussions with local stakeholders revealed that they wanted the study to generate information related to three broad areas:

- the users of POPP schemes;
- the 'processes of care' within the POPP;
- the impact of the POPP for service users.

The range of issues to be covered by the evaluation meant that it needed to draw on a variety of study designs and research methods. The primary methods used are detailed below for each of the three areas.

Users of POPP schemes

A descriptive design was used to collect data about all users of POPP schemes over a period of two years. Data were collected about the demographic characteristics of service users, how and why they requested services from a POPP scheme, and whether or not they actually received support from the scheme. Managers of the POPP schemes were required to complete and submit such data on a quarterly basis.

'Processes of care' within the POPP

The term 'processes of care' embraces a number of operational dimensions and areas of activity. The broad issues covered were those relating to: delivery processes; perceived scheme effectiveness; levels of participation within and partnership arrangements between stakeholder organizations; and stakeholder attitudes to the mechanisms used to monitor the progress of the POPP. Within an evaluation framework, the investigation of such issues captures the strengths and weaknesses of operational process and the extent to which it is adequately integrated with related schemes and services, issues that are crucial to the overall success of a scheme.

A qualitative research design supported this aspect of the evaluation with semi-structured interviews being used to collect data in three phases. The first phase of interviews was conducted with staff responsible for managing POPP schemes, the second with staff engaged in the direct delivery of POPP schemes and the third with staff from agencies with a key stakeholder interest in the POPP (for example, General Practitioners and intermediate care staff, as they might refer individuals to a POPP scheme, and staff from Commissioning Organizations as they might be required to provide financial support for a scheme). Sample questions from the Managers' interview schedule, illustrating the types of issues that were explored, are given in Box 16.1.

In addition to the interviews, two workshops were held with POPP providers and stakeholders. The first was used to explore further issues covered by the phase 1 semi-structured interviews, and the second by the phase 2 and 3 semi-structured interviews. To illustrate the function of the workshops, the schedule for the second workshop is given in Table 16.2.

Impact of the POPP for service users

Two types of impact were explored: Service users' assessments of the services that they had received from a POPP scheme, and the impact that the services offered by POPP schemes had had on their health status, well-being and quality of life (an aspect of the study that was done

Box 16.1   Interview Questions

Delivery Processes

How many referrals are made to your scheme weekly/monthly?
Roughly, what proportion of referrals are accepted by your scheme?
Is there a pattern regarding the referrals?
What are the challenges your scheme is facing in delivery?
How is information managed?
Are there any issues regarding information flows (to and from the scheme)?

Effectiveness

How acceptable do you think the scheme is to clients overall?
How do you think the scheme is perceived by other services?
How well do **you** consider the scheme is working, that is, does it meet its own objectives?
What are the scheme's areas of strength?
What are the scheme's areas of weakness?
How could the scheme be improved?
Is the scheme sustainable?
Are you seeing the clients you thought you would see/the scheme is designed to see?

Participation, Citizenship and Partnership

Do you have links to other schemes? Who are your partners?
How did these links evolve?
How do partnerships work within the POPP initiative?
How do partnerships work beyond the POPP initiative?
What are the benefits of partnership working?
What are the weaknesses of partnership working?
What are the challenges of partnership working?
What is the scope for developing partnerships (further)?
Do you feel that your service is developing and changing as the POPP project develops?
Do you feel part of POPP?
Do you feel that you are gaining enough information/guidance from the POPP?
Are you gaining information useful to service development?

Monitoring Processes of Care

Why is this important?
How should this activity be done in the future?
What has been the value of this interview?
Do you have any other comments?

Table 16.2 A Workshop to Explore Processes of Care Findings relating to POPP Schemes and their Partners.

Programme		
9.30 a.m.	Welcome and Introduction to Workshop	Wanda Russell
9.45 a.m.	Processes of Care: Key Findings relating to POPP Schemes and their Partners	Wanda Russell
10.00 a.m.	**Group Work:** ***In your groups, spend approx. 10 minutes discussing each point below, recording the group's views on the flip chart provided.*** 1. ***Delivery processes:*** • Nature of the partnerships • Understanding of the POPP project: what are the key issues? 2. ***Effectiveness:*** • The POPP schemes have a very positive image regarding their acceptability to clients; but how can the effectiveness of meeting scheme objectives be improved? • What are the key factors that contribute to a scheme's sustainability? What are the obstacles? Do POPP partners have a role in contributing to sustainability?	Facilitators: Wanda Russell Michelle Russell Roger Beech Brenda Roe
10.45 a.m.	Coffee	
11.00 a.m.	Group Work contd.: 3. ***Partnerships:*** • How important is the POPP identity to the individual POPP schemes? • What are the main challenges of working in partnership with services outside of POPP and how can these challenges be addressed? • How can partnerships be strengthened and improved? • What have been the main changes in 'ways of working' that have emerged from working in partnership with others?	Facilitators: Wanda Russell Michelle Russell Roger Beech Brenda Roe
11.45 a.m.	Feedback and discussion	All
12.30 p.m.	Lunch (Two course hot and cold buffet)	
1.00 p.m.	Close	

in collaboration with colleagues who were undertaking a national evaluation that covered all POPP sites across the country (PSSRU, 2008).

The main method used was a postal questionnaire sent to service users who agreed to be contacted. For ease of completion, most questions were closed (Table 16.3) and the questionnaire was on a single side of A4. However, respondents were invited to provide free text comments at the foot of the main questionnaire or overleaf. Validated instruments were used to assess changes in the health status, well-being and quality of life of service users (Bowling, 2005; Dolan *et al.*, 1995; Ryff, 1996). Respondents were asked to complete the questionnaire at two time points: when they first accessed a scheme and six weeks later when their use of the scheme had ended.

Table 16.3   Results of Council survey of user satisfaction with the POPP (low level cluster of schemes n = 744).

Question posed	Response *n* (%)
Was the service you used suitable for your needs?	Yes 694 (93.3)
Did the service you received help you?	Yes 691 (92.9)
Do you think this service should continue?	Yes 716 (96.2)
Would you recommend this service to other people?	Yes 700 (94.1)
How satisfied were you overall with this service?	Extremely/Very 583 (78.3)
	Satisfied 110 (14.8)
	Somewhat/Not 41 (5.5)
	No response 10 (1.4)

Time and other resource constraints meant that it was not feasible to cover all POPP schemes in this aspect of the study, so those to be included were selected in collaboration with research partners from the Council. The three schemes selected for detailed study were the Gardening scheme, the Counselling scheme and the Assistive Technology scheme. They were chosen because they were seen as targeting service users with different types of needs.

Data analysis

Basic frequency distributions and cross tabulations of variables were used to analyse the quantitative data collected about POPP service users. To provide a richer understanding of the differing roles of schemes, they were also grouped into three clusters according to the perceived main purpose of the scheme and the intensity of 'care' provided.

The 'low level' cluster included the Black and Minority Ethnic (BME) Carers and Mental Health scheme, the Stop and Lock scheme, the Gardening scheme and the Stepping Out scheme. The main aim of these schemes was to improve the well-being and quality of life of users. To achieve this aim, those delivering the POPP scheme acted mainly 'on behalf of' service users rather than 'actively with' service users.

The 'intermediate level cluster' included the Time Limited Contact scheme, Handyperson scheme and Care and Repair scheme. Again these schemes were aiming to improve the well-being and quality of life of service users but in addition they also aimed to prevent or reduce an older person's requirement for more costly interventions such as treatment in a hospital. For example, the Care and Repair scheme fitted grab rails with the aim of preventing falls, and the Time Limited Contact scheme offered help with shopping and cleaning for individuals returning from hospital. Hence, schemes were placed in this cluster because of their broader remit and because they were seen as targeting individuals with increased levels of vulnerability.

The 'high level cluster' included the Counselling scheme, the Rapid Intervention scheme, the Holistic Home Assessment scheme and the Assistive Technology scheme. Like the intermediate level cluster, these schemes were aiming to improve the well-being and quality of life of service users and to reduce or prevent their demands for more costly services. For example, the Rapid Intervention scheme provided support for 'cared for' individuals when their carers required hospital care. Relative to the other clusters, they involved more intensive inputs from those delivering the services offered and more active engagement with those receiving services as, for example, in the Counselling scheme.

Content analysis was used to interrogate the field notes generated during the processes of care interviews, with any dominant themes being reported in the final project report. Also reported were any issues that were regarded as important but which were less frequently raised.

Finally, frequency distributions of variables and before and after relationships were used to analyse the data collected by the standardized instruments for measuring the health, well-being and quality of life of service users.

Evaluation results

Given the breadth and depth of this evaluation, it is not possible within this chapter to present all the results generated by the study. Instead, selected results are presented to illustrate the value of a mixed method design when evaluating service initiatives of this type. The strand of enquiry chosen for this illustration explores the extent to which POPP schemes deliver services that:

- promote older people's health, well-being and independence;
- prevent or delay older people needing acute hospital treatment, which is both higher intensity and more costly.

Results are presented in turn for each of the three areas of data collection and analysis.

Users of POPP schemes

Over the period May 2007 to January 2008, there were 7577 referrals to the Council's POPP schemes. The outcome of the referral was documented for 6318 individuals: 5429 (85.9%) received services from a POPP scheme; 312 (4.9%) were regarded as not being suitable for POPP care; and 577 (9.1%) decided not to receive the services from a POPP scheme (for some schemes, individuals had to make a financial contribution for services and this represented a barrier to uptake).

These initial results indicate that the majority of individuals thought that the services offered by a POPP scheme were relevant to their needs at the point at which their referrals were accepted. Remaining results presented focus on the characteristics of referrals to the three clusters of POPP schemes.

There were 3480 referrals to the low level cluster, 2324 to the intermediate level cluster and 1768 to the high level cluster (the destination of seven referrals was unknown). Results allowed comparisons of the characteristics of users by scheme cluster in terms of their ages, living circumstances, referral sources and the recent changes that had affected their lives. Increasing age and living alone both increase the likelihood of a person needing admission to an institution such as a hospital if they suffer an 'acute' event. The data on referral sources and recent changes affecting individuals was used to explore further the 'vulnerability' of service users.

Relative to other scheme clusters, the low level cluster of schemes attracted a younger mix of referrals (33.5% of total referrals were aged 70 and above) and a lower proportion of individuals who lived alone (23.9% of total referrals, although there were a high number of missing data for this variable and cluster). Although a high number of referrals came via Primary Care (37.5% of total referrals), this reflected the fact that most referrals were to the exercise programmes offered by the Stepping Out scheme and individuals needed the approval of their GP before commencing. A desire to become more active and a perceived risk to well-being were the main issues that were raised by referrals. Such findings indicate that, in the short term, this cluster of schemes are unlikely to result in major reductions in client demands for more intensive and costly services for health and social care. However, their impacts from the perspectives of service users are considered later.

Referrals to the intermediate cluster of schemes were older than the low level cluster (70.6% of total referrals were aged 70 and above) and a higher proportion lived alone (59.9% of total referrals). In addition, although numbers were low, a higher proportion of referrals came from services that address higher level needs for care, such as adult services, intermediate care and hospitals (6.1% of all referrals). Clients having higher level needs are also indicated by the fact that recent changes affecting these referrals include coming out of hospital and accident or illness (22.9% of total referrals). Such findings indicate that, although probably small, this cluster of schemes is likely to be having some impact in the short term on client demands for more intensive and costly services for health and social care. Again, impacts from the perspectives of service users are considered later.

Finally, referrals to the high level cluster of schemes were the most elderly (78.1% of total referrals were aged 70 and above) and contained the greatest proportion living alone (66.7% of total referrals). Referrals from sources such as adult services, intermediate care and hospitals were also more evident (47.8% of all referrals) as were clients having experienced recent changes such as coming out of hospital and accident or illness (31.2% of total referrals). Such findings indicate that this cluster of schemes is already having an impact on client demands for more intensive and costly services for health and social care. Again, impacts from their perspectives are considered later.

'Processes of care' interviews

In total, 61 interviews were undertaken: 17 with POPP scheme leads and managers; 22 with individuals directly involved in delivering a POPP scheme; and 22 with individuals with stakeholder interests in the POPP (12 were health orientated stakeholders, such as General Practitioners, and 10 social care orientated stakeholders, such as individuals working for social services or the voluntary sector). The interviews with the 22 external stakeholders allowed the impacts of the POPP on older people's demands for higher cost services for health and social care organizations to be further explored. Feedback is briefly summarized here.

Both health and social care orientated stakeholders indicated that users had positive attitudes to the POPP. In addition, health orientated partners argued that POPP schemes were helping to reduce older people's demands for hospital care by preventing admissions and facilitating discharge. Some also argued that inputs from POPP schemes were helping to prevent the occurrence of crisis situations that may have resulted in an individual needing hospital care. These stakeholders were likely to have had most awareness of POPP schemes within the high level cluster.

The social care orientated stakeholders highlighted the holistic role of the network of POPP schemes in helping older people to live independently at home for longer. Here they are likely to have been referring to schemes within the intermediate cluster, such as the Care and Repair and the Handyperson scheme.

Hence, the qualitative feedback from the processes of care interviews allowed a deeper understanding of themes that had emerged from the analysis of the quantitative data. These

Table 16.4 Results of Council survey of user satisfaction with the POPP (intermediate level cluster of schemes $n = 454$).

Question posed	Response n (%)
Was the service you used suitable for your needs?	Yes 440 (96.9)
Did the service you received help you?	Yes 437 (96.3)
Do you think this service should continue?	Yes 443 (97.6)
Would you recommend this service to other people?	Yes 439 (96.7)
How satisfied were you overall with this service?	Extremely/Very 376 (82.8)
	Satisfied 59 (13.0)
	Somewhat/Not 14 (3.1)
	No response 5 (1.1)

combined sources of information supported the hypothesis that some POPP schemes, and in particular those in the high level cluster, were helping to reduce older people's demands for high cost services for health and social care.

Impact of POPP for service users

The high levels of uptake indicated positive attitudes amongst users towards the services delivered by the POPP at the time of referral. In total, 3911 satisfaction questionnaires were sent to individuals who agreed to be contacted following their use of a POPP scheme. Of these, 1362 returned the questionnaires, a response rate of 34.8%. Tables 16.3–16.5 present the results of this survey with schemes being clustered as before. Very high user approval ratings are evident, with respondents indicating that POPP schemes delivered a service that was suitable for their 'care' needs.

However, the results of this survey do not allow a direct assessment of whether or not access to a POPP scheme improved the health, well-being and quality of life of service users. Hence the need for using validated instruments for measuring changes directly in these domains. In total, 64 users across the three schemes participated in this aspect of the evaluation and were asked to complete the research instruments for assessing their health status, quality of life and well-being at baseline and six weeks later. Completed questionnaires were returned by 45 individuals at baseline (a response rate of 70.3%) and by 25 at follow-up (a response rate of 39.0%). Only 21 individuals completed the survey instruments at both time points.

Table 16.5 Results of Council survey of user satisfaction with the POPP (high level cluster of schemes $n = 162$).

Question posed	Response n (%)
Was the service you used suitable for your needs?	Yes 160 (98.9)
Did the service you received help you?	Yes 157 (96.9)
Do you think this service should continue?	Yes 159 (98.1)
Would you recommend this service to other people?	Yes 158 (97.5)
How satisfied were you overall with this service?	Extremely/Very 126 (77.8)
	Satisfied 29 (17.9)
	Somewhat/Not 5 (3.1)
	No response 2 (1.2)

Table 16.6 Responses to the question 'Thinking about the good and bad things that make up your life, how would you rate your quality of life as a whole?

Response	At baseline N (%)	Six weeks later N (%)
Very Good	3 (6.7)	2 (8.0)
Good	11 (24.4)	8 (32.0)
Alright	16 (35.6)	8 (32.0)
Bad	10 (22.2)	3 (12.0)
Very Bad	2 (4.4)	1 (4.0)
So bad, it could not be worse	2 (4.4)	0 (0.0)
Missing	1 (2.2)	3 (12.0)
Total respondents	**45 (100.0)**	**25 (100.0)**

The results presented in Table 16.6 report changes in participants' self-reported quality of life when they began to receive services from a POPP scheme and six weeks later. At follow up, 72.0% of the individuals who returned the questionnaire described their quality of life as 'alright, good or very good' compared to 66.7% at baseline. The trend towards an improvement in self-reported quality of life was upheld when responses for individuals who had completed the questionnaire at both time points were compared. At follow-up, 76.1% of respondents rated their quality of life 'alright, good or very good' compared to 66.7% at baseline. Other results from this aspect of the evaluation also demonstrated improvements in the health status of respondents of individuals as a result of them accessing a POPP scheme. However, although positive, the small numbers of respondents covered by the survey meant that none of the changes in quality of life and well-being were statistically significant.

Finally, those who participated in this aspect of the evaluation were invited to record any comments that they had concerning the POPP scheme that they had used. Examples of the types of feedback received are:

> I have only accessed the counselling (scheme). It is a wonderful service and extremely helpful getting me back on track and feeling independent.
> I had a gardening problem of overgrown trees which I requested help with. The team removed them for me and relieved my anxieties. I also intend to request a fire safety check in the near future.

Hence, the assessment of the impacts of the POPP for service users embraced a range of methodologies: satisfaction surveys, the use of standardized outcome measures, and approaches for obtaining qualitative feedback from individuals. Overall, these results indicated that the services provided within the POPP were valued by service users and were generating improvements in their health, well-being and quality of life.

Synthesis of findings

The role of this evaluation was to generate information to guide the development of the Council's POPP schemes. The evidence generated by the differing techniques for assessing the impacts of the POPP, from the perspectives of service users, led local stakeholders to conclude that its network of schemes was promoting improvements in the quality of life and well-being of service users.

It is more difficult to reach general conclusions about the ways in which access to a POPP scheme was affecting older people's demands for higher intensity and more costly care. The results generated about the characteristics of service users and feedback from the processes of care interviews led local stakeholders to conclude that schemes within the 'high level' cluster were already having an impact on older people's demands for such care, and those within the 'intermediate level' cluster some impact. Schemes within the 'low level' cluster were unlikely to be having an impact on older people's demands for more intensive and higher cost care in the short term. However, the aim of schemes such as the 'Stepping Out' scheme is to generate benefits of this type in the longer term.

Conclusion

Guidance from the Medical Research Council (Medical Research Council, 2008) demonstrates that the development and implementation of interventions of this type go through a series of phases: designing the intervention; piloting the intervention; and formally evaluating the intervention. Research can support each of these phases of service development but the research questions to be investigated vary. In turn, this means that a range of methods, both quantitative and qualitative, are needed to investigate these questions.

This chapter has illustrated the purpose, nature and outputs of the differing research methods that were used to evaluate this POPP. The adoption and use of the mixed method design, with a focus on a range of complementary research issues, ensured that the results generated by the study were comprehensive and relevant to the requirements of local service commissioners and providers.

Acknowledgements

The chapter authors would like to acknowledge Wanda Russell, who was also part of this project team.

References

Beech, R., Russell, W., Little, R. and Sherlow, S. (2004) An evaluation of a multidisciplinary team for intermediate care at home. *International Journal of Integrated Care*, (4 October 2004). Retrieved from: http://www.ijic.org/.

Beech, R. (2005) Evidence on the effectiveness of intermediate care, in *Intermediate and Continuing Care: Policy and Practice* (eds B. Roe and R. Beech), Blackwell, Oxford, pp. 106–118.

Beech, R., Roe, B., Russell, W. *et al.* (2008) *Evaluating Wigan's Partnership for Older People Project: End of project report.* Retrieved from: http://www.dhcarenetworks.org.uk/_library/Resources/Prevention/ CSIP_Product/FINAL_EVALUATION_REPORT-3.pdf.

Bowling, A. (2005) *Measuring Health: A Review of Quality of Life Measurement Scales*, 3rd edn, Open University Press, Maidenhead.

Department of Health (2000) The NHS Plan: A Plan for Investment, a Plan for Reform, Department of Health, London.

Department of Health (2006) A New Ambition for Old Age – Next Steps in Implementing the National Service Framework for Older People, Department of Health, London.

Department of Health (2008) Making a Strategic Shift to Prevention and Early Intervention: a Guide, Department of Health, London.

Dolan, P., Gudex, C., Kind, P. and Williams, A. (1995) A social tariff for *EuroQol: results from a UK general population survey*. Discussion paper No. 138. York: Centre for Health Economics, University of York.

Medical Research Council (2008) Developing and Evaluating Complex Interventions: New Guidance, Medical Research Council, London. Retrieved from: http://www.mrc.ac.uk/Utilities/Documentrecord/index.htm?d=MRC004871.

PSSRU (2008) National Evaluation of Partnerships for Older People Projects: Interim Report of Progress. Retrieved from: http://www.dh.gov.uk/en/SocialCare/Deliveringadultsocialcare/Olderpeople/PartnershipsforOlderPeopleProjects/index.htm.

Roe, B. (2005) Service development and evaluation in intermediate care, in *Intermediate and Continuing Care: Policy and Practice* (eds B. Roe and R. Beech), Blackwell, Oxford, pp. 61–77.

Ryff, C.D. (1996) Psychological wellbeing, in *Encyclopaedia of Gerontology: Age, Ageing and the Aged* (ed. J.E. Birren), Academic Press, San Diego CA, pp. 365–69.

Postscript

Paula Roberts and Helena Priest

We are all driven by the need to provide high quality health and social care for our patients and clients, and it is imperative that we have a firm evidence base for this practice. Only through the continuous quest for best practice, use of research findings and reflection, can our practice continually improve. Research is a dynamic phenomenon; its concepts, methods and outputs are continually being refined and are still evolving. Thus, this book can be considered as a starting point for a professional career in health or social care research.

In Part One of this book, we introduced readers to the background to research in health and social care and embarked on a journey through the 'typical' stages of research, to support readers conducting academic assignments, reviewing published research, or undertaking research themselves. In Part Two, we illustrated how research might be put into practice through illustrations from real world research, with a particular focus on involving participants in the research process.

The aims of the book were to:

- Support students and practitioners in academic studies that require the use of research evidence.
- Enable students on research methods modules and programmes to follow a learning journey from appraisal of research evidence through to conducting sound empirical studies of their own.
- Support healthcare practitioners wishing to find, evaluate and use research evidence relevant to their practice.
- Provide a starting point for practitioners wishing to conduct their own empirical research in order to enhance their practice.

By working through the book and its associated action points and reflection points, we hope that you will have:

- Examined the historical and theoretical perspectives of research paradigms.
- Explored the rationale for and process of developing research proposals and developed your own.
- Identified ways to conduct a literature search and review, and practised searching and organizing skills.
- Analysed and critiqued literature and practised critiquing skills.
- Considered the ethical implications, requirements and governance of research proposals, and practised preparing documents for ethical review.
- Appreciated theoretical concepts and identified appropriate research methods for your study, comparing strengths and weaknesses of different approaches.
- Developed academic writing and referencing skills and good academic practice.

- Identified a range of destinations and techniques for disseminating your work, and practised writing abstracts and preparing material for presentation in a number of different modalities.
- Been inspired to undertake further reading of printed and online materials.
- Examined research methods in a range of contexts through real world case illustrations.
- Reflected on your learning and potential application of concepts in your own setting.

Wherever you are in your health or social care career, we hope that the book has laid a firm foundation for your current and future practice, and will have inspired you to seek out best practice and to consider undertaking empirical research. If you are new to your profession, we hope it will mark the beginning of your quest for evidence based practice and your future engagement with research, either through your studies or as part of a research team. If you are an experienced professional, we hope it will have inspired you with new ideas and empowered you to seek improvements to enhance your practice, and possibly go on to further study. You may consider undertaking a postgraduate research methods module, followed by a Higher Degree, which will give you a firm foundation to undertake empirical research as part of a research team. Wherever you are on your journey, we hope that you have found this book both practically relevant and inspiring. Good luck!

Index